Functional Disorders
of the Menstrual Cycle

Functional Disorders of the Menstrual Cycle

Edited by

M. G. Brush
United Medical and Dental Schools,
St Thomas's Campus, London, UK

and

E. M. Goudsmit
London

A Wiley Medical Publication

JOHN WILEY & SONS
Chichester · New York · Brisbane · Toronto · Singapore

Library of Congress Cataloging in Publication Data:

Functional disorders of the menstrual cycle/edited by M.G. Brush and
   E.M. Goudsmit.

   p.   cm.—(A Wiley medical publication)
   Includes index.
   ISBN 0 471 91788 5
   1. Menstruation disorders.   2. Premenstrual syndrome.
3. Menstrual cycle.   I. Series.
   [DNLM: 1. Menstrual Cycle.   2. Menstruation Disorders.
3. Premenstrual Syndrome.   WP 550 F979]
RG161.F84   1988
618.1'72—dc19
DNLM/DLC
for Library of Congress   87-27371
                                                                            CIP

British Library Cataloguing in Publication Data:

Functional disorders of the menstrual
   cycle.
   1. Menstruation disorders
   I. Brush, M.G.   II. Goudsmit, E.M.
   618.1'7   RG161

   ISBN 0 471 91788 5

Typeset by Acorn Bookwork, Salisbury, Wilts.
Printed and bound by Anchor Brendon Ltd, Tiptree, Colchester

Contributors List

D. Asso, Department of Psychology, University of London, Goldsmiths' College, London, SE14 6NW

T. Bäckström, Department of Obstetrics and Gynecology, University of Umeå, S-901, 85 Umeå, Sweden.

M. G. Brush, Department of Gynaecology, United Medical and Dental Schools, St Thomas's Campus, London, SE1 7EH

W. R. Butt, Department of Clinical Endocrinology, Birmingham and Midland Hospital for Women, Showell Green Lane, Sparkhill, Birmingham, B11 4HL.

L. Dennerstein, Department of Psychiatry, University of Melbourne, Austin Hospital, Heidelberg, Victoria 3084, Australia.

S. Franks, Department of Obstetrics and Gynaecology, St Mary's Hospital Medical School, London, W2 1PG.

E. M. Goudsmit, London. Mailing address: Department of Gynaecology, United Medical and Dental Schools, St Thomas's Campus, London SE1 7EH.

C. Hawkridge, Endometriosis Society, 65 Holmdene Avenue, London, SE24 9LD.

R. E. Mansel, Department of Surgery, University of Wales College of Medicine and University Hospital of Wales, Heath Park, Cardiff, CF4 4XN.

W. H. Matta, Academic Department of Obstetrics and Gynaecology, Royal Free Hospital School of Medicine, Rowland Hill Street, London, NW3 2QG.

C. A. Morse, Department of Psychiatry, University of Melbourne, Austin Hospital, Heidelberg, Victoria 3084, Australia.

R. PETTY, Sections of Vascular Biology and Endocrinology, MRC Clinical Research Centre, Northwick Park Hospital, Watford Road, Harrow, Middlesex, HA1 3UJ.

W. J. REA, Environmental Health Center, 8345 Walnut Hill Lane, Suite 205, Dallas, Texas 75231 USA.

M. C. P. REES, Nuffield Department of Obstetrics and Gynaecology, John Radcliffe Hospital, Oxford, OX3 9DU.

G. A. SAMPSON, Department of Psychiatry, Whiteley Wood Clinic, Woofindin Road, Sheffield, S10 3TL.

R. W. SHAW, Academic Department of Obstetrics and Gynaecology, Royal Free Hospital School of Medicine, Rowland Hill Street, London, NW3 2QG.

Contents

Preface

A large number of undesirable events are known to be related to the menstrual cycle and may range from the mildly annoying and inconvenient to extremely serious situations, where the physical and mental pressures lead to extremes of tension with total disruption of lifestyle and the family unit.

It was our intention from the start of this book that much of the space should be devoted to premenstrual syndrome (PMS) and we make no apology for this, not only because it is one of our main research interests but, much more importantly, because we feel that there is a great need for a source of reference suitable for the gynaecologists, psychiatrists and other doctors and professionals in fields allied to medicine whose work brings them into contact with PMS sufferers. We also hope that research workers, whether qualified in medicine or science, will find stimulation in the discussion of the recent research in PMS and allied fields.

Although we were not intending to be comprehensive in coverage of disorders linked to the menstrual cycle, we felt that a number of other topics should be included, e.g. cyclical benign breast disease, menstrually linked migraine, dysmenorrhoea, menorrhagia, hyperprolactinaemia, and last, but by no means least, endometriosis. These are all topics in which there is much recent work to review and much research still to be carried out.

It may be asked why we, as research scientists, have undertaken this book. Our answer is that we feel that the importance of PMS and the other menstrually related conditions goes far beyond the routine clinical situation. A wide range of topics in basic reproductive and psychological science are involved in these studies and without the appropriate interdisciplinary laboratory and other scientific studies, any genuine progress would be difficult, if not impossible. Furthermore, the social implications are now recognized as being far-reaching and there is much public interest in the effects of these conditions on the working and family life of women. Although women with severe PMS are obviously the main sufferers, there may also be genuinely serious effects on partners and children. Nevertheless, we did not feel that it was appropriate to discuss the extremely rare cases where PMS is put forward as a defence in murder and manslaughter cases, as others have covered these cases in great detail, but it has to be acknowledged that actual bodily harm either self-inflicted or inflicted on others can, on rare occasions, be a feature of severe PMS.

It is not often realized that the psychological pressures associated with endometriosis can put a very great strain on the sufferer's personal and family life. Severe mood swings, not always associated with pain, may be difficult for the sufferer and her family to cope with and, in some cases, this may lead to job loss or divorce. Similarly, the other conditions discussed can have effects which reach far beyond the hospital or health centre.

We would like to thank Professor R. W. Taylor for his support in our interest in menstrual cycle disorders and Mrs H. Fry for her efficient and enthusiastic secretarial help. We are indebted to the editorial staff of John Wiley & Sons Ltd. for their help and patience during the preparation of the manuscript. As editors, we are very glad to acknowledge the hard work and friendly co-operation of all our contributors.

M. G. BRUSH
United Medical and Dental Schools,
St Thomas's Campus, London SE1.

ELLEN M. GOUDSMIT
London

June 1987

Functional Disorders of the Menstrual Cycle
Edited by M. G. Brush and E. M. Goudsmit
© 1988 John Wiley & Sons Ltd

CHAPTER 1

General and social considerations in research on menstrual cycle disorders with particular reference to PMS

M. G. BRUSH and ELLEN M. GOUDSMIT
*Department of Gynaecology,
United Medical and Dental Schools,
St Thomas's Campus,
London SE1 7EH*

Before embarking on the detailed consideration of PMS and other menstrual cycle-related disorders in the following chapters, it may be helpful to review briefly some general aspects and consider the effects on individual women in various age groups and life styles.

Introduction

There has been growing interest in menstrual cycle disorders during the past decade and this is partly due to the increasing tendency for women to wish to be in control of their own reproductive systems, rather than having their working and personal lives disrupted by menstrually related events. These changing attitudes have also attracted the attention of the media but not always with very helpful results. In the face of this lay interest, it is important that doctors, scientists, nurses and other professionals have convenient access to up-to-date information on menstrual cycle problems. Unfortunately, some aspects are still controversial and, at times, thoroughly confusing. This is particularly true of premenstrual syndrome (PMS), but endometriosis also presents many problems in management, albeit very different ones. It is salutary to remember that not long ago dysmenorrhoea was regarded as a psychogenic condition but now, with the discovery of the crucial role of prostaglandins, a clear-cut cause and treatment has been established. The earlier belief that any condition with psychological symptoms was also

1

psychological in origin, was responsible for sufferers being dismissed as inadequate personalities unable to cope with everyday life.

For some years there has, rightly, been considerable much needed research into the possible underlying physical causes of PMS and other menstrually-related conditions, but now there is a resurgence of interest in the psychosocial influences which may exacerbate the physical condition. This tendency deserves balanced scrutiny as in the wrong hands it could lead to trivialization of the sufferer's distress.

We are all too well aware of the many problems confronting both clinicians and research scientists when embarking on research in this field. Besides providing an up-to-date source of general reference, we hope that the multidisciplinary approach of this book will identify some of the sources of confusion and controversy and, therefore, provide a useful basis for future research. We have also tried hard to avoid any sexist attitudes which would only add to the prejudices about women which still exist in some quarters, even at professional levels.

In addition to the obvious hormonal and psychological aspects, we felt that it would be helpful to include examples of other approaches, such as clinical ecology, cognitive therapy and patient–doctor communication studies. However, we make no claim to be comprehensive and acknowledge that there are other views and other topics that we have been unable to include due to lack of space.

As PMS is such an important and complex problem, we felt it right to include a majority of chapters on this topic. Our contributors have attempted to explore the current state of research and clinical practice, and, not surprisingly, it is clear that a complete consensus is still some way off. Unfortunately, the lack of common ground has confused professionals outside menstrual cycle research and has probably contributed to the dearth of research funding from official sources.

There is also uncertainty in both medical and lay circles caused by failure to distinguish between mild symptoms and those which grossly disrupt all aspects of the sufferer's life. The former are often regarded as a variation of the normal, whereas the severe sufferer deserves all the medical and other help that she can obtain. It is unfortunate that some men, and even some women, attempt to trivialize the very real distress and suffering of very large numbers of women. We hope that our contributors, who include a high proportion of women (not an accident), will go some way to establishing to a wider audience the reality of the suffering from menstrually related disorders that exists world wide.

The History of the Definition of Premenstrual Syndrome

Premenstrual symptoms have been recognized since the days of Hippocrates but it was not until 1931 that they were formally identified as a clinical entity.

In the first paper on what became known as premenstrual tension, American physician Robert Frank referred to women who complained of 'a feeling of indescribable tension', 'unrest, irritability', 'like jumping out of their skin' and 'a desire to find relief by foolish and ill-considered actions'. He noted that these, and other symptoms arose ten to seven days preceding the menstruation and continued until the time that the menstrual flow occurred (Frank, 1931).

In the same year, psycho-analyst Karen Horney published an article on *Die prämenstruellen Verstimmungen* which she ascribed to physiological and psychological causes (Horney, 1967). The term premenstrual tension was used until 1953 when Greene and Dalton argued that the term premenstrual tension was unsatisfactory since tension was only one of the many components of the syndrome and that its use had probably led to a failure to recognize the disorder when tension was absent or was overshadowed by a more serious complaint. They rejected the term 'menstrual syndrome' because it could create the impression that the symptoms only occurred during menstruation and proposed the name premenstrual syndrome, even though they recognized that it was slightly misleading since some symptoms began around ovulation and continued into the menstruation. In their study they limited themselves to women whose symptoms occurred during the premenstrual phase, during ovulation or menstruation and at the time of a missed period. All women had been symptom-free at other times. Moreover, the 'attacks' had occurred during each of the preceding three menstrual cycles so that 'any chance coincidence between the attack and menstruation was eliminated' (Greene and Dalton, 1953).

In 1964, Dalton called the premenstrual syndrome an ambiguous phase and defined it as a wide variety of cyclical symptoms which regularly recur at the same phase of each menstrual cycle, usually during the premenstrual phase or early menstruation, but occasionally also at ovulation.

However, in 1980, following much controversy, she focussed on the importance of a strict definition and she proposed that this should be:

'the recurrence of symptoms on or after ovulation, increasing during the premenstruum and subsiding during menstruation, with complete absence of symptoms from the end of menstruation to ovulation' (Dalton, 1980)

In her opinion, women had to be free from symptoms for at least seven days following the end of menses and if they were not, their symptoms should be described as menstrual distress. In 1984, she reiterated the need for a strict definition and described the premenstrual syndrome as 'the recurrence of symptoms in the premenstruum with absence of symptoms in postmenstruum'. She stressed that symptoms should occur 'exclusively during the second half of the menstrual cycle' and that they should increase in severity as the cycle progressed. Furthermore, they should always be relieved by the onset of the full menstrual flow; they should be absent in the postmenstruum and present for at least three consecutive menstrual cycles.

Dalton has continued to use the term premenstrual tension for the psychological symptoms of tension, irritability, lethargy and depression but believes that failure to adhere to a strict definition of PMS is probably the reason for the high placebo response noted in many controlled trials of drugs.

Several researchers have adopted or adapted Dalton's definition and inclusion criteria e.g. Haskett *et al*. (1980), Goudsmit (1983) and Dennerstein *et al*. (1985). However, Dalton's definition has also been criticized. For instance, both Clare (1980) and Abplanalp (1983) have pointed out that symptoms which make up the syndrome are not uncommon and tend to occur intermittently in women of childbearing years so that premenstrual syndrome should refer to a significant increase in symptoms during the premenstrual phase. Others see the premenstrual syndrome as several different syndromes, each consisting of a cluster of symptoms (e.g. Halbreich and Endicott, 1982) and state that where PMS is seen as one syndrome, all symptoms are given equal weight. Few have addressed the issue of the severity of symptoms included in the syndrome although several people have challenged the view of PMS as something pathological and statistically abnormal. For example, Sutherland and Stewart (1965) claimed that the term premenstrual syndrome implied the existence of a pathological syndrome which required treatment. This they felt, was unsatisfactory because many women only experience one premenstrual symptom and not all the symptoms experienced require treatment. They also noted that some symptoms could occur in the absence of menstruation (after a hysterectomy) and around ovulation, so that the word premenstrual was too restrictive. They preferred a term which emphasized physiology rather than pathology and suggested the terms 'cyclical syndrome' and 'cyclical tension state', the latter replacing the term premenstrual tension. However, these terms have not met with acceptance.

Review of Current Definitions of PMS

There are still major disagreements in the literature about the definition of PMS. The problems are discussed in more detail in Chapter 3 but it may be useful at this point to mention the basic problems.

Some writers take a somewhat detached and negative view and merely report the apparent lack of consensus as they see it (Bancroft and Backstrom, 1985; Keye, 1985; Abraham, 1984; Clare, 1983; Rubinow and Roy-Byrne, 1984). However, there are now a number of opinions which are in close agreement (Dalton, 1977; Haskett *et al*., 1980; Brush, 1979, 1984; Budoff, 1983; Norris, 1983; Dennerstein *et al*., 1985; Goudsmit, 1983; Pariser *et al*., 1985). In particular, it is agreed by these workers that the definition of PMS should include three main criteria (some authors do not mention the third criterion separately, but it does follow from the first and second criteria):

1. Symptoms occur only in the second half (luteal phase) of the cycle, starting at ovulation or varying times after ovulation.
2. Symptoms are relieved by the onset of menstruation with complete absence of symptoms within two to three days after the start of the menstrual flow.
3. PMS is associated with a symptom-free time in the follicular phase lasting at least seven clear days and often nine to ten days.

Further points often mentioned are that symptoms should occur every month though not necessarily to the same degree of severity and that symptoms should worsen in the last few days before the start of menstruation.

If even one or two symptoms persist throughout the cycle, despite the disappearance of the other symptoms, the condition cannot be considered to be true PMS and must be categorized as a form of 'menstrual distress', as defined by Dalton (1977). In many such cases the symptom(s) which exist in the first half of the cycle will show marked exacerbation in the second half.

It is important to note that other authors use different nomenclature for menstrual distress despite the definition being essentially the same, e.g. Harrison (1985) uses the term premenstrual magnification (PMM) but describes the condition in essentially the same way as Dalton (1977).

In our experience, there are some cases where conditions 1 and 3 above are met but the sufferer reports symptoms which persist throughout menstruation. On close enquiry, these menstrual symptoms often prove to be not identical with those noted before menstruation and may represent a form of reaction to the distress of severe PMS and its secondary consequences in the family (see p. 59).

Another area of controversy is the listing of the main symptoms characteristic of PMS when they occur in the cyclical manner described above. An amazing number of symptoms have been reported as part of PMS (Dalton, 1964, 1977; Moos, 1968) but, clearly, only a few of these have a high incidence and many of the so-called symptoms are poorly defined with little clinical significance. Others are not part of PMS at all and represent examples of menstrual distress. However, there is a useful consensus of opinion (Brush, 1979, 1984; Reid and Yen, 1981; Norris, 1983; Abraham, 1983; Harrison, 1985) supporting the following as having significantly high incidence: irritability (sometimes extreme), depression, anxiety, breast swelling and pain, headaches, abdominal bloating, poor concentration, poor co-ordination, food cravings, lethargy, weight gain, and change in libido.

Other symptoms with definite correlation with PMS but much lower incidence, include acneiform skin eruptions, constipation, mouth ulcers, idiopathic bruising, swelling of fingers and ankles, insomnia, and backache.

Factors Associated with the First Onset of Significant PMS

Significant PMS can occur in teenage girls (see pp. 9–10) and there have even been documented instances of 'PMS-like symptoms' occurring immediately before the onset of the menarche. Brush *et al*. (1987) found that in 32.9 per cent of a series of 304 PMS sufferers, the condition started at or close to the menarche. However, there seems to be agreement with the report of Dalton (1977) that the largest number of cases start soon after childbirth. Brush *et al*. (1987) noted a 46.7 per cent association between preceding childbirth and PMS onset. If normal breast feeding is undertaken, PMS is unlikely to develop until the menstrual cycle restarts just before or just after lactation ceases; but if periods recommence rapidly in the absence of breast feeding, then PMS may start just a few weeks after delivery. The effect of a pregnancy in precipitating PMS is not correlated with the first or any particular subsequent pregnancies and the reasons for any individual pregnancy being followed by PMS are not known. Indeed, there is no specific information as to why pregnancy in general should be liable to produce this effect. Once PMS has occurred, it is highly likely that any subsequent pregnancy will also be followed by PMS.

Other factors which have been associated with the onset or worsening of PMS include, tubal ligation, hysterectomy with conservation of ovaries, and stopping the oral contraceptive pill. These are discussed later on pp. 60–61 and 58 respectively. Brush *et al*. (1987) found an association with the above preceding events of 2 per cent, 0.7 per cent and 4.0 per cent respectively. In 13.8 per cent of cases, careful enquiry failed to elicit any significant event preceding PMS onset.

It has also been reported that PMS may become a significant problem when menstruation resumes after a period of amenorrhoea.

Incidence

There is little doubt that large numbers of women between the ages of twelve and 50 suffer significant distress from premenstrual syndrome (PMS), but there are widely differing estimates of the percentage incidence. Several factors serve to compound the problem, including differences in definition of significant PMS and small numbers in the samples assessed. Some of the estimates clearly include anyone complaining of any mildly unpleasant premenstrual phenomenon and others go to the other extreme by reporting very low incidences.

It has to be admitted that none of the current estimates can be considered reliable in a statistical sense. Unfortunately, the resources needed to undertake a reliable survey of PMS incidence in the general female population would be too great in the present financial climate.

Our own extrapolation (Brush, 1979, 1984) from various sources suggests that 40 per cent of women between twelve and 50 who are not on the pill, suffer significant PMS symptoms which they would definitely like to be without, and that 5–10 per cent experience severe symptoms which cause very significant discomfort and disruption of working and family life. The latter estimate is in agreement with the estimates of Backstrom *et al*. (1983), Woods *et al*. (1982), Abplanalp *et al*. (1980).

A general estimate of 50 per cent incidence is given by Hargrove and Abraham (1982), while Reid and Yen (1981) state that 70–90 per cent of women report regular premenstrual symptoms and 20–40 per cent suffer some degree of temporary mental or physical incapacitation.

Effects of PMS on Work

Mild PMS, lasting two to three days and involving slight irritability, weepiness, tiredness and swollen abdomen, is unlikely to have a significant effect on a woman's performance at work and may not be noticed by the senior staff and colleagues. A very different situation may exist in severe PMS, lasting ten to fourteen days in each cycle. The effects of the mental symptoms, such as irritability, tension and depression, may be quite noticeable to colleagues and may prejudice working efficiency. The physical discomforts of swollen abdomen and breasts may add to the general feeling of being premenstrual. Weeping bouts are not uncommon and may cause great embarrassment. The lack of co-ordination which is often seen, may greatly reduce efficiency in jobs involving manual skills, such as typing, machine-operating, and driving. Concentration may also suffer whether or not headaches are present.

Partly because of the natural reluctance of women to admit to problems which may adversely affect their employment prospects, little statistical information is available.

If the situation is both severe and long-term, considerable loss of confidence may occur and this may lead to the PMS sufferer being unable to accept promotion.

In certain extreme cases, incidents may occur which lead to threatened or actual dismissal, or the sufferer may resign rather than face the difficulties of coping with PMS at work.

A useful general discussion of PMS problems in relation to work is given by Lauersen and Stukane (1983).

PMS and Marital Problems

The effects of PMS on domestic life are very far-reaching, but it is important to distinguish between specifically marital problems, those affecting children directly, and general effects on home life.

The irritability, tensions and anxieties experienced by the PMS sufferer may often be hidden at work or otherwise outside the home but are frequently released at home, particularly when in the company of the husband or other partner. This may lead to rows, often about trivial matters which would normally be ignored and to other apparently irrational and out of character behaviour. If the partner is unable or unwilling to understand the nature of the PMS problem, some serious marital problems may be caused or existing problems aggravated.

In women who may have a latent tendency to violent behaviour, the tensions of PMS may release the inhibitions which normally keep the violence under control, and assaults on partners are by no means uncommon. Where the husband is unable to restrain his wife or avoid her violent activity, serious injury may result. The converse is the heavily built husband who, exasperated by the verbal or physical violence of his wife, retaliates with excessive violence causing serious injury.

It is extremely difficult to obtain reliable statistics about the use of violence in the marriage because of the obvious reluctance to admit to antisocial and, possibly, illegal behaviour. In particular, the PMS sufferer may afterwards be bitterly ashamed of her actions and experience prolonged bouts of weeping. She may then wish to blot out the incident from her mind as much as possible.

A frequently reported PMS symptom is change in sexual interest. Usually there is a marked decrease, but much less frequently there is a sharp increase in sexual interest just before menstruation. The latter is not very likely to cause trouble in the marriage unless the partners are very poorly matched, but the decrease in interest can lead to very great strains on the marriage, especially if the husband does not appreciate the nature of the PMS problem and has normal levels of sexual interest. In severe cases, there may be complete loss of interest in sex from mid-cycle until menstruation ensues. If followed by further abstinence due to menstruation, there may be only about seven days per month in which sexual activity is tolerated. If the tensions and rows generated by this problem have been severe, the PMS sufferer may become increasingly tense all the time and sexual activity may cease altogether. In some cases, this may lead to the breakdown of the marriage and subsequent divorce.

The reasons for the loss of sexual interest and activity may be varied and complex. Physical discomfort may play an important role, particularly if the breasts are swollen and sore, and also if the abdomen is swollen with a tight stretched skin.

In one case (M. G. Brush, unpublished) in which abdominal swelling was extremely noticeable, the woman was convinced that her husband did not love her when she was 'swollen and ugly', and at these times avoided his possible advances by staying up very late watching television, etc.

Possibly, a more common cause of loss of sexual interest is the underlying tension and irritability which preclude the relaxation necessary for enjoyment of sex. A further factor is the very marked tiredness associated with PMS despite normal daily activities.

If the treatment of PMS is successful in other respects, it is likely that sexual interest will greatly improve, although progress may be slow at first if the earlier problems caused marked psychological distress.

Effects of PMS on the Family

The milder degrees of PMS may pass unnoticed among the usual ups and downs of family life. Some degree of irritability, for example, can hardly be described as unusual in women who lead a hectic life looking after a home and several young children.

When PMS is severe, the situation is very different and the effects of PMS on the family may be drastic. When irritability and tension are extreme, children may become frightened of their mother and this may affect their relationships with others or even induce stress-related illnesses. Similarly, if depression and withdrawing from normal life is marked, the effect on the family as a whole may be very severe.

The physical symptoms may also affect the family. Physical contact, such as hugging, may be refused due to very sore breasts, or even swollen abdomen in some cases, and this may lead to misunderstandings and unhappiness. The effects of lack of co-ordination, such as breaking of crockery or ornaments, may precipitate family rows which add to the tension.

The above account is based on our own experience in counselling studies, but is in accord with Harrison (1985) and other authors.

Apart from the psychological effects of PMS on the family, there is a small but definite risk of dangerous violence to children, leading to risk of serious injury and consequent conflict with the law.

Treatment of the violent PMS sufferer is not always easy. Many of the standard treatments, both hormonal and nutritional (see Chapters 5 and 7), do not give adequate help when given alone, but certain combinations may be helpful, such as dydrogesterone 10 mg twice daily on days five to 26 and pyridoxine 100–150 mg, or evening primrose oil 6–8 capsules daily plus pyridoxine 100–150 mg day^{-1}. In extremely severe cases of irritability, it may be necessary to use a sedative in conjunction with PMS treatment in order that the extremes of agitation and violence may be avoided.

Premenstrual Problems in Teenage Girls

There is no doubt that PMS can occur in young girls even from the first onset of menstruation, but the incidence in this age group (12–18 years) is probably quite low. Unfortunately, few accurate statistics on incidence in teenagers are available, apart from interesting studies from Finland (Kantero and Widholm, 1971; Widholm and Kantero, 1971) showing a 40 per cent incidence of PMS in adolescents with irritability, tension and fatigue as main symptoms, and a low incidence of oedematous symptoms. Several groups have reported general experience of PMS in young girls or well documented single cases (Williams and Weeks, 1952; Wenzel, 1960; Teja, 1976; Berlin *et al.*, 1982; Harrison, 1985).

It is quite likely that a number of cases are missed due to confusion with teenage moodiness, psychological problems associated with adjustment to the onset of menstruation, and similar ill-defined concepts. Furthermore, dysmenorrhoea may present in a more dramatic and pressing manner leading to PMS being ignored.

In our experience, mental symptoms, such as irritability, anxiety, confusion, and poor concentration, are the most common in teenagers but physical symptoms, such as sore breasts, headaches, and food cravings, also occur. Bloating of the abdomen, fingers and ankles appears to be very uncommon in teenagers, in agreement with Widholm and Kantero (1971).

It is very important to identify and treat PMS in this age group as if the teenager is left without help, the effects on her work, sport and social life may be very far-reaching. As before, the best proof of the existence of PMS is the correct use of a suitable menstrual chart, preferably a version simplified for use with this age group. If the teenager refuses co-operation in chart keeping or other recording, it may be possible for the parents to keep a chart of the more obvious symptoms, particularly if the teenager is prepared to mention the dates of her periods.

In all cases, treatment is probably best started by counselling and dietary adjustment, if necessary followed by the use of low doses of pyridoxine $(40-80 \text{ mg day}^{-1})$ (see p. 71). In more severe cases with correct body weight for age and general physical maturity, it may be appropriate to increase to adult dose levels of pyridoxine or evening primrose oil, as necessary.

For both physical and psychological reasons, it is inadvisable to use hormonal treatment for PMS in this group, especially in the younger girls. Sometimes, the combined contraceptive pill is given to quite young girls for treatment of dysmenorrhoea but this should be carefully monitored for side-effects. Sometimes side-effects of the 'pill', especially depression, bloating, and headaches may be confused with PMS. Occasionally the 'pill' will induce migraine of a prolonged and frightening nature.

Effect of Individual Attitudes and Expectancies on PMS

So far, this discussion has focussed on the negative consequences of PMS on the life of women. However, PMS, like most other illnesses, is itself susceptible to outside influences, including the existence of concurrent stressful events and cognitive factors such as knowledge, attitudes and expectancies about the illness.

There have been an increasing number of studies focussing on the relationship between premenstrual symptoms and attitudes, and some of these are discussed in Chapter 10. It is noticeable, however, that many of these studies have limited themselves to the investigation of negative attitudes on symptom-reporting, usually in a group of young healthy volunteers. There is also lack of longitudinal studies, to assess the permanence of 'altered' attitudes and the possibility that the experimentally-induced changes in symptom-reporting, could be further manipulated by imparting positive information. It is for these reasons that we have been reluctant to discuss this aspect of premenstrual symptomatology in more detail. The danger of much of the existing research in this field is that, because the findings obtained in a small group of women, usually college students, have been generalized by implication to what is arguably a different group of women, suffering from PMS, an impression has been created that women in general, and women with PMS in particular, are suggestible, thus reinforcing old myths and distorting the experience of many PMS sufferers. This, we believe, is most regrettable but easily rectifiable.

References

Abplanalp, J. M. (1983). Premenstrual syndrome: a selective review, *Women and Health*, **8**, 107–123.

Abplanalp, J. M., Haskett, R. F. and Rose, P. M. (1980). The premenstrual syndrome, *Psychiatric Clinics of North America*, **3**, 327–347.

Abraham, G. E. (1983). Nutritional factors on the etiology of the premenstrual tension syndromes, *Journal of Reproductive Medicine*, **28**, 446–464.

Abraham, S. (1984). Premenstrual or postmenstrual syndrome? *Medical Journal of Australia*, **141**, 327–328.

Bäckström, T., Baird, D. T., Bancroft, J., Bixo, M., Hammarbäck, S., Sanders, D., Smith, S. and Zetterlund, B. (1983). Endocrinological aspects of cyclical mood changes during the menstrual cycle or the premenstrual syndrome, *Journal of Psychosomatic Obstetrics and Gynaecology*, **2**, 8–20.

Bancroft, J. and Bäckström, T. (1985). Premenstrual syndrome, *Clinical Endocrinology*, **22**, 313–336.

Berlin, F. S., Bergey, G. K. and Money, J. (1982). Periodic psychosis of puberty: a case report, *American Journal of Psychiatry*, **139**, 119–120.

Brush, M. G. (1979). *Premenstrual Syndrome and Period Pains*, Womens Health Concern, London.

Brush, M. G. (1984). *Understanding Premenstrual Tension*, Pan, London.

Brush, M. G., Bennett, T. and Hansen, K. (1987). *A retrospective report on the use of pyridoxine in the treatment of premenstrual syndrome (PMS) at St Thomas's Hospital and Medical School 1976–1983* (submitted for publication).

Budoff, P. W. (1983). The use of prostaglandin inhibitors for the premenstrual syndrome, *Journal of Reproductive Medicine*, **28**, 469–478.

Clare, A. W. (1980). Progesterone, fluid and electrolytes in the premenstrual syndrome (letter). *British Medical Journal*, **281**, 810–811.

Clare, A. W. (1983). Psychiatric and social aspects of premenstrual complaint, *Psychological Medicine*, Monograph Supplement, **4**, 1–58.

Dalton, K. (1964). *The Premenstrual Syndrome*, Heinemann, London.

Dalton, K. (1977). *Premenstrual Syndrome and Progesterone Therapy*, Heinemann, London.

Dalton, K. (1980). Progesterone, fluid and electrolytes in the premenstrual syndrome, (letters) *British Medical Journal*, **281**, 61, 1008.

Dalton, K. (1984). *The Premenstrual Syndrome and Progesterone Therapy*, (2nd edition), Heinemann, London.

Dennerstein, L. Spencer-Gardner, C., Gotts, G., Brown, J. B., Smith, M. A. and Burrows, G. D. (1985). Progesterone and the premenstrual syndrome: a double blind crossover trial. *British Medical Journal*, **290**, 1617–1621.

Frank, R. T. (1931). The hormonal causes of premenstrual tension, *Archives of Neurology and Psychiatry*, **26**, 1053–1057.

Goudsmit, E. M. (1983). Psychological aspects of premenstrual symptoms, *Journal of Psychosomatic Obstetrics and Gynaecology*, **2**, 20–26.

Greene, R. and Dalton, K. (1953). The premenstrual syndrome, *British Medical Journal*, **i**, 1008–1014.

Halbreich, U. and Endicott, J. (1982). Classification of premenstrual syndrome, in *Behaviour and the Menstrual Cycle*, (Ed. R. Friedman) Dekker, New York, pp. 243–265.

Halbreich, U., Endicott, J. and Lesser, M. (1985). The clinical diagnosis and classification of premenstrual changes, *Canadian Journal of Psychiatry*, **30**, 489–497.

Hargrove, J. T. and Abraham, G. E. (1982). The incidence of premenstrual tension in a gynecologic clinic, *Journal of Reproductive Medicine*, **27**, 721–726.

Harrison, M. (1985). *Self-help for Premenstrual Syndrome*, (2nd edition) Random House, New York.

Haskett, R. F., Steiner, M., Osmun, J. N. and Carroll, B. J. (1980). Severe premenstrual tension: delineation of the syndrome, *Biological Psychiatry*, **15**, 121–139.

Horney, K. (1967). Premenstrual tension, in *Feminine Psychology*. (Ed. H. Kelman) Norton, New York, pp. 99–106.

Kantero, R.-L. and Widholm, O. (1971). Correlation of menstrual traits between adolescent girls and their mothers, *Acta Obstetrica et Gynecologica Scandinavica*, **Suppl. 14**, 30–36.

Keye, W. R. (1985). Medical treatment of premenstrual syndrome, *Canadian Journal of Psychiatry*, **30**, 483–488.

Lauersen, N. H. and Stukane, E. (1983). *Premenstrual Syndrome and You*, Pinnacle, New York.

Moos, R. H. (1968). Typology of menstrual cycle symptoms, *American Journal of Obstetrics and Gynecology*, **103**, 390–402.

Norris, R. V. (1983). Progesterone for premenstrual tension, *Journal of Reproductive Medicine*, **28**, 509–516.

Pariser, S. F., Stern, S. L., Shank, M. L., Falko, J. M., O'Shaughnessy, R. W. and Friedman, C. I. (1985). Premenstrual syndrome: concerns, controversies and treatment, *American Journal of Obstetrics and Gynecology*, **153**, 599–604.

Reid, R. L. and Yen, S. C. (1981). Premenstrual syndrome, *American Journal of Obstetrics and Gynecology*, **139**, 85–104.

Rubinow, D. R. and Roy-Byrne, P. (1984). Premenstrual syndrome: overview from a methodologic perspective, *American Journal of Psychiatry*, **141**, 163–172.

Sutherland, H. and Stewart, I. (1965). A critical analysis of the premenstrual syndrome, *Lancet*, **i**, 1180–1183.

Teja, J. S. (1976). Periodic psychosis of puberty, *Journal of Nervous and Mental Disease*, **162**, 52–57.

Wenzel, U. (1960). Periodical twilight states in puberty. *Archiv fur Psychiatrie und Nervenkrankheiten*, **201**, 133–150.

Widholm, O. and Kantero, R.-L. (1971). Menstrual patterns of adolescent girls according to the chronological and gynecological ages, *Acta Obstetrica et Gynecologica Scandinavica*, **Supplement 14**, 19–29.

Williams, E. Y. and Weeks, L. R. (1952). Premenstrual tension associated with psychotic episodes: preliminary report, *Journal of Nervous and Mental Diseases*, **116**, 321–329.

Woods, N. J., Most, A. and Dery, G. K. (1982). Prevalence of perimenstrual symptoms, *American Journal of Public Health*, **72**, 1257–1264.

Functional Disorders of the Menstrual Cycle
Edited by M. G. Brush and E. M. Goudsmit
© 1988 John Wiley & Sons Ltd

CHAPTER 2

Physiology and psychology of the normal menstrual cycle

DOREEN ASSO
Department of Psychology,
University of London Goldsmiths' College
London SE14 6NW

Introduction

The menstrual cycle is an integral part of the normal existence of women throughout nearly 40 years of reproductive life. The current attention to the premenstrual days has served to maintain a clinical image of the cycle and this book emphasizes that the cycle is subject to a wide range of disorders. In contrast there has been much less awareness of the continuous, and mainly positive, physiological and psychological changes of the reproductive cycle. During the reproductive years, the internal climate is different from day to day and a host of variables are at different points in their rhythmic activity at any given time. This chapter will discuss the present knowledge of the normal rhythmic patterns through the cycle. Insofar as the discussion can be structured in terms of distinct phases, the cycle will be divided into five, based on a notional 28-day rhythm, day one being the first day of bleeding:

Phase	Day
Menstrual	1–5
Follicular	6–12
Ovulatory	13–15
Luteal	16–23
Premenstrual	24–28

This categorization, together with many other similar ones, is based on the changes in the ovarian and pituitary hormones and the effects of those changes on the reproductive organs. The different oestrogenic hormones will be referred to as oestrogen. The main oestrogen produced by the ovary is

15

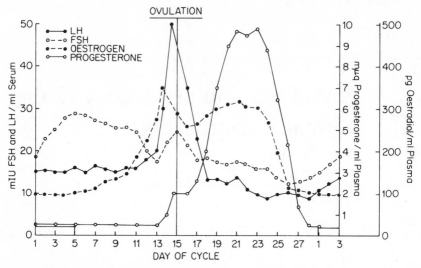

Figure 1. Levels of oestrogen, progesterone, luteinizing hormone, and follicle stimulating hormone through the menstrual cycle. Reproduced by permission of The C. V. Mosby Co from Taymor, M. L., Berger, M. J., Thompson, I. E., and Karam, K. S. (1972). Hormonal factors in human ovulation. *American Journal of Obstetrics and Gynecology*, **114**, 445–453

oestradiol. Oestrone is produced in smaller amounts. Oestriol and other oestrogenic metabolites are excreted in the urine. Progesterone is the progestational hormone which is usually measured and, less frequently, 17α-hydroxyprogesterone. The rhythmic fluctuations in oestrogen, progesterone, follicle stimulating hormone (FSH) and luteinizing hormone (LH) are well documented (see Figure 1); but it is increasingly clear that they are part of a larger pattern of cyclical changes which have far-reaching effects. More details are emerging of a number of neurophysiological variables which change systematically throughout the cycle. It is no longer surprising that the search for a simple relationship between the ovarian and pituitary hormones on the one hand, and the psychological and behavioural manifestations of the cycle on the other, has proved fruitless (Bancroft and Bäckström, 1985; Clare, 1985). A complete understanding of the normal menstrual cycle, and of its malfunctions, will come from elucidation of the complex inter-relationships of cyclical changes in the nervous and endocrine systems, which influence feelings and behaviour. The reproductive process is a highly complicated, finely balanced series of events, which takes place in a context of many other biological functions.

The Classical View of the Reproductive Cycle

The essential events which have traditionally defined the normal reproductive cycle are well known and will be briefly outlined here. A rather longer account is given in Asso (1983) and for more detailed elaboration see Linkie (1982).

The timing of the menstrual cycle is determined by the inherent rhythmicity of the ovaries. This is achieved by positive and negative feedback of oestrogen, modulated by progesterone in the luteal phase, on levels of the pituitary hormones FSH and LH. These gonadotrophins are controlled by gonadotrophin releasing hormone (GnRH) from the hypothalamus. Although it is useful and functionally appropriate to refer to the onset of bleeding as day one, the beginning of a cycle, the events of the new cycle have already been set in train one or two days before, in the previous cycle. The premenstrual fall in oestrogen stimulates secretion of GnRH from the hypothalamus to the pituitary; this starts a rise in FSH which increases during menstruation. The arrival of FSH at the ovaries stimulates the growth of several follicles which in turn become a source of oestrogen. One function of this early rise of oestrogen is the reconstruction and regrowth of the endometrium, shed during menstruation, which within two to three days of oestrogen secretion is transformed from a disrupted, torn state to one of complete renewal. The rising levels of oestrogen, through a negative feedback effect on the hypothalamus and the pituitary, then cause a decline in FSH. This decline is normally survived by only the largest follicle; by virtue of its size it produces the most oestrogen. Since oestrogen facilitates the uptake and binding of FSH, this large follicle would be best able to offset the decline in FSH by taking up more of it. The other follicles, more vulnerable to the drop in FSH, go into an atretic degradation process but in so doing, in response to tissue loss, they form stromal tissue which secretes small amounts of androgens, particularly androstenedione, which rises to a 15 per cent higher level than at any other time in the cycle. Apart from aromatization to oestrogen, it is presumed that the function of androgens in the late follicular phase is to induce atresia in all but one of the follicles. Progesterone, and possibly 17α-hydroxyprogesterone, appear to modulate the feedback of oestrogen; these hormones are secreted in very small amounts by the follicles just before the mid-cycle LH surge and may serve to stimulate both the LH and the FSH surge. The part played by FSH in ovulation is unknown. It is LH which appears to be critical to ovulation and to subsequent luteinization of the ovulatory follicle. The importance of FSH seems to be in the preparation for ovulation; it stimulates follicle growth and probably, more specifically, the maturation of the one successful follicle. It may contribute to optimal conditions at ovulation, rather than being essential to the process.

Ovulation occurs about 30–36 h after the LH peak which causes the surviving follicle to burst and to release the mature egg. Prostaglandins, which rise sharply before ovulation, are probably of prime importance in expelling the ovum, which is transported towards the uterus both by contractions of the fallopian tube and by the rhythmic beating of the cilia within the tube. The rupture in the vacated follicle is quickly healed and the cells which line the follicle proliferate and luteinize and the follicle becomes the corpus luteum, a process which depends on certain minimal levels of LH. The luteal cells in turn provide the progesterone and the oestrogen of the luteal phase. If there is no fertilization, the oestrogen, with prostaglandins, causes the corpus luteum to regress which then results in a sharp fall in oestrogen and progesterone. These low levels, together with the action of prostaglandins, lead to the end of the cycle, and to the endometrium being shed in the menstrual flow. The decline of oestrogen and progesterone also causes a gradual rise in FSH which begins the development of a new set of follicles, thus initiating the events of another cycle.

If the ovum is fertilized the corpus luteum remains functional, due to the secretion from the placenta of human chorionic gonadotrophin (hCG). This ensures that the corpus luteum will produce progesterone until the placenta itself can secrete that hormone, about six to eight weeks after conception.

Various changes in the reproductive organs, notably the vagina and the uterus, also define the menstrual cycle. The mucus membrane layer of the vagina changes with the hormonal changes of the cycle. There are characteristic morphological changes in response to oestrogen during the follicular phase and immediately after the LH surge the pyknotic process, which has been taking place in the vaginal cells, is at a maximum before steadily declining to the end of the cycle. The mucus of the cervix also begins to change early in the cycle and becomes most copious before the LH surge, giving the highest spinnbarkeit reading just before ovulation. This reading is an index of the length of the mucus threads which create channels through which spermatozoa can pass. There is also maximal ferning, brought about by crystallization which makes a fern-like pattern on a dried film of the mucus material. A new endometrium, the inner membrane of the uterus, starts to form under the influence of the oestrogen which is produced by the growing follicles. Later in the cycle, it is progesterone which completes the preparation of the endometrium for pregnancy, a process which, if no fertilization takes place, is nullified.

A Broader View of the Events of the Menstrual Cycle

Other systematic changes with the menstrual cycle, in many variables, have been established with differing degrees of certainty. Table 1 gives a simplified view of the available information on various hormones and neurotransmitters. For some of them consistent findings are sparse; many other variables which are undoubtedly important in the reproductive process, are omitted from the

Table 1. Neuroendocrine changes

	Menstrual Days 1–5	Follicular Days 6–12	Ovulatory Days 13–15	Luteal Days 16–23	Premenstrual Days 24–28
Oestrogen	Low	Rising to peak	Falling	Rising	Falling sharply
Progesterone	Low	Low	Starting to rise	Rising to peak	Falling sharply
Luteinizing hormone	Low	Low	Rise to and fall from peak	Low	Low
Follicle stimulating hormone	Raised	Low	Rise to and fall from peak	Low	Rising
Androstenedione	Low	Raised	Raised	Falling	Low
Testosterone	Low	Rising	Raised	Falling	Low
Prolactin[a]	Low	Rising	Peak	Falling then rising	Raised
Renin[a]	Low	Low	Rising	Rise to and fall from peak	Low[b]
Angiotensin[a]	Low	Low	Rising	Raised	Low
Aldosterone[a]	Low	Low	Low	Rising to peak	Raised then falling
CNS activation	Low[a]	Rising[a]	High	Falling	Low
β-Endorphin[a]	Low	Low	Rising	Rising to peak	Abrupt fall
Noradrenaline[a] (peripheral)	Unknown	Low	Raised	Raised	Unknown
Adrenaline[a] (peripheral)	Unknown	Low	Raised	Raised	Unknown
MAO (peripheral)[a]	Raised	Raised	Raised then falling	Low	Rising

[a] Based on limited findings.
[b] A minority of women may have peak around day 28.

table because so little is known about cyclical changes in them. This is true, for example, of several neurotransmitters, prostaglandins and melatonin. Where any of these have been measured at some point in the cycle, this will be mentioned. It has to be emphasized that the purpose of the table is simply to give some idea of the rhythms in some important variables within the cycle. Also, discussion in this chapter of the neurochemistry of the menstrual cycle is necessarily tentative because we are only just on the threshold of detailed knowledge of this topic. Table 2 gives a simplified picture of the psychological and sensory changes which have been most studied, as well as of sexuality

Table 2. Psychological, sensory and sexuality changes

	Menstrual Days 1–5	Follicular Days 6–12	Ovulatory Days 13–15	Luteal Days 16–23	Premenstrual Days 24–28
Positive feeling	Rising	Raised	High	Raised	Low
Anxiety	Falling[a]	Low	Low	Low	High
Tension/irritability	Falling[a]	Low	Low	Low	High
Hostility	Falling	Low	Low	Low	High
Depression	Insufficient information	Low	Low	Insufficient information	Inconclusive findings
Sexual Arousal[a]	Low	High	Falling	Falling	Raised
Sexual activity[c]	Low	High	Falling (but increased autosexual)	Low	Slightly raised
Vision	Rising	Rising	High	Low	Low
Audition	Rising	Rising	High	Low	Rising
Touch[d]	Rising	High	High	Low	Low
Olfaction	Low	Raised	High	Raised	Raised

[a] Rate of fall probably related to presence and duration of pain.
[b] Based on slightly inconsistent findings.
[c] Differs across cultural groups; other social factors also influence, see pp. 30–31.
[d] Tactile sensitivity of the breast highest immediately premenstrual, and after ovulation.

through the cycle. Findings from studies of women with frank disorders of the cycle are omitted from the tables. Relevant aspects of the variables in the two tables, and other less documented ones, will be summarized in nine broad categories: ovarian and pituitary hormones; androgens; prolactin and prostaglandins; adrenocortical hormones; the nervous system; positive feelings; negative feelings; sexual response; and sensory response. The question of the relationships between the variables will be examined; most of these relationships have been shown to be temporal, correlational or plausible, rather than demonstrably causal.

Ovarian and Pituitary Hormones

The activities of these hormones have been extensively investigated because of their fundamental role in the reproductive process. This has been outlined above, and the levels of these hormones in each phase of the cycle are shown in Table 1. As the cycle begins, levels of oestrogen, progesterone and LH are at their lowest; FSH is raised. In the follicular phase, FSH falls, oestrogen rises to a peak, progesterone stays low and begins to rise only right at the end of the phase, as do LH and FSH. The peaks of LH and FSH occur in the ovulatory phase though FSH is also at least equally high at the end of menses, oestrogen falls, but not to its lowest point, and progesterone begins a rather steep rise. Both progesterone and oestrogen are high in the luteal phase. Premenstrually, LH remains low, oestrogen and progesterone decline sharply and, towards the end of this phase, FSH starts to rise.

There are no precise relationships between individual levels of these hormones and measures of mood and behaviour at any point in the normal menstrual cycle (Backstrom et al., 1983; Clare, 1985). The most clear-cut temporal relationship is between the reported negative feelings of the premenstrual phase and the sharp decline in levels of oestrogen and progesterone at that time although in some women the onset of mood changes precedes the fall in steroids. There are no other obvious temporal relationships between the hormones and psychological variables (Bancroft and Bäckström, 1985). It is clear that there are crucial questions to be answered about the possible intermediary mechanisms, or co-factors, which underlie the ways in which each individual experiences the menstrual cycle and this will be discussed in the following sections.

Androgens

Testosterone and androstenedione levels show considerable individual variation during the cycle but the mean levels (Figure 2 and Table 1) are just above baseline in the menstrual phase, rising through the follicular phase to a higher plateau which is maintained through the ovulatory phase, starting to fall thereafter down to baseline level by the end of the cycle (Judd and Yen, 1973; Bancroft et al., 1983). These changes, though statistically significant, are quite small and some women show no mid-cycle rise. Androgens are secreted from the adrenal cortex and the ovary and are thought to contribute not only to the basic reproductive process (see page 17 above) but also to other cyclical manifestations of the menstrual cycle, especially in terms of their association with sexuality. Sanders and Bancroft (1982), reporting that sexuality is low when testosterone is high at mid-cycle, suggest that the behavioural effects of testosterone may be of relatively long latency, but other clarifications are needed and have been suggested. For example, Bancroft et al. (1983) found that sexuality which was independent of a relationship (e.g. masturbation) was positively associated with testosterone levels during the cycle but that there was a negative association as regards sexuality in the context of relationships.

Schreiner-Engel et al. (1981) used photoplethysmographic recordings of vaginal vasocongestion to measure physiological sexual arousal to erotic stimuli in the laboratory with no partner present. The group figures showed lower arousal during the ovulatory phase compared with the follicular and luteal phases. Correlation between physiological arousal and oestradiol and progesterone levels were low and negative. However, correlations between testosterone levels and the vaginal measure of arousal were positive and significant during the ovulatory phase.

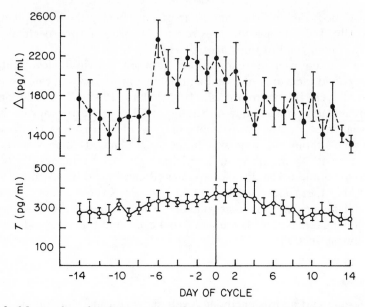

Figure 2. Mean value of androstenedione ($\triangle$) and of testosterone (T). O is ovulation day. The vertical bars represent one S.E.M. For both hormones, levels in the middle third of the cycle were significantly higher than in the first or last thirds. Reproduced by permission of the Endocrine Society, from Judd, H. L. and Yen, S. S. C. (1973). Serum androstenedione and testosterone levels during the menstrual cycle. *Journal of Clinical Endocrinology and Metabolism*, 36, 475–481. © The Endocrine Society 1973

Sanders and Bancroft (1982) suggest the possibility that if, in spite of the sexually-enhancing effects of testosterone, other effects (of testosterone) produce dissatisfaction or conflict with the partner, some women might adopt lifestyles (e.g. homosexuality or living alone) in which their testosterone-induced sexuality would not be in conflict with their testosterone-influenced personalities. Androstenedione, a much weaker androgen which varies with the cycle in a similar way to testosterone, with an even more marked rise in the ovulatory phase, may also contribute effects similar to those of testosterone described above. There is a case to be made for androgens being one biological basis for certain aspects of sexuality, but other biological, psychological, and social factors are doubtless also important (see section on 'Sexual response' below).

Prolactin and Prostaglandins

Prolactin shows a menstrual pattern, provided time of day effects are controlled for. Following earlier conflicting findings, Vekemans *et al.* (1977) showed that levels are low before ovulation, when there is a small peak; then they fall again before rising and staying higher than the early follicular phase level until the onset of menstruation (Table 1). In the reproductive process, prolactin is involved in the growth of follicles and in corpus luteum function. Very high levels of prolactin produce anovulation, either through some action at the hypothalamic and pituitary levels, which produces abnormal oestrogen feedback or through direct effects at the ovarian level (see Chapter 13). This effect is probably partly mediated by melatonin (Cutler and Garcia, 1980). Oestrogen is known to promote the synthesis of prolactin and its release by the pituitary (Yen and Jaffe, 1978). Prolactin has a mutually antagonistic relationship with progesterone and, like progesterone, it can affect fluid balance (Brush, 1977). It is reasonable to assume that prolactin contributes to any emotional effects of the cycle, for the following reasons:

1. Prolactin is inhibited by various neurotransmitters and increased by monoamine oxidase activity, which are all related to emotion.
2. Levels of prolactin rise markedly after stress (Yen and Jaffe, 1978).
3. The effects of prolactin on ovulation are at least in part mediated by melatonin (through the effects of light) and there is evidence that melatonin is controlled by sympathetic neurones of the autonomic nervous system, which is closely involved in emotional responsiveness.

Although the influence of prolactin on ovulation through, among other factors, emotional reactions, is very likely, any part it may play in premenstrual syndrome is not clear (Steiner et al., 1984; see Chapters 6 and 8).

Prostaglandins play a crucial role in the reproductive process; they are not included in the Table 1 because there is so little precise information about cyclical changes in them. Neither are the mechanisms of action of prostaglandins entirely clear. They appear to have an intermediary role in the integration of endocrine function. They are found in the brain, and oestrogen is presumed to modulate the pulsatile pattern of the release of prostaglandins in the central nervous system (see Coulam, 1981). More specifically, ovarian prostaglandins rise sharply before ovulation and seem to be important in the expulsion of the ovum from the follicle (Cutler and Garcia, 1980). They also, in conjunction with oestrogen-primed effects of progesterone, probably bring about the demise of the corpus luteum. The prostaglandin which serves this purpose is produced by the endometrium which has been primed by the corpus luteum. The luteal regression causes the decline in oestrogen and progesterone and the subsequent menstrual bleeding; prostaglandins appear also to be involved in the vasospasm which precedes the breakdown and shedding of the endometrium. Certainly, high levels of prostaglandins are found in the endometrium before menstruation, and in menstrual blood (Yen and Jaffe, 1978). In addition they play a part in the uterine contractions during the menstrual flow and may modulate the amount and duration of bleeding (see Chapter 15). One or more of the prostaglandins may, for example through a central effect, or by increasing fluid retention, be a basis for psychological and physical changes during the cycle. This possibility is reinforced by the fact that γ-linolenic acid, which is a precursor of prostaglandin E_1, appears to be effective in some cases of premenstrual syndrome (Brush, 1982; Bancroft and Bäckström, 1985). At least one mechanism in this effect might be the intermediary role played by prostaglandins in the integration of neuroendocrine function, and specifically as modulators of the autonomic nervous system (see Coulam, 1981).

Adrenocortical Hormones

Renin activates angiotensin, which in turn stimulates the secretion of aldosterone. Table 1 shows that all three fluctuate roughly in parallel through the menstrual cycle, with low levels in the menstrual and follicular phases, rising from ovulation to a peak in the luteal phase, after which they fall back to low levels (Rausch and Janowsky, 1982). It is not clear whether these hormones are important mechanisms in some of the cyclical effects of ovarian hormones. Oestrogen stimulates renin activity, leading to higher levels of angiotensin and aldosterone secretion and excretion; but there is some evidence that the slight, transient, salt- and water-retaining effect of oestrogen is independent of its ability to enhance aldosterone production. Progesterone appears to have an indirect relationship with aldosterone in that the salt and water loss caused by progesterone is compensated for by parallel changes in renin and aldosterone levels (Reid and Yen, 1981).

The renin–angiotensin–aldosterone system has been the subject of a great deal of study, particularly because of its salt- and water-retaining properties; these properties have been thought to make it a possible basis for some of the physical and psychological changes of the cycle, but clear evidence for this has failed to materialize (Reid and Yen, 1981; Bancroft and Bäckström, 1985). The possibility nevertheless remains that the mineralocorticoid system is an intermediary mechanism in some of the cyclical manifestations, and this may be clarified with improved techniques (Janowsky and Rausch, 1985). As regards fluid retention specifically, the findings on cyclical change are inconsistent. It seems that the common fluctuations in bloating and distension cannot be satisfactorily explained by water retention (Bancroft and Bäckström, 1985).

Cortisol does not appear in Table 1 because there are insufficient consistent findings on changes with the cycle. It may be that cortisol does not systematically fluctuate directly with the cycle, but rather as a result of cyclical changes in reactivity to stress (Collins *et al.*, 1985) and see pp. 124–125.

The Nervous System

The close reciprocal relationship between the nervous and the endocrine systems in general is obvious. It is evident throughout the reproductive process, where the hypothalamus, through gonadotrophin releasing hormone, exerts control over the pituitary hormones in their interaction with the ovarian hormones. There is a wide range of evidence that oestrogen increases and progesterone decreases central nervous system activity. It is therefore inevitable that many of the effects of cyclical hormone change are mediated by the nervous system. Individual differences in reactivity of the nervous system to hormone levels is probably an important variable in determining other changes with the cycle.

Although there is at present no way of measuring directly the responsiveness of hormonal target areas in the nervous system, there are many other indices of various aspects of nervous system functioning through the different phases of the reproductive cycle. There are several measures of levels of activity, such as EEG changes in α-frequency, EEG photic driving responses, contingent negative variation, two-flash fusion, and sensory after-effect. Also highly relevant is the activity of the neurotransmitters which are involved in the release of hormones and, reciprocally, are affected, in their content and turnover, by different hormones (see Coulam, 1981). In addition to the importance of levels of nervous system activity and reactivity, and of neuro-transmitters, to feelings and behaviour, Gandelman (1983) has pointed out that, more specifically, one effect of gonadal hormones on the nervous system is to alter the way in which incoming stimuli are processed. This would be a mechanism in, for example, the changes within the menstrual cycle in sensory response and in related behaviour. Not only the central nervous system but also the peripheral autonomic nervous system is an important intermediary mechanism in the hormonal effects of the cycle, particularly as regards psychological and behavioural manifestations. In work on the menstrual cycle, only a few attempts have been made to measure central and peripheral processes separately. In general, the frequently different patterns of activity in the two systems have been demonstrated and, more specifically, with the menstrual cycle there appear to be differential changes in certain aspects of the activity and reactivity of the two systems, measured both objectively and by individual self-report (Asso, 1986). Autonomic activity, not shown on the tables because of incomplete information on changes through the whole cycle, will be referred to again later.

A general point is that, given the neurophysiological and functional complexities of nervous system activity, not all aspects of cortical function, nor all components of the autonomic nervous system, would be equally implicated as intermediary mechanisms in the effects of hormonal changes.

Table 1 shows changes through the cycle in central nervous system activation, based on studies which used a variety of measures. Central arousal rises, probably during the follicular phase to a peak around ovulation, and thereafter falls and remains low to the end of the cycle (see Asso, 1983). This pattern corresponds temporally with the increasingly positive, buoyant mood of the first half of the cycle, through the quieter, more contented luteal phase, to the reported negative mood at the end.

Levels of just one brain opioid, β-endorphin, have been measured through the reproductive cycle, and the rather tentative information currently available is shown on Table 1; low levels at the beginning of the cycle, rising through the ovulatory phase to a peak in the luteal phase, before an abrupt decline premenstrually. In an understanding of the diverse manifestations of the menstrual cycle, the endorphins are highly relevant since they modulate not only sensitivity to pain, but also the intensity of certain emotions, as well as various aspects of reward and memory. They appear in addition to regulate certain arousal responses, both in the central and in the autonomic nervous systems (see Panksepp, 1986).

Noradrenaline is certainly involved in the control of gonadotrophin release, though the mode of action is not clear. Like the other monoamine neurotransmitters, noradrenaline has overlapping effects with oestrogen and progesterone, both in facilitating ovulation and as regards behavioural effects (see Rausch and Janowsky, 1982). Table 1 suggests that noradrenaline is raised in the ovulatory and luteal phases of the cycle (see Collins, et al., 1985). These authors' findings on noradrenaline and adrenaline, are consistent with the patterns shown in Table 1, insofar as the results of the first of two cycles studied by them are concerned. For the present purpose, the first cycle is the most relevant, since it was free of any attenuation of effects by repetition.

Adrenaline, not much in evidence in the central nervous system, is secreted from the adrenal medulla in response to fear and anxiety and brings about increases in blood pressure and cardiac input. Adrenaline levels throughout the cycle have not been unequivocally established but, as shown on Table 1, may well rise steadily through the cycle to a high by the end of the luteal phase (see Collins et al., 1985).

Not shown on the table, because of inadequate information, are other neurotransmitters which are involved in the control of hypothalamic hormone-releasing mechanisms and which are also important in mood and behaviour. They are known to change at certain points in the cycle, but the precise cyclical patterns are not clear. Of those in the central nervous system which have been studied in this context, dopamine and serotonin have been shown to be influenced by ovarian hormones, and there is a little evidence of changes in peripheral levels which parallel the ovarian hormone changes (see Rausch and Janowsky, 1982).

Monoamine oxidase, which inactivates the monoamine neurotransmitters, is also directly affected by steroid hormone activity. Although the findings are slightly equivocal, during the cycle peripheral monoamine oxidase (see Table 1) seems to be raised up to ovulation, falling thereafter to a low in the middle of the luteal phase, after which it rises again (see Baron et al., 1980; Bancroft and Bäckström, 1985).

Neurotransmitters are closely involved in every aspect of the reproductive cycle, and they are also vital in all aspects of human functioning; for example they are involved in mood, emotion, sleep, sexual activity, motivation and sensory response. The autonomic nervous system also has a reciprocal relationship with the endocrine system. An important mediator in this relationship is noradrenaline, which is one of the main effectors of sympathetic innervation and hence has important influence on emotional response. Measurement of autonomic nervous system activity is notoriously difficult because different components of the system react differentially within and among individuals and in varying situations. Bearing firmly in mind that findings have to be interpreted with caution, it nevertheless appears that certain aspects (not all) of autonomic reactivity (as opposed to levels), and certain other indices of autonomic functioning, are high premenstrually and low at midcycle (see Asso, 1983). These changes, and probably individual perception of them, play an important part in other manifestations of the cycle (see Asso, 1986).

Findings in the next two sections, on positive and negative feelings, rely on self-report methods. There is controversy about the relative accuracy of retrospective and of daily self-reports; also about whether the reports reflect the 'true' state rather than social attitudes towards menstruation. Conclusive evidence for or against these points of view is difficult to establish but it seems reasonable to conclude that, where all steps are taken to ensure representative groups, reliable and valid questionnaires and careful instructions, the majority of well-conducted studies of self-reports of the experience of the menstrual cycle are fairly accurate versions of biological and psychological realities. There are various justifications for this conclusion (see, for example, Asso, 1983; Bancroft and Bäckström, 1985). It also has to be noted that, when objective measures of, say, negative changes premenstrually, are made (for example, attempted suicide; secretion of cortisol which is a physiological response to stress), women who do not report negative change have similar, or sometimes higher, scores than those who do; this seems to indicate that some women, even though they experience increased distress premenstrually, do not attribute it to the cycle, or possibly do not feel it noteworthy or appropriate to mention it on a non-menstrual questionnaire. The important point to emerge from this controversy is the need for rigorous standards of methodology and of interpretation of findings.

Positive Feelings

Positive feelings through the cycle have been less frequently studied than negative feelings. This has contributed to the somewhat distorted lay view of the menstrual cycle. In the 'Positive feeling' category on Table 2 studies have included well-being, pleasantness, cheerfulness, energy, elation, vigour, affectionateness. The table shows that feelings such as these are reported to increase through the menstrual and the follicular phases to reach a high point around ovulation, to remain quite high through the luteal phase, and to decline premenstrually. The findings of predominantly positive feelings in non-clinic women in the follicular, ovulatory and luteal phases are virtually unanimous (see Asso, 1983; Sanders *et al.*, 1983).

As regards the premenstrual phase, although reports of positive feelings are unusual, this might not be quite as marked if women were more often asked about positive moods at that time. For example, Halbreich and Endicott (1982) point out that some women have increased feelings of well-being, are more efficient and have more energy premenstrually. They found that, in a group of 154 women receiving no treatment for any menstrual disorder, 17 per cent qualified for inclusion in a premenstrual category of increased well-being syndrome. There are other reports of positive feelings co-existing with negative ones premenstrually (e.g. Abplanalp *et al.*, 1980; Awaritefe *et al.*, 1980). Clinical reports, too, are often of labile mood at this time. Also, with due regard to the wide individual and cultural differences, group figures usually show a small premenstrual rise in sexual arousal and sexual activity. In the menstrual phase some studies find an easing of negative feelings and increased relaxation, others find continuing negative mood. There are wide individual differences in the extent to which, and the speed with which, negative feelings are replaced by positive ones in the course of menstruation. It seems likely that one important determinant of these individual differences is the amount of pain and discomfort in this phase (see below). There seems to be no doubt that women report positive feelings for the greater part of the reproductive cycle and perhaps, for some women some of the time, even in the premenstrual phase. This is in spite of the fact that they have only rarely been asked questions specifically about positive states.

Negative feelings

Anxiety, tension, irritability and hostility are shown on Table 2 to be on the decrease (from a premenstrual high) during the menstrual phase and to remain low until the last, premenstrual, phase of the cycle. Depression, though frequently cited as a premenstrual or menstrual symptom, is not unequivocally established as a widespread feature of the premenstrual phase (see Asso, 1983). There may often be a tendency to cry or to feel low as part of one or other of the clusters of premenstrual symptoms, but there are no consistent findings of the characteristics of current clinical descriptions of depression. There is insufficient information to draw conclusions about depression in the menstrual phase. As mentioned above, the amount of negative feeling experienced during the menstrual phase may be a function of the amount of pain and discomfort experienced (Paige, 1971; Abplanalp et al., 1979; Beumont et al., 1975; Golub and Harrington, 1981). It is assumed that, in affected women, on the abatement of pain or discomfort, usually after one or two days, there is a move to the positive mood climate which normally lasts through to the start of the next premenstrual phase. Reports of premenstrual negative feelings are extremely frequent (see Asso, 1983; Bancroft and Bäckström, 1985; Halbreich and Endicott, 1985), but there is a small minority of studies which found no significant cyclical variation in some moods. Such studies are listed here with some information about subjects studied and questionnaires used, though it is not clear whether differences in design and methods of assessment could explain these divergent results:

1. Abplanalp et al. (1979), 33 participants recruited in a medical centre, all currently in a stable heterosexual relationship; Profile of Moods States (POMS) with two moods added.
2. Parlee (1980), seven medical centre employees; POMS [Both of these studies found no significant variations with the cycle on the POMS, not designed to measure menstrual changes, although significant fluctuations were found on the Menstrual Distress Questionnaire (MDQ)].
3. Lahmeyer et al. (1982), eleven staff and students of a medical centre; MDQ and state anxiety scores raised premenstrually, but not statistically significant.
4. Sanders et al. (1983), one only of three groups recruited, this group pre-selected for reporting no cyclical changes in well-being in physical state; non-significant fluctuations, on Mood Adjective Check List and Visual Analogue Scale.
5. Slade (1984), 118 student nurses; author's own modifications of and additions to the MDQ; cyclical physical symptoms were noted but no significant mood changes.
6. Zimmerman and Parlee (1973), fourteen students with regular cycles; ad hoc self-rated symptom scale.

There seems no doubt that there are significant changes in feelings associated with the menstrual cycle. The great majority of studies have shown this using a variety of measures: self report measurement by retrospective, daily, menstrually-related and non-menstrually related questionnaires; objective measures of behaviour and stress; psychophysiological measures; or well-documented clinical and anecdotal accounts. Each of the changes can occur independently of the cycle, but the patterns referred to here are specifically related to the reproductive cycle; for example, they are attenuated, abolished or changed by the combination pill and, on the rare occasions when the studies have included a group of men for control purposes, the men do not show similar cyclical fluctuations. There are variations in the cyclical patterns, within and across individuals; changes in some feelings are more clear-cut than in others; but all are best seen as tendencies which create a varying psychological climate and which can be enhanced or diminished for any individual by other states and other events at the time. One possible view of these changes has been put by Sanders *et al*. (1983). They suggest, with some supporting evidence, that the most salient cyclical variation is in the general state of well-being, with negative feelings varying in impact from one individual to another. Asso (1986), using both a self-report index of cortical arousal reflected in feelings such as buoyancy, vigour, and a psychophysiological measure of neural sensitivity, i.e. cortical alertness, found these indices were high inter-menstrually and were low premenstrually, and that, within individuals, low premenstrual levels on these measures were significantly related to negative feelings. Little and Zahn, in 1974, in a study using a variety of psychophysiological measures and an adjusted questionnaire measure of 'positive activation', concluded that normal women suffer premenstrually and at the beginning of menstruation, not so much from pronounced cyclical shifts in negative feeling as from a lack of positive energy and 'warmth'. This withdrawal of buoyancy, alertness and vigour would presumably be a biological by-product of the events in the second half of a non-fertilized reproductive cycle; the effect of this would combine with other biological factors at that time (e.g. sharp decline in β-endorphin) and with very significant psychological and social factors, to produce the experience of the end of the cycle for each individual.

Sexual Response

Approximate estimates of cyclical variations in sexual arousal and activity are shown on Table 2 with some reservations. Some of the information is inconclusive, but it seems certain that in most women there are fluctuations with the cycle. The precise pattern appears to depend on cultural differences; also on whether the feeling or activity is 'autosexual' and, if not, whether it is woman- or man-initiated. Results are clearer and somewhat different when ovulation is accurately established (Udry and Morris, 1977). With these reservations, a frequent overall pattern appears to be of sexual arousal being low at the beginning of the cycle, highest in the follicular phase, and falling during the ovulatory and luteal phases, rising somewhat premenstrually. Sexual activity follows a somewhat similar, though not entirely identical, pattern. Within this oversimplified picture a much more complex situation prevails.

There is no evidence of a direct relationship between female ovarian hormones and sexuality (Sanders and Bancroft, 1982). The only suggestion of a temporal relationship is the frequent finding of raised sexuality in the follicular phase, when oestrogen is rising. This is not a very close temporal association since the increase in sexuality in usually reported to start post-menstrually, probably somewhat before the rise in oestrogen is appreciable.

In the adrogens section on page 21, several studies were cited which suggest that sexuality in women appears to be related to androgen levels only under certain circumstances; namely sexuality that is independent of a relationship or is woman- rather than man-initiated. Androgen levels were not measured in a study by Adams *et al.* (1978) but it was a rare attempt to distinguish between heterosexual and autosexual activity and fantasy, and between man- and woman-initiated sexual behaviour. Women experienced an increase in woman-initiated heterosexual behaviour and in auto-sexual behaviour and fantasy at ovulation (which corresponds to raised androgen levels in the woman). There is another study (Matteo and Rissman, 1984) which did not measure androgen levels, but which casts some light on these complexities. It involved seven lesbian couples whose sexual responses were independent of interaction with men and of contraception. It was found that activity increased at mid-cycle and decreased in the luteal phase. There was no reduction or increase in sexual activity before, during or after menstruation. The authors suggest that their mid-cycle findings may reflect biologically adaptive factors such as heightened sensory acuity and the possible facilitation by orgasm of sperm transport. They make no mention of the higher androgen levels, which are at least arguably relevant.

There are detailed accounts of cyclical fluctuations in sexuality in Sanders and Bancroft (1982) and in Morris and Udry (1982). From the work outlined in this chapter it seems possible that there is a biologically-based increase in sexual feelings and activity in women in the middle of the menstrual cycle, i.e. attributable to hormones and heightened sensory perception. This manifests itself particularly in auto-erotic thoughts and behaviour, and possibly in increased initiation of sexual activity by the woman. No mid-cycle rise is reported in man-initiated sexual activity. Where individual levels of androgens are measured, these are related to indices of sexuality which are independent of a relationship (for example, masturbation, vaginal response to erotic stimuli in the laboratory); sexuality in a relationship seems to be much more a function of the relationship and of the social context than of biological factors. Variables such as inhibitions about intercourse during menstruation which may produce pre- and postmenstrual peaks and the influence of contraceptive methods, may obscure the biological effects. It is likely that many physiological and social variables contribute to the pattern of sexuality even in any one individual.

Sensory Response

This topic will be discussed briefly, in the context of the part it plays in wider psychological and behavioural changes with the cycle. The acuity of all the senses changes with the menstrual cycle and the topic has been reviewed in detail by Parlee (1983) and Gandelman (1983). There are no simple statements to be made about precise cyclical patterns with each sense, since these differ somewhat with different stimuli. Table 2 shows a generalized view of changes in vision, audition, touch and smell. There are insufficient consistent findings on taste. The four senses on the table appear to reach a peak of sensitivity around ovulation; vision, audition and touch all very broadly rise in the first half of the cycle to the ovulatory peak and decline thereafter. Smell is different in that sensitivity seems to be low then rising before ovulation and remaining fairly high to the end of the cycle.

As mentioned, within any sensory modality, the cyclical variations are specific to certain stimuli. For example, olfactory sensitivity varies to a greater or lesser extent in response to different odorants. This mechanism appears to reflect rather finely the purpose of increasing the likelihood of reproduction; the changes are greatest for exaltolide which resembles muscone, a mammalian sex-attractant. The variations which are found cannot be attributed to non-sensory factors, since these are usually controlled for by the use of signal detection methods.

The repercussions of these sensory variations on other changes with the cycle are considerable, and more knowledge of them would contribute to a better understanding of, for example, the psychological and behavioural fluctuations. The perception of stimuli from the environment is fundamental to responses of all kinds; and the hormones must change the manner of processing of incoming information, both by a direct effect on relevant structures and through the intermediary of the central nervous system (Gandelman, 1983).

Conclusions

The complexities of the menstrual cycle continue to emerge, and some of the direct and intermediary mechanisms of these manifestations are becoming clearer. There are well-known fundamental changes in the ovarian and pituitary hormones and in the reproductive organs which normally occur in a cyclical fashion through the reproductive years of each woman. In each ovulatory cycle the early stages of the procreative process are enacted. There are many other neuroendocrine changes with the cycle. Some are an essential part of reproduction; some are an incidental outcome of that process. There is no reason to doubt that there are inherent psychological and behavioural concomitants of the natural plan which ensure the continuation of human life.

These inherent psychological factors are the specific tendencies or predispositions to feelings and behaviour which are appropriate to the reproductive endeavour. Overlaid on the biologically-determined changes are acquired psychological and social effects. Also, environmental factors and events at the time have considerable influence.

There has been no demonstration of a direct relationship between individual levels of ovarian and pituitary hormones on the one hand, and mood and behaviour on the other. Nevertheless, these hormones are in a close functional relationship with the nervous system. Many studies have shown the direct effects of oestrogens and progesterone on the amount of activation in various parts of the brain; there have also been indications of a general effect on brain activity of FH and LSH. It is therefore clear that, with the fluctuations in the levels of these hormones, there will be changes in levels of nervous system activity; this is particularly relevant given the influence of nervous system activity on feelings and behaviour. The reproductive hormones also mediate the effects of other hormones (such as prolactin and prostaglandins), and they have important reciprocal relationships with the neurotransmitters which have been shown to be closely implicated in all forms of psychological and behavioural response.

There are few details of the ways in which androgens, which vary with the cycle, are involved in the reproductive process. Androgens may be an important biological component in the changes with the cycle in some aspects of sexuality, notably sexual feeling and activity which is independent of a partner. Prolactin is closely involved with reproductive functions; various neurotransmitters and the ovarian hormones have regulatory effects on prolactin, which in turn changes fluid balance and possibly emotional reactions. The release of prostaglandins in the central nervous system is thought to be regulated by oestrogen. Conversely, prostaglandins combine with the ovarian hormones to play a determining role in the reproductive process. They are also possibly implicated in emotional response by a different route, namely the autonomic nervous system which seems to be modulated in some way by prostaglandins.

The activities of the renin–angiotensin–aldosterone system vary systematically with the cycle, but the precise role of this system in other changes with the cycle is not clear, though it is assumed to have effects, at least through its salt- and water-retaining properties. The central and autonomic nervous systems play an important part in the widespread manifestations of the menstrual cycle. Some of the details will await the development of new techniques, but it is already clear that many aspects of nervous system activity provide the mechanisms of cyclical change; for example, through their reciprocal relations with ovarian and other hormones, through their control over the ways in which incoming information is processed, and through their regulation of the internal environment which is a basis of psychological responses of all kinds. A background tendency to positive feelings prevails through most of the cycle. The tendency towards changes in mood throughout the cycle is in general appropriate to the reproductive process which unfolds. As fluid retention and pain decline after the onset of menstruation, and as a new set of follicles grows, a mood of progressively greater relaxation and easing of emotional tensions starts and gradually moves, through the follicular into the ovulatory phase, which is a more energetic, assertive, state of well-being where appropriate sensory functions are most acute and cortical arousal is raised; all of which is conducive to conception. In the early luteal phase, when the endometrium is being prepared for pregnancy, the psychological climate tends rather towards a more passive, inward-turning, contented mood which would favour the safeguarding of a fertilized ovum. If there is no pregnancy, the process is reversed, ovarian hormones decline sharply, cortical arousal is low and within four or five days the endometrium starts to be shed in the menstrual flow, usually with some discomfort and pain in the time leading up to and during the onset of menstruation. It is hardly surprising that positive feelings do not predominate at this time of the cycle.

No simple description of sexuality through the cycle is possible, probably because of strong psychological and social factors which often outweigh the biological ones and have differential effects on individuals and groups. It seems likely that a biological pattern is more often expressed in autonomous sexuality, whereas feelings and behaviour with a partner are influenced by many more or less subtle psychological and social factors which are part of all relationships, and especially where fundamental questions of sexuality and procreation are involved. The idea of a homogeneous model of changes in sexual response with the human cycle has to be abandoned in favour of several models, each of which reflects different personal and cultural elements.

The cyclical changes in sensory response appear to be finely tuned to a biological purpose; in each modality there are varying degrees of change according to the particular stimulus. The gonadal hormones appear to determine these fluctuations, in ways not entirely understood. The effects of the sensory variations are far-reaching since they alter the perception of, and the responses to, incoming information. The growing understanding of the physiological and psychological mechanisms of the reproductive process and of the relationships between them will continue to have considerable theoretical and practical implications.

References

Abplanalp, J. M., Donnelly, A. F. and Rose, R. M. (1979). Psychoendocrinology of the menstrual cycle: I. Enjoyment of daily activities and moods. *Psychosomatic Medicine*, **41**, 587–604.

Abplanalp, J. M., Haskett, R. and Rose, R. M. (1980). The premenstrual syndrome. *Advances in Psychoneuroendocrinology*, 3, 324–347.

Adams, D. B., Gold, A. R. and Burt, A. D. (1978). Rise in female-initiated sexual activity at ovulation and its suppression by oral contraceptives. *New England Journal of Medicine*, 299, 1145–1150.

Asso, D. (1983). *The Real Menstrual Cycle*. John Wiley, Chichester.

Asso, D. (1986). The relationship between menstrual cycle changes in nervous system activity and psychological, behavioural and physical variables. *Biological Psychology*, 23, 53–64.

Awaritefe, A., Awaritefe, M., Diejomaoh, F. M. E. and Ebie, J. C. (1980). Personality and menstruation. *Psychosomatic Medicine*, 42, 237–251.

Bäckström, T., Sanders, D., Leask, R., Davidson, D., Warner, P. and Bancroft, J. (1983). Mood, sexuality, hormones, and the menstrual cycle. II. Hormone levels and their relationship to the premenstrual syndrome. *Psychosomatic Medicine*, 45, 503–507.

Bancroft, J. and Bäckström, T. (1985). Premenstrual syndrome. *Clinical Endocrinology*, 22, 313–336.

Bancroft, J., Sanders, D., Davidson, D. and Warner, P. (1983). Mood, sexuality, hormones and the menstrual cycle. III. Sexuality and the role of androgens. *Psychosomatic Medicine*, 45, 509–516.

Baron, M., Levitt, M. and Perlman, R. (1980). Human platelet monoamine oxidase and the menstrual cycle. *Psychiatry Research*, 3, 323–327.

Beumont, P. J., Richards, D. H. and Gelder, M. G. (1975). A study of minor psychiatric and physical symptoms during the menstrual cycle. *British Journal of Psychiatry*, 126, 431–434.

Brush, M. G. (1977). The possible mechanisms causing the premenstrual tension syndrome. *Current Medical Research and Opinion*, 4, **Supplement 4**, 9–15.

Brush, M. G. (1982). Efamol (evening primrose oil) in the treatment of the premenstrual syndrome in *Clinical Uses of Essential Fatty Acids*, (Ed. D. F. Horrobin) Eden Press, Montreal, pp. 155–162.

Clare, A. W. (1985). Hormones, behaviour and the menstrual cycle. *Journal of Psychosomatic Research*, 29, 225–233.

Collins, A., Eneroth, P. and Landgren, B. M. (1985). Psychoneuroendocrine stress responses and mood as related to the menstrual cycle. *Psychosomatic Medicine*, 47, 512–527.

Coulam, C. B. (1981). Age, estrogens, and the psyche. *Clinical Obstetrics and Gynecology*, 24, 219–229.

Cutler, W. B. and Garcia, C. R. (1980). The psychoneuroendocrinology of the ovulatory cycle of women: a review. *Psychoneuroendocrinology*, 5, 89–111.

Gandelman, R. (1983). Gonadal hormones and sensory function. *Neurosciences and Biobehavioural Review*, 7, 1–17.

Golub, S. and Harrington, D. M. (1981). Premenstrual and menstrual mood changes in adolescent women. *Journal of Personality and Social Psychology*, 41, 961–965.

Halbreich, U. and Endicott, J. (1982). Classification of premenstrual syndromes, in *Behavior and the menstrual cycle*, (Ed. R. C. Friedman), Marcel Dekker, New York, pp. 243–265.

Halbreich, U. and Endicott, J. (1985). Methodological issues in studies of premenstrual changes. *Psychoneuroendocrinology*, 10, 15–32.

Janowsky, D. S. and Rausch, J. L. (1985). Biochemical hypotheses of premenstrual tension syndrome. *Psychological Medicine*, 15, 3–8.

Judd, H. L. and Yen, S. S. C. (1973). Serum androstenedione and testosterone levels during the menstrual cycle. *Journal of Clinical Endocrinology and Metabolism*, **36**, 475–481.

Lahmeyer, H., Miller, M. and DeLeon-Jones, F. (1982). Anxiety and mood fluctuation during the normal menstrual cycle. *Psychosomatic Medicine*, **44**, 183–194.

Linkie, D. M. (1982). The physiology of the menstrual cycle, in *Behavior and the Menstrual Cycle* (Ed. R. C. Friedman), Marcel Dekker, New York, pp. 1–21.

Little, B. C. and Zahn, T. P. (1974). Changes in mood and autonomic functioning during the menstrual cycle. *Psychophysiology*, **11**, 579–590.

Matteo, S. and Rissman, E. F. (1984). Increased sexual activity during the midcycle portion of the human menstrual cycle. *Hormones and Behavior*, **18**, 249–255.

Morris, N. M. and Udry, J. R. (1982). Epidemiological patterns of sexual behavior in the menstrual cycle, in *Behavior and the Menstrual Cycle* (Ed. R. C. Friedman), Marcel Dekker, New York, pp. 129–153.

Paige, K. E. (1971). Effects of oral contraceptives on affective fluctuations associated with the menstrual cycle. *Psychosomatic Medicine*, **33**, 515–537.

Panksepp, J. (1986). The neurochemistry of behaviour. *Annual Review of Psychology*, **37**, 77–107.

Parlee, M. B. (1980). Changes in moods and activation levels during the menstrual cycle in experimentally naive subjects, in *The Menstrual Cycle*, Vol. 1, (Eds. A. J. Dan, E. A. Graham and C. P. Boecher), Springer, New York, pp. 247–263.

Parlee, M. B. (1983). Menstrual rhythms in sensory processes: a review of fluctuations in vision, olfaction, audition, taste, and touch. *Psychological Bulletin*, **93**, 539–548.

Rausch, J. L. and Janowsky, D. S. (1982). Premenstrual tension: etiology, in *Behavior and the Menstrual Cycle* (Ed. R. C. Friedman), Marcel Dekker, New York, pp. 397–427.

Reid, R. L. and Yen, S. S. C. (1981). Premenstrual syndrome. *American Journal of Obstetrics and Gynecology*, **139**, 85–104.

Sanders, D. and Bancroft, J. (1982). Hormones and the sexuality of women and the menstrual cycle. *Clinics in Endocrinology and Metabolism*, **11**, 639–659.

Sanders, D., Warner, P., Bäckström, T. and Bancroft, J. (1983). Mood, sexuality, hormones and the menstrual cycle. I. Changes in mood and physical state: Description of subjects and method. *Psychosomatic Medicine*, **45**, 487–501.

Schreiner-Engel, P., Schiavi, R. C., Smith, H. and White, D. (1981). Sexual arousability and the menstrual cycle. *Psychosomatic Medicine*, **43**, 199–214.

Slade, P. (1984). Premenstrual emotional changes in normal woman: fact or fiction? *Journal of Psychosomatic Research*, **28**, 1–7.

Steiner, M., Haskett, R. F., Carroll, B. J., Hays, S. E. and Rubin, R. T. (1984). Plasma prolactin and severe premenstrual tension. *Psychoneuroendocrinology*, **9**, 29–35.

Udry, J. R. and Morris, N. M. (1977). The distribution of events in the human menstrual cycle. *Journal of Reproduction and Fertility*, **51**, 419–425.

Vekemans, M., Delvoye, P., L'Hermite, M. and Robyn, C. (1977). Serum prolactin levels during the menstrual cycle. *Journal of Clinical Endocrinology and Metabolism*, **44**, 989–993.

Yen, S. S. C. and Jaffe, R. B. (1978). *Reproductive Endocrinology*. W. B. Saunders, Philadelphia.

Zimmerman, E. and Parlee, M. (1973). Behavioral changes associated with the menstrual cycle: an experimental investigation. *Journal of Applied Social Psychology*, **3**, 335–344.

Functional Disorders of the Menstrual Cycle
Edited by M. G. Brush and E. M. Goudsmit
© 1988 John Wiley & Sons Ltd

CHAPTER 3

Definition of premenstrual syndrome and related conditions

GWYNETH A. SAMPSON
Department of Psychiatry,
Whiteley Wood Clinic,
Woofindin Road,
Sheffield S10 3TL

Menstruation itself is an event marked by the 'shedding of blood' and is therefore observable not only to the woman in whom it occurs but can be demonstrated if need be to others. Even so, there is often uncertainty as to whether bleeding is 'menstrual flow', 'flooding' or 'spotting' and any definition such as, 'menstruation is a time when women require to use sanitary protection' is an arbitrary one. It is therefore not surprising that as we do not have a clear definition of menstruation, we have even less clear definition of all the other reported phenomena which occur before or during the time of bleeding. Our increasing knowledge of the endocrinology of the menstrual cycle has added to the dilemma as bleeding is not always a consequence of the same endocrine profile.

Many phenomena have been reported as related to menstruation, either before, during or after bleeding. However, as the premenstrual and menstrual weeks together comprise half of the life of women in the reproductive years, one would predict half of all reported phenomena would be perimenstrual 'by chance' and thus very accurate definition of terminology is essential in all studies on premenstrual and other menstrually related events.

These phenomena include changes in mood, pain, bloating; some of these problems are reported to cause changes in behaviour or response patterns which would be measurable. There is also some evidence of change in behaviour without 'complaints' (d'Orban and Dalton, 1980).

The menstrual cycle can be sub-divided by time (days) although this requires agreement as to markers, e.g. first day of bleeding, LH surge, 'ovulation'. Unfortunately menstrual cycles even in the same individual are not consistent in terms of length or endocrine changes (Lenton and Landgren, 1985). There is therefore a real problem in choosing how to sub-divide the cycle—by time, by endocrine status, by standardization to 28 days and then sub-dividing into equal parts'.

There have been many definitions of 'premenstrual syndrome' (PMS) but at last a consensus is becoming closer. The essence of all definitions is a group of symptoms, primarily of irritability, depression, breast tenderness and bloating which occur periodically and show a clear relationship between the presence of symptoms and the time of onset of menstruation. Perhaps the most influential of all the definitions of recent years is that of Dalton (1984) who defines PMS 'as the recurrence of symptoms in the premenstruum with absence of symptoms in the postmenstruum. To this she added the following criteria:

1. Symptoms must occur exclusively during the second half of the menstrual cycle.
2. Symptoms must increase in severity as the cycle progresses.
3. Symptoms must be relieved by the onset of the menstrual flow.
4. Symptoms must have been present for at least three consecutive cycles.

'Premenstrual pain' is described either as a facet of PMS but also as a type of dysmenorrhoea. 'Menstrual distress' is a term used by Dalton (1984) for 'the presence of intermittent or continuous symptoms present throughout the menstrual cycle which increase in severity during the premenstruum or menstruation'. She states, 'this definition does not require that the recurrence of symptoms always be at the same time in each menstrual cycle'. Dennerstein et al. (1984) defines 'menstrual distress' as the presence of symptoms of a diagnosable psychiatric disorder which are of at least moderate intensity throughout the cycle with exacerbation in the premenstruum. Abraham (1984) suggests the term 'postmenstrual syndrome' to describe the relative increase in efficiency and performance, heightened sense of well-being and elevation of mood occurring in some women from the end of menstruation until ovulation. However, these positive changes are not 'symptoms' and the use of 'syndrome' in this connection is inappropriate.

In the Sheffield clinic one-third of referrals have a significant increase in well-being postmenstrually, thus showing that this state is not common to all women in this category. The term 'perimenstrual' covers symptoms linked to either or both the premenstrual and menstrual phases. The term 'syndrome' typically refers to a group of symptoms that occur together and characterize a medical or 'abnormal' condition. In PMS it is often used in a more general sense to refer to an inter-related set of experiences that form an identifiable pattern.

Symptoms

Dalton (1984) states that 'the symptoms that can occur in the syndrome are of extraordinary diversity and include many of the commonest symptoms in each medical speciality'. She reports that the commonest reported symptoms at first visit are depression (in 71 per cent of women); irritability (56 per cent); tiredness (35 per cent); headache (33 per cent); bloatedness (31 per cent) and breast tenderness (21 per cent). Sampson and Prescott (1987) found the commonest reported symptoms were irritability (98 per cent); tension (95 per cent); depression (93 per cent); bloatedness (86 per cent); loss of energy (86 per cent) and problems with concentration (85 per cent). Other authors (O'Brien and Symonds, 1985; Rubinow et al., 1984) also find psychological rather than somatic symptoms commoner, although most workers report both psychological and somatic symptoms.

Moos' Menstrual Distress Questionnaire is a list of such symptoms (see Table 1) which has been widely used and adapted by research workers in several countries (Moos, 1985). It was devised from several lists of symptoms which were given and rated on a group of younger women (mean age 25.2 years). The data for 47 symptoms for a sample of 839 women was then intercorrelated and factor analysed to produce eight factor scales composed of an empirically inter-related group of items. No premenstrual symptoms are specific to the condition—they can be experienced by men, children and non-menstruating women, and are symptoms which can be considered either 'normal' or 'ill'. The psychological symptoms are common in happiness, grief, anxiety states, reactive depression and formal psychiatric illness.

We do not yet know whether it is 'normal' for most women to experience some premenstrual symptoms which they do not 'complain' of, i.e. women 'complaining of PMS' are one end of the spectrum of those women who experience premenstrual symptoms. An alternative hypothesis is that PMS is a clear-cut condition which women either have or have not, i.e. a circumscribed illness. Only large epidemiological studies of complete populations will elucidate this dilemma.

Timing of Symptoms

The key to the diagnosis of PMS is not the presence of symptoms but the time relationship of these symptoms to menstruation. Although the onset of bleeding is usually considered to be the end of the premenstrual phase, studies on perimenopausal and hysterectomized women (Bäckström et al., 1981) demonstrate the presence of premenstrual symptoms without bleeding.

Several patterns of premenstrual symptom timing have been described, some starting at midcycle and others occurring just premenstrually. There has as yet been no prospective epidemiological study with daily ratings to provide

Table 1. Symptom scales from the Moos Menstrual Distress
Questionnaire

1. Pain 　5. Muscle stiffness 　9. Headache 　16. Cramps 　22. Backache 　25. Fatigue 　37. General aches and pains	5. Water retention 　1. Weight gain 　10. Skin disorders 　30. Painful breasts 　34. Swelling
2. Concentration 　2. Insomnia 　6. Forgetfulness 　7. Confusion 　24. Lowered judgement 　29. Difficulty concentrating 　33. Distractible 　35. Accidents 　42. Lowered Motor 　co-ordination	6. Negative affect 　3. Crying 　11. Loneliness 　21. Anxiety 　27. Restlessness 　36. Irritability 　38. Mood swings 　40. Depression 　45. Tension 7. Arousal 　13. Affectionate 　14. Orderliness
3. Behavioural change 　4. Lowered school or work 　performance 　8. Take naps; stay in bed 　15. Stay at home 　20. Avoid social activities 　41. Decreased efficiency	18. Excitement 　31. Feelings of well-being 　47. Burst of energy, activity 8. Control 　12. Feeling of suffocation 　19. Chest pains 　32. Ringing in ears
4. Autonomic reactions 　17. Dizziness, faintness 　23. Cold sweats 　26. Nausea, vomiting 　28. Hot flushes	39. Heart pounding 　43. Numbness, tingling 　46. Blind spots, fuzzy vision 9. 44. Appetite change

normative data for the usual pattern and timing of symptoms; traditionally they are described as increasing in severity as menstruation approaches, peaking immediately premenstrually and diminishing with the onset of bleeding. Many authors report a substantial number of women with symptoms which are not confined to the premenstrual phase but persist into menstruation.

Recording of Symptoms

When to Record

Retrospective Rating　There have been many studies drawing attention to a discrepancy between recalled data and information obtained daily throughout the cycle. This was first pointed out by McCance *et al.* (1937) and Altman *et al.* (1941). May (1976) studied women throughout the menstrual cycle, recording mood in several ways and at a later interview obtained a retrospective rating of physical discomfort and mood. He found no relation between a woman's interview report of her mood changes and those changes as actually reported at the differing phases of the menstrual cycle. Metcalf and Hudson (1985) compared retrospective recall on a PMS Self Evaluation Questionnaire and daily records using a visual analogue scale over six cycles and found daily reports showed less severe symptoms than those described at the initial rating.

Retrospective rating ascertains if a woman 'complains of premenstrual syndrome' but does not then differentiate between those who 'complain of premenstrual syndrome and on prospective rating show an increase in symptoms premenstrually and those who 'complain but do not have an increase in symptoms premenstrually'.

However, several authors still use retrospective rating, especially in epidemiological studies. In one study a postal questionnaire was used with a table listing 26 symptoms on which women were asked to indicate:

1. Those which they experienced before menstruation.
2. The duration in days of those symptoms.
3. Whether the symptoms troubled them 'a little', 'moderately', or 'much' (I.H.F. Report, 1979).

As such surveys only produce retrospective reports of 'complaining' it is debatable as to whether they are of value epidemiologically although they may be helpful for studying the relationship between symptom complaints and other factors which could provide a basis for further studies.

Some other problems associated with retrospective studies are that they cannot assess the variance of symptoms during the cycle or the relationship of symptoms to life events. Moreover, there may not be adequate distinction between symptoms occurring before and during bleeding. They may well reflect beliefs about the menstrual cycle and therefore produce a culturally-based biased response (Abplanalp, 1983). There is evidence that they overestimate the presence and severity of symptoms. However, they are of value in screening a population who can then be screened prospectively; they also estimate the incidence of 'complaining' and, as 'complaining' is related to seeking consultation and taking medication, could be used to plan service and other requirements.

Measuring at several fixed times in the cycle   Measurements made at one time in the cycle do not allow an assessment of baseline complaining—e.g., if symptoms are only recorded, albeit prospectively, in the premenstrual phase there is no means of assessing periodicity. In some studies although data is collected at several points during the cycle only one measurement—usually premenstrual—is used in the final data analysis (Graham *et al.*, 1978).

Prospective daily ratings Most authors now conclude that daily prospective rating is the most reliable method of assessing symptoms of PMS (Sampson and Prescott, 1981; Rubinow *et al.*, 1984). Daily ratings may be self-recorded or observed.

Symptom Severity

Although most rating methods list similar symptoms there are a diversity of means of recording the severity of the symptoms. The symptoms are not specific to PMS and may occur with normal or abnormal life stress or minor physical disorders. It is the rise and fall in intensity paramenstrually which is diagnostic.

Forms such as the menstrual chart described by Dalton (1984) and the PMTS Self Rating Scale (Steiner *et al.*, 1980) rate only presence of symptoms.

The Moos Menstrual Distress Questionnaire (Moos, 1985) initially rated symptoms from one (no reaction at all) through to six (acute or partially disabling) whilst the more recent version of the questionnaire rated zero (none) through four (present severe). The Daily Symptom Rating Scale (Taylor, 1979) rates from zero (not at all) through five (very large amount).

Halbreich *et al.* (1982) note that severity ratings made in comparison to a base rate are often more sensitive to differences between groups than are 'absolute severity' ratings of the same clinical feature. They give instructions to rate the severity of change described in each item compared with the usual non-premenstrual score as 'not applicable' (e.g. 'missed work' if unemployed), 'no change' (feature not present at all or did not change in severity), 'minimal change' (only slightly apparent to you, others would probably not be aware of change), 'mild change' (definitely apparent to you and/or others who know you well), 'severe change' (very apparent to you and/or others who know you well), 'extreme change' (degree of change or severity is so different from your usual state that it is very apparent to you or even people who do not know you well might notice).

Several studies use visual analogue scales (Rubinow *et al.*, 1984; Metcalf and Hudson, 1985) which allow for changes in symptom intensity; one advantage is that they do not restrict the user to preset arbitrary categories.

Clearly recording of severity is subjective but whilst it is of value to compare a woman's Monday headache with her Friday one, the value of comparing severity scores between individuals is debatable. It has been reported that a high proportion of women presenting for help with PMS are self-diagnosed and that frequently this diagnosis is not supported by subsequent daily prospective recording. This could theoretically lead to comparable symptoms being rated more severely by these women than by those who do not 'complain' of PMS (Sampson, 1983).

Recording the Base Line

As PMS is an increase in symptom intensity it is important to record the base line, ideally this is done by daily prospective rating. The base line is likely to fluctuate with life stress; in one study an unpredictable peak occurring in several women was finally explained by examination of the actual rather than menstrual date—December 24!

How to Record

Observed events   Although there is a large but debatable literature concerning observable events related to the menstrual cycle (suicide attempts, accidents, assaults upon people or property) in clinical reality these are very rare and therefore unsuitable for assessing changes in symptomatology.

Assessment by rater   One of the earliest assessments of affective change during the menstrual cycle was by a 'rater' analysing dreams (Benedek and Rubenstein, 1939). Silbergeld *et al.* (1971) used a half-hour unstructured interview given by a trained rater who rated on a nine point scale fourteen categories of behaviour and affect (interview rating test).

Self rating   Many authors have devised methods for self rating premenstrual symptoms, some designed for one trial only, others validated on a larger population. All scales record presence of psychological and physical symptoms, they vary as to whether they assess symptom severity. Some scales are designed for prospective use, others for retrospective surveys.

Some workers use self rating scales devised to measure anxiety and depression in a general population, e.g. Modified Beck Depression Scale (Beaumont *et al.*, 1975).

The most widely used questionnaire is the Moos Menstrual Distress Questionnaire (MDQ; Moos, 1985). There are two forms of the MDQ, Form C (over-all cycle)—originally Form A—enables a woman to report her menstrual cycle experiences in three phases of her most recent cycle, i.e. retrospectively. Form T (today) enables a woman to describe her reactions or symptoms for one or more specific days. Form T is suitable for repeated assessment and has been shown to have no evidence of instrument deterioration (Wilcoxon *et al.*, 1976). The MDQ has been revised both in terms of order of items and scales; the original MDQ rates one through to six, the current MDQ zero through to four.

The Premenstrual Assessment Form (PAF) developed by Halbreich et al. (1983) is a retrospective measure. It consists of 95 items descriptive of premenstrual changes in specific kinds of mood, behaviour and physical condition with each item rated on a six point scale of severity of change from usual condition. Women are asked to report their perceptions of each of the symptoms for their last three menstrual cycles. The PAF focusses on degree of change in symptoms rather than on the intensity of the symptom occurrence. The analysis of the PAF data provides a more detailed description of different kinds of retrospectively recalled symptoms than other scales. When the PAF is compared with prospective recording it is reported that women tend to describe their 'worst cycle' on the initial PAF but after one month of daily ratings women tend to score somewhat lower in describing the past cycle on the PAF. The authors comment that the more severe the premenstrual changes described on the PAF the more likely they were to be confirmed by daily ratings.

A menstrual symptom questionnaire devised by Hargrove and Abraham (1982) consists of nineteen symptoms each rated on a four point scale retrospectively for the week following and week preceding menses. Rubinow and Roy-Byrne (1984) note that as the scale was not constructed using standard psychometric procedures that would ensure internal consistency, reliability, reduction of redundancy and cohesiveness of sub-groups, the sensitivity and specificity of the constructs used are questionable.

Metcalf and Hudson (1985) point out the value of a two-tailed visual analogue scale with negative moods always tied to appropriate positive moods; they suggest the positive and negative ends of the scale be reversed in successive questions. They feel a 'normal to dreadful' scale may induce more of a negative response than a 'very good to dreadful' scale.

Several studies use 100 mm visual analogue scales (Metcalf and Hudson 1985; Rubinow et al., 1984).

The self rating scale for premenstrual tension syndrome (PMTS Self Rating Scale) devised by Steiner et al. (1980) is developed from the MDQ with 36 symptoms rated on a yes/no response. It may be used as a daily questionnaire or retrospectively. Maddocks et al. (1986) use the PMTS Self Rating Scale although they comment on the lack of normative data for the scale when used prospectively.

The Daily Symptom Rating Scale (DSRS) (Taylor, 1979) was constructed from items previously used in questionnaires and rating scales measuring menstrual symptoms and has been tested for reliability and validity. It consists of seventeen items rated on a zero through five rating scale and has been demonstrated to produce similar results to the MDQ.

The Prospective Record of the Impact and Severity of Menstrual Symptomatology (PRISM) developed by Reid and Maddocks (Reid, 1985) consists of a 49 day one page calendar listing symptoms to rate one through three; recording lifestyle impact, life events and medications.

The daily dairies used by Dalton were designed for use by GPs and are not specific enough to be used in research.

It has been pointed out by Metcalf and Hudson (1985) that information obtained at interview or by retrospective questionnaire is of limited value in predicting the severity of subsequent episodes of PMS. Metcalf and Hudson feel that it is only when information obtained at interview is combined with information from daily records during untreated and placebo treated cycles that the predictive accuracy of the reliability of a PMS diagnosis is good. They make an interesting point that the daily questionnaire should not be too cumbersome lest it hampers the 'normal' daily symptoms it is recording.

Correlating Symptoms with the Menstrual Cycle

Unfortunately for research workers women do not demonstrate either personal or between women consistency of length of menstrual cycle so a simple numerical relationship of symptoms to cycle day is inappropriate. The presence of daily symptoms may be plotted and a simple calculation of their presence and distribution at arbitrary phases added and a mean per phase calculated. Some workers count back from menstruation (M−1, M−2, etc).

Where symptom intensity as well as presence is recorded a graph may be plotted of symptom intensity against time, likewise symptom clusters (see Figure 1) or visual analogue scale scores.

However, for comparison of groups of women and treatments studied over several cycles, numerical data has to be provided to allow cycle comparisons. The commonest method is to sub-divide the cycle into phases and add the symptom score for each phase. There is no agreed definition of menstrual cycle phases so different authors use differing phases. For example, O'Brien *et al*. (1979) divide the cycle into four phases, Beaumont *et al*. (1975) into a different four; Silbergeld *et al*. (1971) into six phases and Dalton (1977) into seven phases.

When the phase scores are used to produce data many authors only use scores from two or three phases. The phase before menstruation (which varies in studies from five to fourteen days); menstruation (which varies from five to seven days) and a time after menstruation. This latter time varies, and should ideally be adaptable for varying cycle lengths. Taylor (1979) uses all of the cycle apart from menstruation and seven premenstrual days; Rubinow *et al*. (1984) a week after the cessation of menstruation and Metcalf and Hudson (1985) days five to fourteen. The commonest method to produce a 'hard' figure for PMS is to use the difference between the premenstrual score and the score of the 'time after menstruation'.

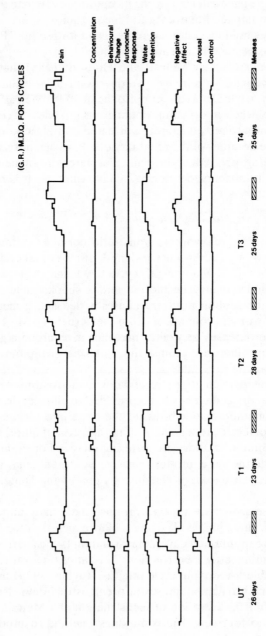

Figure 1. A graph of Moos' Symptom Clusters against time plotted for one subject over five cycles

Sampson and Jenner (1977) describe a method using a least mean square method of fitting sine waves to daily data. This gives a measure of the variation of complaining due to the menstrual cycle, a mean measure of complaining throughout the cycle and the time of the maximal value of the best fit wave compared with the onset of menses. The method can assess whether the increase in symptoms is statistically significant and it can cope with variable cycle lengths.

Abraham et al. (1985) fix the day of ovulation and menstruation and average the days between ovulation and menstruation into seven points such that each point on a computer print-out is the average of one to three days. This is then repeated between menses and ovulation. The data are then computer plotted, which gives a sine wave if there is a premenstrual increase. They report that the advantages are that large volumes of data can be reduced without loss of information and that statistical inferences based on averages become more valid than those based on raw data. These latter two methods use data from all the cycle rather than a limited number of days.

Comparison Between Cycles

Cycles from one individual will require comparison in treatment studies, and in aetiological or epidemiological studies cycles from many individuals need comparing.

Several authors standardize scores to a scale with a mean of zero and a standard deviation of one. Moos (1977) transforms MDQ raw scores into standard scores with a mean of 50 and standard deviations of ten for each scale. This transformation makes it possible to compare scales with each other within one phase, to compare scales across different phases, to compare women with each other across scales and to draw 'menstrual symptom profiles' which graphically depict women's symptom complaints.

The increasing interest amongst research workers in differentiating subgroups of PMS sufferers requires reliable methods of cycle comparison from daily plotted data; there is as yet no standard method for doing this.

Comparison Between PMS Sufferers' Cycles and 'Normal' Control Cycles

If one is able to diagnose the presence of PMS it seems appropriate to be able to diagnose an absence of PMS. Women without premenstrual symptoms could theoretically act as a 'normal' control group—however, the use of the word 'normal' for a woman without premenstrual symptoms implies PMS is 'abnormal', and we have as yet no information as to whether PMS is a clear-cut phenomenon or one end of a spectrum disorder which the majority of women experience. If most women have premenstrual symptoms it is the 'control without premenstrual symptoms' who is statistically abnormal!

Those authors who include 'controls' (Sampson and Jenner, 1977; Dennerstein *et al.*, 1986) often find the 'controls' have cyclical symptoms in relation to menstruation although they may not 'complain of premenstrual syndrome'. It would seem appropriate to have at least two 'control' groups:

1. Those women who do not complain of premenstrual symptoms and do not demonstrate cyclical symptoms.
2. Those who do not complain of PMS but demonstrate cyclical symptoms on prospective rating.

The Value of Defining PMS

PMS means different things to different people—women, their families, general practitioners, research workers, the media and marketing organizations. If a woman visits her general practitioner saying 'I've got PMS' and the doctor feels she has not, their problem is one of differing definitions. This semantic difficulty can cause equal frustration and distress to women who feel they cannot communicate with their doctors and research workers who feel most of the patients they see have not got PMS by their rigidly defined criteria.

Women

Women who are aware of changes in themselves in relation to menstruation may feel it important to have a label—'time of the mcnth', 'the curse' are common labels. In a recent survey inquiring of ex-patients what they found helpful when attending the Sheffield PMS Clinic, 'having a PMS label' was important as it 'made others realize there was a problem'. Women may use the label to describe several conditions—and 'hormones' or 'periods' can be perceived as the cause of symptoms which are due to relationship difficulties or life stress. However, there is no good evidence to refute the fact that the majority of women with premenstrual symptoms lasting a few days use the label appropriately and find it a convenient way of describing their experiences, predicting their presence and adapting their life to the symptoms.

Clinicians

The majority of medical management of PMS is carried out by general practitioners; there are very few specialist clinics in the UK although there has been a recent proliferation of PMS clinics in the USA. A recent postal survey of general practitioners' views on PMS (Alexander *et al.*, 1986) reports that 81 per cent believed they were usually successful in treating PMS. These doctors had clearly made a diagnosis they considered satisfactory—over half the group viewed medication as the most appropriate method of dealing with symptoms. We do not know how the majority of general practitioners make a diagnosis of PMS, or how strict their criteria are. The majority will have had no formal undergraduate or postgraduate teaching on the topic; there are no standard guidelines and their only information may have come from the media, advertising or patients themselves.

It would seem appropriate for a general practitioner, when faced with a woman complaining of PMS, to evaluate her complaints and to exclude other differential diagnoses—the commonest being anxiety states, 'stress', reactive depression and gynaecological conditions producing pain.

General practitioners have a limited time available at the initial interview when the problem may be raised, and because of this the following management scheme may be appropriate.

At the presenting interview the type and duration of symptoms are recorded and the woman is given daily record forms, chosen from the several types currently available. She should be instructed how to complete the daily diary, preferably filling it in every evening from the time of the initial visit. It is often helpful to ask her to stop any treatment she is currently taking. An appointment should be made for a second interview at which gynaecological history and examination, and a full obstetric, psychiatric, personal and medication (prescribed and 'over the counter') history is taken. The question 'why have you come for help *now*' may produce valuable information. At the second visit her charts should be assessed to see if they are being correctly completed and the patient encouraged to continue using them. The majority of women are happy to wait for 'treatment' if they understand the need for a full assessment. In some practices this second visit is linked to a 'Well Woman', family planning or smear clinic. The third visit must be at least two complete menstrual cycles after the first visit as it is important to have at least two cycles of prospective daily dairies for the woman and her doctor to assess. At this visit the doctor should in most cases have enough information to decide if PMS is a primary diagnosis or if there is an alternative gynaecological or psychological diagnosis. If the diagnosis is unclear, further daily prospective charting for two months often elucidates the diagnostic dilemma.

Other secondary health care specialists such as gynaecologists and psychiatrists could follow a similar management scheme although there may be more time available in an out-patient clinic to combine the first and second interviews.

Medico-legal

Menstrual problems as a defence to crime long predate the recognition of PMS (Smith, 1981). Recent cases have required evidence dating from before the offence which shows cyclic symptoms in relation to menstruation, e.g.

daily diaries, observed reports (d'Orban, 1983). It would seem inappropriate to diagnose PMS on retrospective evidence produced after a crime had been committed.

Research

Many of the diagnostic tools used in producing a research worker's definition of PMS have already been described in this chapter. There is a consensus opinion amongst research workers that the majority of women they screen do not have symptoms which occur only premenstrually and which persist over several cycles (Rubinow *et al.* 1984; Steiner *et al.*, 1980; Sampson and Prescott, 1981; Metcalf and Hudson, 1985). Clearly research workers have the 'strictest' definition of PMS and other paramenstrual complaints.

Summary

There does appear to be a group of disorders which produce real distress for women which are related to the menstrual cycle. Although there is a blurring of categories the disorders include primary dysmenorrhoea, premenstrual pain and PMS. Unfortunately the menstrual cycle is sometimes blamed for other real problems which are not directly related to it. The psychological symptoms of PMS are ubiquitous and need differentiating from anxiety states, depression and stress-induced disorders, the physical symptoms from gynaecological or gut disorders. The definition is not a simplistic 'PMS or no PMS' as many psychological or medical disorders may show an increase in symptoms premenstrually. It may also be appropriate to sub-divide 'PMS' into sub-groups of symptom complexes. Proposals for such sub-groups have been put forward (Abraham, 1983) but are not yet generally accepted. Only long-term epidemiological studies will establish definitive sub-groups of PMS. These studies will be complex as, of course, the 'presenting complaint' is dependent upon the ethnic, cultural, socio-economic and psycho-dynamic condition of the woman as well as her menstrual cycle.

At present it may be helpful to record:

1. Is the woman 'complaining' that she has premenstrual symptoms (a PMS reporter)?
2. On prospective charting does she have consistent premenstrual symptoms? (If yes—a PMS reporter with menstrually-linked symptoms. If no—a PMS reporter with no menstrually-linked symptoms).
3. Is there a premenstrual increase of symptoms of a different disorder (premenstrual increase of X disorder)?
4. Do her symptoms interfere with her home, work or social life?

Acknowledgement

I wish to thank Gillian Gill and Elsa Forsythe for their help.

References

Abplanalp, J. M. (1983). Psychological components of the premenstrual syndrome. Evaluating the research and choosing the treatment. *Journal of Reproductive Medicine*, 28, 517–524.

Abraham, G. E. (1983). Nutritional factors in the etiology of the premenstrual tension syndrome. *Journal of Reproductive Medicine*, 28, 446–464.

Abraham, S. (1984). Premenstrual or postmenstrual syndrome? *Medical Journal of Australia*, 141, 327–328.

Abraham, S., Mira, M., McNeil, D., Vizzaro, J., Fraser, I. and Llewellyn Jones, D. (1985). Changes in mood and physical symptoms during the menstrual cycle, in *Premenstrual Syndrome and Dysmenorrhea*, (Eds. M. Y. Dawood, J. L. McGuire and L. M. Demers) Urban and Schwarzenberg, Baltimore, pp. 41–50.

Altman, M., Knowles, E. and Bull, H. D. (1941). A psychosomatic study of the sex cycle in women. *Psychosomatic Medicine*, 3, 199–225.

Alexander, D. A., Taylor, R. J. and Fordyce, I. D. (1986). Assessing our record with PMS. *Journal of the Royal College of General Practitioners*, 36, 10–12.

Bäckström, C. T., Boyle, H. and Baird, D. T. (1981). Persistence of symptoms of premenstrual tension in hysterectomized women. *British Journal of Obstetrics and Gynaecology*, 88, 530–536.

Benedek, T. and Rubenstein, B. B. (1939). The correlations between ovarian activity and psychodynamic processes. Part 2. (The menstrual phase). *Psychosomatic Medicine*, 1, 461–485.

Beaumont, P. J. V., Richards, D. H. and Gelder, M. G. (1975). A study of minor psychiatric and physical symptoms during the menstrual cycle. *British Journal of Psychiatry*, 126, 431–434.

Dalton, K. (1977). *The Premenstrual Syndrome and Progesterone Therapy*, 1st edition, Heinemann, London.

Dalton, K. (1984). *The Premenstrual Syndrome and Progesterone Therapy*, 2nd edition, Heinemann, London.

Dennerstein, L., Morse, C., Brown, J., Smith, M., Oats J. and Burrows, G. (1986). Hormonal treatment for premenstrual complaints, in *Frontiers of Hormonal Research* (Ed. A. Genazzani) Parthenon Press, Carnford.

Dennerstein, L., Spencer Gardner, C., Brown, J. B., Smith, M. A. and Burrows, G. D. (1984). Premenstrual tension—hormonal profiles. *Journal of Psychosomatic Obstetrics and Gynaecology*, 3, 35–51.

d'Orban, P. T. and Dalton, J. (1980). Violent crime and the menstrual cycle. *Psychological Medicine*, 10, 353–359.

d'Orban, P. T. (1983). Medicolegal aspects of the premenstrual syndrome. *British Journal of Hospital Medicine*, 30, 404–409.

Graham, J. J., Harding, P. E., Wise, P. N. and Berriman, H. (1978). Prolactin suppression in the treatment of premenstrual syndrome. *Medical Journal of Australia*, 2, **Special Supplement 3**, 18–20.

Halbreich, U., Endicott, J. and Nee, J. (1983). Premenstrual depressive changes. *Archives of General Psychiatry*, 40, 535–542.

Halbreich, U., Endicott, J., Schacht, S. and Nee, J. (1982). The diversity of premenstrual changes as reflected in the premenstrual assessment form. *Acta Psychiatrica Scandinavica*, **65**, 46–65.

Hargrove, J. T. and Abraham, G. E. (1982). The incidence of premenstrual tension in a gynaecological clinic. *Journal of Reproductive Medicine*, **27**, 721–724.

I.H.F. Report (1979). *The Premenstrual Syndrome—A Report from the International Health Foundation*, I.H.F., Geneva.

Lenton, E. A. and Landgren, B. M. (1985). The normal menstrual cycle, in *Clinical Reproductive Endocrinology*, (Ed. R. P. Shearman) Churchill Livingstone, Edinburgh, pp. 81–108.

Maddocks, S., Hahn, P., Moller, F. and Reid, R. L. (1986). A double blind placebo controlled trial of progesterone vaginal suppositories in the treatment of premenstrual syndrome. *Americal Journal of Obstetrics and Gynecology*, **154**, 573–581.

May, P. R. (1976). Mood shifts and the menstrual cycle. *Journal of Psychosomatic Research*, **20**, 125–130.

McCance, R. A., Luff, M. C. and Widdowson, E. H. (1937). Physical and emotional periodicity in women. *Journal of Hygiene (London)*, **37**, 571–611.

Metcalf, M. G. and Hudson, S. M. (1985). The premenstrual syndrome. Selection of women for treatment trials. *Journal of Psychosomatic Research*, **29**, 631–638.

Moos, R. H. (1977). *Menstrual Distress Questionnaire Manual*, Social Ecology Laboratory, Stanford University, California.

Moos, R. H. (1985). *Perimenstrual Symptoms: A Manual and overview of Research with the Menstrual Distress Questionnaire*, Social Ecology Laboratory, Department of Psychiatry and Behavioural Sciences, Stanford University, California.

O'Brien, P. M. S., Craven, D., Selby, C. and Symonds, E. M. (1979). Treatment of premenstrual syndrome by spironolactone. *British Journal of Obstetrics and Gynaecology*, **86**, 142–147.

O'Brien, P. M. S. and Symonds, E. M. (1985). The premenstrual syndrome, in *Clinical Reproductive Endocrinology*, (Ed. R. P. Shearman) Churchill Livingstone, Edinburgh, pp. 599–620.

Reid, R. L. (1985). Premenstrual syndrome, In *Current Problems in Obstetrics, Gynecology and Fertility*, Vol. 8, (Ed. J. M. Leventhal) Year Book Medical Publishers, Chicago, Illinois.

Rubinow, D. R. and Roy-Byrne, P. (1984). Premenstrual syndrome: Overview from a methodologic perspective. *American Journal of Psychiatry*, **141**, 163–172.

Rubinow, D. R., Roy-Byrne, P., Hoban, C., Gold, P. W. and Post, R. M. (1984). Prospective assessment of menstrually related mood disorders. *American Journal of Psychiatry*, **141**, 684–686.

Sampson, G. A. (1983). Stress and premenstrual syndrome, in *The Premenstrual Syndrome*, (Ed. R. W. Taylor) Medical News Tribune Ltd., London, pp. 43–49.

Sampson, G. A. and Jenner, F. A. (1977). Studies of daily recording from the Moos Menstrual Distress Questionnaire. *British Journal of Psychiatry*, **130**, 265–271.

Sampson, G. A. and Prescott, P. (1981). The assessment of the symptoms of premenstrual syndrome and their response to therapy. *British Journal of Psychiatry*, **138**, 399–405.

Sampson, G. A. and Prescott, P. (1987). 'I've got PMS doctor'—A review of those women who seek help in Premenstrual Syndrome Clinics (in press).

Silbergeld, S., Brast, N. and Noble, E. P. (1971). A double blind study of symptoms, mood and behaviour and biochemical variables using Enovid and placebo. *Psychosomatic Medicine*, **33**, 411–427.

Smith, R. (1981). *Trial by Medicine. Insanity and Responsibility in Victorian Trials*, Edinburgh University Press, Edinburgh.

Steiner, M., Haskett, R. F. and Carroll, B. J. (1980). Premenstrual tension syndrome—the development of research diagnostic criteria and new rating scales. *Acta Psychiatrica Scandinavica*, **62**, 177–190.

Taylor, J. W. (1979). The timing of menstruation related symptoms assessed by a daily symptom rating scale. *Acta Psychiatrica Scandinavica*, **60**, 87–105.

Wilcoxon, L., Schrader, S. and Sherif, C. (1976). Daily self reports on activities, life events, moods and somatic changes during the menstrual cycle. *Psychosomatic Medicine*, **38**, 399–417.

Functional Disorders of the Menstrual Cycle
Edited by M. G. Brush and E. M. Goudsmit
© 1988 John Wiley & Sons Ltd

CHAPTER 4

The role of specialized investigations in the management of the more unusual spontaneous and iatrogenic disorders of the menstrual cycle

M. G. BRUSH
Department of Gynaecology
United Medical and Dental Schools, St Thomas's Campus,
London SE1 7EH

Not all disturbances of function in the menstrual cycle fit easily into the classical definitions of PMS, dysmenorrhoea, menorrhagia, etc.

Some of these less typical problems occur spontaneously and are relatively rare, i.e. mid-cycle problems, anovulatory cycles with premenstrual difficulties and the so-called 'postmenstrual' syndrome. Rather more common are the disturbances which appear to be a consequence of medical treatment, e.g. PMS-like conditions while on the oral contraceptive pill, and problems after tubal ligation and hysterectomy. Other specialized situations include premenstrual deterioration of allergic conditions and the special problems of premenstrual breast conditions, especially if aggravated by fibrocystic breast disease.

In all these situations it may be difficult, if not impossible, to apply orthodox PMS treatment, and investigation may be an essential preliminary to any attempt at treatment. In this chapter these specialized situations are considered, and appropriate investigations and action are suggested.

Mid-cycle Problems

It has been recognized by many authors that PMS can start at midcycle (Israel, 1938; Harrison, 1982; Labrum, 1983; Norris, 1983; Reid and Yen, 1983; Brush, 1984) though this has been denied or ignored by many other writers.

Quite frequently symptoms begin to appear from the approximate time of ovulation and build up steadily to a peak just before the onset of menstruation. Alternatively, there may be an unpleasant two to three days of PMS around the time of ovulation followed by a return to a reasonable state until typical PMS shows itself in the five to seven days before menstruation (Reid and Yen, 1983).

It may be very important to establish the time of ovulation as precisely as possible, particularly if it is occurring early. Many women may be unaware that it is not very uncommon for ovulation to occur from days eight to eleven rather than days 12 to 14, as commonly believed. If an unequivocal answer is not obtained from temperature charts or observation of cervical mucus, serial blood samples for oestradiol, LH, FSH and progesterone may be justified to attempt to catch the ovulation peak or, failing that, detect the first rise in progesterone levels. An alternative method of detecting ovulation may be frequent ultrasound tests (Hackelöer et al., 1979; Queenan et al., 1980, Sallam et al., 1982), but this is usually impractical except for those women living close to major hospitals. Failure to identify the time of ovulation may lead to delay in starting appropriate treatment, which may greatly reduce its effectiveness and may also cause unnecessary worry to the PMS sufferer.

Other Midcycle Situations

Mittelschmerz (ovulation pain)   Ovulation pain is usually regarded as within the range of normal by gynaecologists but may be very frightening to the women who suffer from it, unless they are used to it. It usually lasts only a few hours but may be very sharp. If pain is present for longer than 48 hours there may be other factors involved and gynaecological advice is needed, especially if the pain is severe. If the sufferer is concerned to have proof that the pain is associated with ovulation, hormone tests to establish the midcycle peaks of oestradiol, LH and FSH may be helpful, especially if carried out in association with ultrasound and cervical mucus studies.

Recent work, using ultrasound and hormone measurements, has shown conclusively that true mittelschmerz is a pre-ovulatory phenomenon (O'Herlihy et al., 1980).

Treatment of midcycle pain may be difficult unless total suppression of ovulation can be justified. Quite good results can often be obtained by giving dydrogesterone, 10 mg twice daily from day five to day 26. This may be especially appropriate if dysmenorrhoea or severe PMS is also present as these problems may also be improved. Dydrogesterone is not contraceptive in action but appears to alter the characteristics of the ovulation to a more acceptable form.

If the ordinary contraceptive pill can be accepted by the patient, a good result may also be obtained.

Midcycle Migraine   Another event which may confuse the situation at mid-cycle is the rather rare condition of 'midcycle migraine' which last up to two or three days.

Menstrually-linked migraine accounts for 20–25 per cent of all migraine in women and occurs just before or just after the start of menstruation (see Chapter 14). In a small proportion of menstrual migraine sufferers, there is also an attack of migraine at midcycle (Lance and Anthony, 1966; Adams, 1977; Migraine Trust, 1979). Even more rarely, midcycle migraine may occur separately with no association with menstrual migraine.

The characteristics of midcycle migraine are similar to those of other types of migraine and the usual methods of symptomatic relief can be used (see Chapter 14). It is certainly very unwise to attempt to use the contraceptive pill to suppress ovulation in midcycle migraine sufferers, as it is likely to make the migraine situation much worse. Similarly, any attempt to use synthetic progestogens, including dydrogesterone, should be undertaken with great caution in case marked deterioration of migraine occurs.

Anovulatory Cycles

Controversy exists over the possible occurrence of premenstrual symptoms in women with anovulatory cycles (Bancroft and Bäckström, 1985). Orthodox opinion suggests that if ovulation does not take place, it is impossible for true PMS to occur due to the absence of progesterone on the second half of the cycle, as this is thought to preclude the hormonal environment which is believed to act as the final trigger to the symptoms of PMS. However, certain brief preliminary reports have suggested that PMS-like problems may occur in proven anovulatory cycles (Adamopoulous *et al.*, 1972; Andersen *et al.*, 1977; Bäckström *et al.*, 1983), but firm evidence for this appears to be lacking.

Due to the unreliability of basal body temperature charts in a high percentage of cases, it is not easy to get satisfactory evidence of anovulatory cycles unless plasma progesterone measurements or high resolution ultra-sound are used. Ideally, plasma progesterone should be measured on several occasions in the second half of the cycle, but this is rarely possible outside the research clinic. However, it is easier to obtain a progesterone value between days 20–22 in a 28-day cycle and, for this purpose, a single value may be perfectly adequate, particularly if the value is clearly undetectable or clearly high (Israel *et al.*, 1972; Radwanska *et al.*, 1981; Hull *et al.*, 1982; Wathen *et al.*, 1984).

Further studies on the incidence of PMS-like conditions in women with anovulatory cycles would be very useful, especially if supported by detailed endocrine studies. At present it is not possible to give firm recommendations for treatment where 'PMS' is suspected in anovulatory cycles but it would be worth trying orthodox nutritional approaches.

PMS-like Problems While Using Oral Contraception

It is sometimes suggested that oral contraception is a suitable treatment for PMS but experience suggests that this is not so, especially if the PMS is severe. However, it is true that PMS-like problems are very unlikely to occur while on the pill if there has been no PMS before. On stopping the pill, it is not uncommon for PMS to start in women who have not suffered from it before. Various aspects of PMS and the pill have been reviewed by Brush (1985).

If cyclical problems, similar to PMS, are seen in a woman on the pill, it is important to assess whether the situation is due to side-effects of the pill (Guillebaud, 1980; Spence, 1981) or to a PMS-like syndrome. Genuine pill side-effects are likely to be present throughout the time that the pill is taken and, in the case of depression, it may be fairly easy to control the situation with pyridoxine treatment (Baumblatt and Winston, 1970; Adams et al., 1973; Winston, 1973; Applegate et al., 1979; Miller, 1985).

However, a few cases do occur in which a definite cyclical pattern is claimed starting from day fourteen and continuing until the onset of menstruation. The usual symptoms reported are bloating, irritability and other mood changes. Virtually no experimental studies have been carried out on women on the pill with a 'PMS-like' condition, and it is only possible to speculate on possible mechanisms, such as failure of complete suppression of the events leading up to ovulation or other cyclical events precipitating symptoms in the presence of the continuous oestrogen–progestogen environment.

In a small study on 77 women with PMS who took oral contraceptives, Freeman et al. (1985) reported that 30 per cent became worse, 34 per cent improved, and 36 per cent noted no change. Cullberg (1972) noted a group of PMS sufferers whose symptoms were worse on oral contraceptives with their brief premenstrual episodes of depression being replaced by chronic mild to moderate depression.

Various anecdotal reports assert improvement in PMS symptoms while taking oral contraceptives (Keye, 1985; Smith, 1975; Kutner and Brown, 1972; Nilsson and Solvell, 1967; Herzberg and Coppen, 1970), but well designed trials have reported different findings. Moos (1968) reported no significant difference in the distribution of premenstrual symptoms in a study comparing oral contraceptive users versus controls, and Morris and Udry (1972), in a double-blind placebo controlled study with oral contraceptive users versus controls, showed no significant difference but considerable variability. Herzberg et al. (1970) noted a small increase in severe depression in oral contraceptive users as compared with controls.

Little work has been carried out on the progesterone-only pill (POP) in the treatment of PMS. Anecdotal reports of responses are very variable and it is clear that well designed studies may be needed to establish the value of the POP in PMS.

It is difficult to draw any final conclusions about oral contraception in relation to PMS due to conflicting reports and lack of detailed biochemical studies. However, there seems to be a need for caution and regular monitoring if oral contraception is used in women with a known history of severe PMS.

Postmenstrual PMS

Very occasionally women may claim that they suffer from PMS-like symptoms throughout menstruation, or starting in mid-menstruation and continuing until about day twelve of the cycle. Obviously, this is outside the accepted definition of PMS, but as the history may strongly suggest a cyclical phenomenon, it may be of value to consider the possibilities.

When ordinary PMS appears to continue until the end of menstruation, a careful history will often show that the symptom pattern changes within 24–48 h of the onset of menstruation and the main complaints are tiredness and depression with little or no sign of bloating, breast problems or food cravings. In some cases, the symptoms are mainly due to reaction and, possibly, guilt feelings arising from events caused by the PMS, especially if extreme mental and family stress has been present. In severe cases of this 'menstrual PMS', it may be necessary to carry out routine investigation, including haemoglobin and free thyroxine measurements. Normal results in these tests, combined with strong reassurance, may encourage the sufferer to co-operate with further counselling and nutritional help. It is helpful to recommend that nutritional help is continued throughout menstruation rather than stopping on day two of the cycle. A strong multivitamin and mineral supplement can be added to any existing treatment, such as vitamin B_6 and/or γ-linolenic acid.

In the extremely rare cases in which a cluster of symptoms similar to PMS occurs between days three and twelve on a regular basis, it may be necessary to carry out a full endocrine screening and, possibly, a clinical chemistry screen to exclude other conditions. If results are completely normal and psychological stresses appear to be absent, it may be helpful to start continuous vitamin and mineral supplements on a trial basis. Any other action is best decided on an individual basis. Suppression of ovulation has been tried but should probably be regarded as a last resort.

Claims for 'PMS' in Pregnancy, Menopause, etc.

Some writers about PMS carry to extremes their belief in its importance by asserting that 'PMS' or a PMS-like condition can occur in situations where the ovarian cycle does not exist, such as pregnancy and both natural and surgical menopause (Gray, 1941; Morton, 1950; Dalton, 1984; Labrum, 1983;

Janowsky and Rausch, 1985). They claim to have observed symptoms occurring in a regular monthly pattern and assert that it represents a type of PMS. This seems to make a nonsense of definitions now generally agreed. The only possible explanation of such events could be some residual cyclical activity in the pituitary–ovarian axis which had not been entirely obliterated by pregnancy or the menopause. No endocrine or other scientific evidence has ever been advanced in support of these assertions and they will not be considered further in this contribution.

Nearly all recent discussion on the definition of PMS specifically excludes conditions which are not associated with the luteal phase of the cycle (Pariser et al., 1985; Magos and Studd, 1984).

PMS After Hysterectomy

It is common gynaecological practice to conserve both ovaries during a hysterectomy unless they are diseased and, in such situations, ovarian function will usually continue for many years with little or no change (Whitelaw, 1958; Beavis et al., 1969; Doyle et al., 1971). PMS sufferers who are in this position will, therefore, be liable to experience cyclical problems closely similar to those they had before hysterectomy but without the menstrual flow to act as a marker to the cycle. Relief from the problems of pain and heavy periods which led to the hysterectomy, may produce improvement in mood in some cases, but in the more unlucky sufferers, all the earlier symptoms continue and may, indeed, become significantly worse (Lauersen and Stukane, 1983).

It may be necessary to establish the timing of the ovarian cycle by means of at least four blood samples over four weeks analysed for oestradiol, progesterone, LH and FSH. Once the timing of the cycle is known, it becomes much easier to arrange suitable treatment and there is considerable psychological reassurance for the patient in knowing the precise nature of the situation.

An interesting study on seven women with PMS before and after hysterectomy, carried out by Bäckström et al. (1981) showed clearly that cyclical physical and mental symptoms previously associated with PMS persisted after hysterectomy. Unfortunately, the study was only continued for two cycles after hysterectomy. Some small improvements in PMS symptoms were noted after hysterectomy but these could be accounted for by various short-term psychological factors associated with the successful outcome of the operation as regards general health.

It is also interesting to note the normal cyclical ovarian activity seen by Fraser et al. (1973) in two women with congenital absence of uterus, fallopian tubes, and vagina.

Tubal Occlusion and PMS

Several authors have noted adverse changes in menstrual pattern and ovarian function after sterilization by tubal ligation (Muldoon, 1972; Radwanska *et al.*, 1979, 1982; Hargrove and Abraham, 1981). Sterilization by electro-coagulation or tubal ring is often said to have no adverse effects (Stock, 1978; Lawson *et al.*, 1979; Kwak *et al.*, 1980; Bhiwandiwala *et al.*, 1982). Corson *et al.*, 1981 found no significant difference in progesterone and oestradiol levels after sterilization as compared with control values.

It has been suggested that PMS may start or become more severe after tubal ligation (Hargrove and Abraham, 1981) but, although the data are rather limited, it was not unreasonable to suggest that the considerable interference with the blood supply to the fallopian tubes and ovaries, as can happen in surgical sterilization, might affect ovarian secretory activity. This, in turn, might alter the ovarian signals which are involved in the final pathway to the onset of PMS. However, De Stefano *et al.* (1985), in a large study on sterilized women and controls, were unable to find a significant difference in PMS incidence between the two groups.

As it would appear that laparoscopic sterilization by clips or cautery is less likely to interfere with the cycle than tubal ligation, it would be helpful to have more evidence on the incidence of PMS after all forms of sterilization, and also more data on any endocrine changes that may be noted.

In individual cases, it may be helpful to measure mid-luteal progesterone levels together with oestrogen, FSH and LH values.

Premenstrual Deterioration of Allergic Conditions

It is now slowly being recognized that a variety of allergic conditions may show marked worsening in the premenstrual phase of the cycle (Wraith, 1982). Strictly speaking, this should be regarded as another example of 'menstrual distress', as discussed earlier (Chapter 1), but will be considered here as it could be mistaken for PMS in some circumstances. It can also occur simultaneously with PMS (Atton-Chamla *et al.*, 1980) and cause considerable confusion. In particular, allergic symptoms will be unaffected by all the commonly used treatments for PMS, thereby causing anxiety about the future outlook for the sufferer's condition.

Although not all asthma is of allergic aetiology, it is interesting that Gibbs *et al.* (1984) found that 40 per cent of asthmatic women showed significant premenstrual deterioration. Unfortunately, the authors did not consider the allergic history of their patients.

In common with all other medical consultations, a good consultation about PMS should include a brief dietary and allergy history. If this raises any suspicion of a significant allergic background, enquiry should be extended to cover a much more detailed background and include discussion of possible chemical sensitivities which are rarely included in orthodox medical histories. If there is any hint of the common allergies to house dust, pollen, moulds, animal hair, etc., an IgE test should be taken to give some idea of the severity of the condition. Atton-Chalma *et al.* (1980) found very high levels of IgE in 27 per cent of their PMS patients, but the study was a small one and further information would be valuable. An IgE level may also be helpful in less well defined conditions and may point to the need for more specialized allergic investigations.

There are many allergies and sensitivities which do not react in the IgE test and there are no generally recognized laboratory tests available for the investigation of these conditions. It may be necessary to refer the sufferer to an expert in allergy or clinical ecology but in some cases of food allergy a simple exclusion diet followed by a challenge with suspected foods may be sufficient to identify the offending substances. If only one or two simple groups of food, such as wheat products or milk products, are involved, it may be possible to recommend a diet which will give great improvement without any danger of lack of balance or vitamin deficiency in the diet. However, if a number of different food allergies are involved, specialist help is very important as inexpert attempts at dietary manipulation can lead to further ill health in some cases.

Premenstrual Breast Conditions

There is considerable overlap between various types of breast discomfort which form part of PMS and benign breast disease occurring quite separately from PMS (the latter is discussed at length in Chapter 12).

In some cases of moderate to average breast swelling and discomfort occurring solely as part of a well defined PMS with several symptoms, it is almost certainly not necessary to undertake any special investigations in the first instance. It is usually preferable to undertake a therapeutic trial of pyridoxine, evening primrose oil, or both together (see Chapter 5), and only consider investigations if no satisfactory response is obtained. In the majority of less severe cases, the response to pyridoxine or evening primrose oil is good (Brush, 1982, 1984).

In severe cases of breast discomfort, or in milder cases where preliminary therapy has been unsuccessful, it is important that the clinician carries out routine breast examination to detect the possible presence of fibrocystic breast disease as, if this is present, the future management may be rather different. The next step is to measure serum prolactin levels and, if possible, carry out a general hormone profile including oestradiol, mid-luteal progesterone, LH and FSH, and thyroxine, to exclude the presence of more general endocrine disease.

Even in severe cases of premenstrual breast discomfort and in PMS co-existing with fibrocystic breast disease, prolactin levels may often be quite normal (Cole *et al.*, 1977; Mansel *et al.*, 1978; Blichert-Toft *et al.*, 1979; Watt-Boolsen *et al.*, 1981), in which case the sufferer can be reassured that no serious hormone disorder is present and that orthodox nutritional treatment is likely to succeed in the next eight to twelve weeks. However, hyperprolactinaemia has been reported in benign breast disease (Cole *et al.*, 1976) but our experience would suggest that this is quite unusual.

If the prolactin levels are raised up to 100 per cent above the upper limit of the normal range (say, 800 mU 1^{-1} where the normal range is 70–380 mU 1^{-1}, a skull X-ray may be considered desirable together with a therapeutic trial of a low dose (1.25–2.5 mg day $^{-1}$) of bromocriptine. If prolactin levels are reduced into the normal range by bromocriptine, it is probable, but by no means certain, that the breast discomfort will be relieved, particularly if no fibrocystic condition is present.

Where the prolactin levels are raised to more than 100 per cent above the upper limit of the normal range, the clinician may wish to carry out more detailed tests to exclude serious pituitary disease. These may include pituitary tomographs or CAT scan and visual field investigations. Frequent monitoring of the prolactin levels during bromocriptine therapy may be desirable.

If a severe fibrocystic condition is present, it may take at least four months, and sometimes much longer, before any form of treatment is successful even if prolactin levels have been reduced to normal by bromocriptine. If response is delayed, it may be valuable to carry out a regular check of prolactin levels to ensure that the dose of bromocriptine is still adequate.

On an experimental basis, TRH and LH-RH tests have been employed in a few cases of severe cyclical mastalgia (Kumar *et al.*, 1984). The release of prolactin, LH and FSH was significantly greater in these patients than in controls. These results are discussed in detail in Chapter 12. It would be very useful if TRH and LH-RH tests could be carried out in well defined cases of PMS which include breast problems.

It is very unusual for other hormone changes to be seen in cyclic breast conditions (Kumar *et al.*, 1984) but if abnormalities are found, investigations should be carried out on an individual basis. It was suggested by Sitruk-Ware *et al.* (1977) that progesterone deficiency in the luteal phase and the consequent unopposed oestrogen activity was a cause of benign breast disease. However, this has not been confirmed by other studies (Swain *et al.*, 1973; England *et al.*, 1975; Kumar *et al.*, 1984; M. G. Brush, unpublished).

Although London *et al.* (1983), in a double-blind study of vitamin E versus placebo in PMS patients, failed to find significant improvement in premenstrual breast conditions, these authors still advocate the use of 600 u day^{-1} dl-α-tocopherol in fibrocystic breast disease on the basis of open studies (London *et al.*, 1978, 1981; Sundaram *et al.*, 1981). They were unable to detect any significant difference in vitamin E levels between patients and controls, but the numbers involved were small. It would, therefore, be very valuable if more detailed studies of vitamin E levels and metabolism could be carried out in women with various types of menstrually-linked breast conditions.

The work of Minton *et al.* (1979a, b, 1981) suggested that women with fibrocystic breast disease may benefit by stopping all caffeine-containing drinks, but the methodology involved is open to considerable criticism. The conflicting results of subsequent studies, whether prospective or case control, are reviewed in detail by Levinson and Dunn (1986), who conclude that there is little evidence to support an association between caffeine consumption and fibrocystic breast disease. Further work with rigorous methodology and studies on metabolism and excretion of caffeine and other methyl xanthines would be helpful in resolving this problem, although in a preliminary study, Sundaram *et al.* (1982) found no significant difference in serum methyl xanthine levels between patients with fibrocystic breast disease and controls.

References

Adamopoulous, D. A., Loraine, J. A., Lunn, S. F., Coppen, A. and Daly, R. (1972). Endocrine profiles in premenstrual tension. *Clinical Endocrinology*, 1, 283–292.

Adams, P. W., Rose, D. F., Folkard, J., Wynn, V., Seed, M. and Strong, R. (1973). Effect of pyridoxine hydrochloride (vitamin B_6) upon depression associated with oral contraception, *Lancet*, i, 897–904.

Adams, R. D. (1977). Headache in *Harrison's Principles of Internal Medicine* (8th edition) McGraw Hill, New York, p. 23.

Andersen, A. B., Larsen, J. F., Steenstrup, O. R., Svenstrup, B. and Nielsen, J. (1977). The effect of bromocriptine on the premenstrual syndrome. A double-blind clinical trial, *British Journal of Obstetrics and Gynaecology*, 84, 370–374.

Applegate, W. V., Forsythe, A. and Bauernfeind, J. B. (1979). Physiological and psychological effects of vitamins E and B_6 on women taking oral contraceptives. *International Journal of Vitamin and Nutrition Research*, 49, 43–50.

Atton-Chamla, A., Favre, G., Goudard, J.-R., Miller, G., Rocca Serra, J.-P., Teitelbaum, M., Vallette, C. and Charpin, J. (1980). Premenstrual syndrome and atopy: a double-blind clinical evaluation of treatment with a gamma-globulin/histamine complex. *Pharmatherapeutica*, 2, 481–486.

Bäckström, C. T., Boyle, H. and Baird, D. T. (1981). Persistence of symptoms of premenstrual tension in hysterectomized women. *British Journal of Obstetrics and Gynaecology*, 80, 530–546.

Bäckström, T., Sanders, D., Leask, R., Davidson, D., Warner, P. and Bancroft, J. (1983). Mood, sexuality, hormones, and the menstrual cycle. II. Hormone levels and their relationship to the premenstrual syndrome. *Psychosomatic Medicine*, 45, 503–507.

Bancroft, J. and Bäckström, T. (1985). Premenstrual syndrome. *Clinical Endocrinology*, 22, 313–316.

Baumblatt, M. J. and Winston, F. (1970). Pyridoxine and the pill. *Lancet*, i, 832–833.

Beavis, E. L. G., Brown, J. B. and Smith, M. A. (1969). Ovarian function after hysterectomy with conservation of the ovaries in pre-menopausal women. *Journal of Obstetrics and Gynaecology of the British Commonwealth*, 76, 969–978.

Bhiwandiwala, P. P., Mumford, S. D. and Feldblum, P. J. (1982). Menstrual pattern changes following laparoscopic sterilization. A comparative study of electro coagulation and the tubal ring in 1025 cases. *Journal of Reproductive Medicine*, 27, 249–255.

Blichert-Toft, M., Andersen, A. N., Henriksen, O. B. and Mygind, T. (1979). Treatment of mastalgia with bromocriptine: a double-blind cross-over study. *British Medical Journal*, i, 237.

Brush, M. G. (1982). Efamol (gamma-linolenic acid) in the treatment of the premenstrual syndrome, in *Clinical Uses of Essential Fatty Acids*, (Ed. D. F. Horrobin) Eden, Montreal, pp. 151–161.

Brush, M. G. (1984). *Understanding Premenstrual Tension*, Pan, London.

Brush, M. G. (1985). The premenstrual syndrome before and after pregnancy. *Maternal and Child Health*, 10, 19–25.

Cole, E. N., England, P. C., Sellwood, R. A. and Griffiths, K. (1976). Prolactin in benign and malignant breast disease. *Journal of Endocrinology*, 69, 49–50P.

Cole, E. N., Sellwood, R. A., England, P. C. and Griffiths, K. (1977). Serum prolactin concentrations in benign breast disease throughout the menstrual cycle. *European Journal of Cancer*, 13, 597–603.

Corson, S. L., Levinson, C. J., Batzer, F. R. and Otis, C. (1981). Hormonal levels following sterilization and hysterectomy. *Journal of Reproductive Medicine*, 26, 363–370.

Cullberg, J. (1972). Mood changes and menstrual symptoms with different gestagen-estrogen combinations. A double-blind comparison with placebo, *Acta Psychiatrica Scandanavica*, Supplement 236, 1–86.

Dalton, K. (1984). *The Premenstrual Syndrome and Progesterone Therapy*, Heinemann, London.

De Stefano, F., Perlman, J. A., Peterson, H. B. and Diamond, E. L. (1985). Long-term risk of menstrual disturbances after tubal sterilization. *American Journal of Obstetrics and Gynecology*, 152, 835–841.

Doyle, L. L., Barclay, D. L., Duncan, G. W. and Kirton, K. T. (1971). Human luteal function following hysterectomy as assessed by plasma progestin. *American Journal of Obstetrics and Gynecology*, 110, 92–97.

England, P. C., Skinner, L. G., Cottrell, K. M. and Sellwood, R. A. (1975). Sex hormones in breast disease. *British Journal of Surgery*, 62, 806–809.

Fraser, I. S., Baird, D. T., Hobson, B. M., Michie, E. A. and Hunter, W. (1973). Cyclical ovarian function in women with congenital absence of the uterus and vagina. *Journal of Clinical Endocrinology and Metabolism*, 36, 634–637.

Freeman, E. W., Sondheimer, S., Weinbaum, P. J. and Rickels, K. (1985). Evaluating premenstrual symptoms in medical practice. *Obstetrics and Gynecology, N.Y.*, 65, 500–505.

Gibbs, C. J., Coutts, I. I., Lock, R., Finnegan, O. C. and White, R. J. (1984). Premenstrual exacerbation of asthma. *Thorax*, 39, 833–836.

Gray, L. A. (1941). The use of progesterone in nervous tension states. *Southern Medical Journal*, 34, 1004–1006.

Guillebaud, J. (1980). *The Pill*, Oxford University Press, Oxford, pp. 55–119.

Hackelöer, B. J., Fleming, R., Robinson, H. P., Adam, A. H. and Coutts, J. R. (1979). Correlation of ultrasonic and endocrinologic assessment of human follicular development. *American Journal of Obstetrics and Gynecology*, 135, 122–148.

Hargrove, J. T. and Abraham, G. E. (1981). Endocrine profile of patients with post-tubal-ligation syndrome. *Journal of Reproductive Medicine*, 26, 359–362.

Harrison, M. (1982). *Self-help for Premenstrual Symptoms*, Random House, New York, p. 66.

Herzberg, B. and Coppen, A. (1970). Changes in psychological symptoms in women taking oral contraceptives. *British Journal of Psychiatry*, **116**, 161–164.

Herzberg, B. N., Johnson, A. L. and Brown, S. (1970). Depressive symptoms and oral contraceptives. *British Medical Journal*, **4**, 142–145.

Hull, M. G. R., Savage, P. E., Bromham, D. R., Ismail, A. A. A. and Morris, A. F. (1982). The value of a single progesterone measurement in the mid-luteal phase as a criterion of a potentially fertile cycle ('ovulation') derived from treated and un-treated conception cycles. *Fertility and Sterility*, **37**, 355–360.

Israel, R., Mishell, D. R., Stone, S. C., Thornycroft, I. H. and Ayer, D. L. (1972). Single luteal phase serum progesterone assay as an indicator of ovulation. *American Journal of Obstetrics and Gynecology*, **112**, 1043–1046.

Israel, S. L. (1938). Premenstrual tension. *Journal of the American Medical Association*, **110**, 1721–1723.

Janowsky, D. S. and Rausch, J. (1985). Biochemical hypotheses of premenstrual tension syndrome. *Psychological Medicine*, **15**, 3–8.

Keye, W. R. (1985). Medical treatment of premenstrual syndrome. *Canadian Journal of Psychiatry*, **30**, 483–488.

Kumar, S., Mansel, R. E., Scanlon, M. F., Hughes, L. E., Edwards, C. A., Woodhead, J. S. and Newcombe, R. G. (1984). Altered responses of prolactin, luteinizing hormone and follicle stimulating hormone secretion to thyrotrophin-releasing hormone/gonadotrophin-releasing hormone stimulation in cyclical mastalgia. *British Journal of Surgery*, **71**, 870–873.

Kutner, S. J. and Brown, W. L. (1972). Types of oral contraceptives, depression and premenstrual symptoms. *Journal of Nervous and Mental Disorders*, **155**, 153–162.

Kwak, H. M., Chi, I. C., Gardner, S. D. and Laufe, L. E. (1980). Menstrual pattern changes in laparoscopic sterilization patients whost last pregnancy was terminated by therapeutic abortion: a two year follow-up study. *Journal of Reproductive Medicine*, **25**, 67–71.

Labrum, A. H. (1983). Hypothalamic, pineal and pituitary factors in the premenstrual syndrome. *Journal of Reproductive Medicine*, **28**, 438–445.

Lance, J. W. and Anthony, M. (1966). Some clinical aspects of migraine. A prospective survey of 500 patients. *Archives of Neurology*, **15**, 356–361.

Lauersen, N. H. and Stukane, E. (1983). *Premenstrual Syndrome and You*, Pinnacle, New York, pp. 75–76.

Lawson, S., Cole, R. A. and Templeton, A. A. (1979). The effect of laparoscopic sterilization by diathermy or silastic bands on post-operative pain, menstrual symptoms and sexuality. *British Journal of Obstetrics and Gynaecology*, **86**, 659–663.

Levinson, W. and Dunn, P. M. (1986). Non-association of caffeine and fibrocystic breast disease. *Archives of Internal Medicine*, **146**, 1773–1775.

London, R., Solomon, D., London, E. *et al.* (1978). Mammary dysplasia: clinical response and urinary excretion of 11-desoxy-17-ketosteroids and pregnanediol following alpha-tocopherol therapy. *Breast*, **4**, 19.

London, R. S., Sundaram, G. S., Schultz, M., Nair, P. P. and Goldstein, P. J. (1981). Endocrine parameters and alpha-tocopherol therapy in patients with mammary dysplasia. *Cancer Research*, **41**, 3811–3813.

London, R. S., Sundaram, G. S., Murphy, L. and Goldstein, P. J. (1983). Evaluation and treatment of breast symptoms in patients with the premenstrual syndrome. *Journal of Reproductive Medicine*, **28**, 503–508.

Magos, A. L. and Studd, J. W. W. (1984). PMS—a new approach to cause and cure, *Contemporary Obstetrics and Gynecology*, **24**, 85–91.

Mansel, R. E., Preece, P. E. and Hughes, L. E. (1978). A double-blind trial of the prolactin inhibitor bromocriptine in painful benign breast disease. *British Journal of Surgery*, **65**, 724–727.

Migraine Trust (1979). *Understanding Migraine*, The Migraine Trust, London, pp. 18–19.

Miller, L. T. (1985). Oral contraceptives and vitamin B_6 metabolism, in *Vitamin B_6: Its Role in Health and Disease*, (Eds. R. D. Reynolds and J. E. Leklem) A R Liss, New York, pp. 243–255.

Minton, J. P., Foecking, M. K., Webster, D. J. T. and Matthews, R. H. (1979a). Response of fibrocystic disease to caffeine withdrawal and correlation of cyclic nucleotides with breast disease. *American Journal of Obstetrics and Gynecology*, **135**, 157–158.

Minton, J. P., Foecking, M. K., Webster, D. J. T. and Matthews, R. H. (1979b). Caffeine, cyclic nucleotides and breast disease. *Surgery*, **86**, 105–109.

Minton, J. P., Abou-Issa, H., Reiches, N. and Roseman, J. M. (1981). Clinical and biochemical studies on methylxanthine-related fibrocystic breast disease. *Surgery*, **90**, 299–304.

Moos, R. H. (1968). Psychological aspects of new contraceptives. *Archives of General Psychiatry*, **19**, 87–94.

Morris, N. M. and Udry, J. R. (1972). Contraceptive pills and day by day feelings of well being. *American Journal of Obstetrics and Gynecology*, **113**, 763–765.

Morton, J. H. (1950). Premenstrual tension. *American Journal of Obstetrics and Gynecology*, **60**, 343–352.

Muldoon, M. J. (1972). Gynaecological illness after sterilization. *British Medical Journal*, **1**, 84–85.

Nilsson, L. and Solvell, L. (1967). Clinical studies of oral contraceptives—a randomised, double-blind crossover study of 4 different preparations. *Acta Obstetrica Gynecologica Scandanavica*, **46**, Suppl. 8.

Norris, R. V. (1983). Progesterone for premenstrual tension. *Journal of Reproductive Medicine*, **28**, 509–516.

O'Herlihy, C., Robinson, H. P. and De Crespigny, L. J. C. (1980). Mittelschmerz is a pre-ovulatory symptom. *British Medical Journal*, **280**, 986.

Pariser, S. F., Stern, S. L., Shank, M. L., Falko, J. M., O'Shaughnessy, R. W. and Friedman, C. I. (1985). Premenstrual syndrome: concerns, controversies and treatment. *American Journal of Obstetrics and Gynecology*, **153**, 599–604.

Queenan, J. T., O'Brien, G. D., Bains, L., Collins, P. O., Simpson, J., Collins, W. P. and Campbell, S. (1980). Ultrasound scanning of ovaries to detect ovulation in women. *Fertility and Sterility*, **34**, 99–105.

Radwanska, E., Burger, G. S. and Hammond, J. (1979). Luteal deficiency among women with normal menstrual cycles, requesting reversal of tubal sterilization. *Obstetrics and Gynecology, N.Y.*, **54**, 189–192.

Radwanska, E., Hammond, J. and Smith, P. (1981). Single mid-luteal progesterone assay in the management of ovulatory infertility. *Journal of Reproductive Medicine*, **26**, 85–89.

Radwanska, E., Headley, S. K. and Dmowski, P. (1982). Evaluation of ovarian function after tubal sterilization. *Journal of Reproductive Medicine*, **27**, 376–384.

Reid, R. L. and Yen, S. S. C. (1983). The premenstrual syndrome. *Clinical Obstetrics and Gynecology*, **26**, 710–717.

Sallam, H. N., Marinho, A. O., Collins, W. P., Rodeck, C. H. and Campbell, S. (1982). Monitoring gonadotrophin therapy by real-time ultrasonic scanning of ovarian follicles. *British Journal of Obstetrics and Gynaecology*, **89**, 155–159.

Sitruk-Ware, A. R., Sterkers, N., Mowszowicz, I. and Mauvais-Jarvis, P. (1977).

Inadequate corpus luteum function in women with benign breast diseases. *Journal of Clinical Endocrinology and Metabolism*, **44**, 771–774.

Smith, S. L. (1975). Mood and the menstrual cycle in *Topics in Psychoneuroendocrinology*, (Ed. E. J. Sacher) Grune & Stratton, New York, pp. 19–58.

Spence, A. M. (1981). Contraception, in *Gynaecology in Nursing Practice*, (Eds. M. A. Shorthouse and M. G. Brush) Bailliere, London, pp. 96–124.

Stock, R. J. (1978). Evaluation of sequelae of tubal ligation. *Fertility and Sterility*, **29**, 169–174.

Sundaram, G. S., London, R. S., Manimekalai, S., Nair, P. P. and Goldstein, P. (1981). Alpha-tocopherol and serum lipoprotens. *Lipids*, **16**, 223–237.

Sundaram, G. S., London, R. S., Manimekalai, S., *et al.* (1982). Serum methylxanthine levels in women with fibrocystic disease of the breast (Abst). *Journal of the American Association of Clinical Chemistry*, **28**, 1632.

Swain, M. C., Hayward, J. L. and Bulbrook, R. D. (1973). Plasma oestradiol and progesterone in benign breast disease. *European Journal of Cancer*, **9**, 553–556.

Wathen, N. C., Perry, L., Lilford, R. J. and Chard, T. (1984). Interpretation of single progesterone measurement in diagnosis of anovulation and defective luteal phase: observations on analysis of the normal range. *British Medical Journal*, **288**, 7–9.

Watt-Boolsen, S., Andersen, A. N. and Blichert-Toft, M. (1981). Serum prolactin and oestradiol levels in women with cyclical mastalgia. *Hormone and Metabolic Research*, **13**, 700–702.

Whitelaw, R. G. (1958). Ovarian activity following hysterectomy. *Journal of Obstetrics and Gynaecology of the British Commonwealth*, **65**, 917–932.

Winston, F. (1973). Oral contraceptives, pyridoxine and depression. *American Journal of Psychiatry*, **130**, 1217–1221.

Wraith, D. G. (1982). Asthma and rhinitis, in *Food Allergy* (Eds. J. Brostoff and S. J. Challacombe), Saunders, London, pp. 101–112.

Functional Disorders of the Menstrual Cycle
Edited by M. G. Brush and E. M. Goudsmit
© 1988 John Wiley & Sons Ltd

CHAPTER 5

Vitamins, essential fatty acids and minerals in relation to the aetiology and management of premenstrual syndrome

M. G. BRUSH

Department of Gynaecology,
United Medical and Dental Schools,
St Thomas's Campus,
London SE1 7EH

Introduction

Since the introduction of vitamin B_6 (pyridoxine) as a treatment for PMS about ten years ago, there has been increasing interest in nutritional methods for the management of PMS. At first, the use of these methods was largely empirical but some biochemical evidence regarding aetiology gradually became available.

The use of vitamin B_6 was followed in 1982–83 by the introduction of the essential fatty acid, γ-linolenic acid (GLA), used alone or in combination with vitamin B_6 and sometimes other vitamins and minerals.

In the last few years a number of combined regimes have become popular and both proprietary mixtures and individual regimes have been used. It is usually quite impossible to even attempt to understand their mode of action, except in very general terms, but they can be very useful. Particular attention has been paid to magnesium and zinc in conjunction with vitamin B_6 and GLA as a PMS treatment, but much more evidence is needed before the relative importance of the various minerals can be fully assessed.

This chapter reviews the information available on the possible role of vitamins, essential fatty acids and minerals in the aetiology of PMS and the ways in which nutritional treatments have been carried out.

Vitamins

Vitamin B$_6$

History The first interest in vitamin B$_6$ in the treatment of PMS was undoubtedly stimulated by its successful use in the management of depression associated with the use of the combined oral contraception (Baumblatt and Winston, 1970; Adams *et al.*, 1973; Winston, 1973).

An isolated attempt to study vitamin B$_6$ treatment of PMS was made by Stokes and Mendels (1972) using 50 mg day^{-1} in a double-blind comparison of vitamin B$_6$ and placebo, but the results were inconclusive, probably due to there being only thirteen subjects and the comparatively small dose level of vitamin B$_6$. The use of vitamin B$_6$ in PMS lapsed until Dr P. F. H. Giles (unpublished) carried out studies in Australia in 1974–75, using 50–80 mg day^{-1}. Unfortunately, these results were not published in detail but were sufficiently impressive for Giles to recommend the use of vitamin B$_6$ to the author, who was able to arrange trials in a larger number of patients through colleagues at St Thomas's Hospital, London (Kerr, 1977; Day, 1979). It was found that 80–100 mg day^{-1} vitamin B$_6$ gave good improvement in 50–60 per cent of patients with a further 20 per cent showing useful partial improvement.

In 1980, Abraham and Hargrove carried out a double-blind crossover study on 25 women with PMS who were given a placebo or a 500 mg capsule of a long-acting form of vitamin B$_6$ daily for three consecutive cycles each. A significant improvement in PMS symptoms over placebo effect was seen in 21 of these subjects. Despite the high dose of vitamin B$_6$ used, no side-effects were reported.

In a double-blind multiple crossover study, Mattes and Martin (1982) studied one PMS sufferer who correctly identified either 50 mg vitamin B$_6$ or placebo when administered for ten days before each menstruation, and also reported a reduction in premenstrual depression and bloating. Although a very small study, it appears to have been well conducted and the design used could be the basis for more extended studies.

Barr (1984) carried out a double-blind crossover study on 48 women who were given a 100 mg long-acting preparation of vitamin B$_6$ versus placebo for two cycles on each preparation. The results were highly significantly better on the vitamin B$_6$ cycles. Williams *et al.* (1985) also used 100 mg day^{-1} in a large double-blind trial carried out in a general practice setting and found significant over-all improvement as compared with the placebo group. In contrast to the study of Barr (1984), a long-acting preparation was not used and the trial was not of a crossover design.

Quite apart from these academic studies, the use of vitamin B$_6$ at 100–150 mg day^{-1} has become widespread among PMS sufferers (Brush

1982a, b, 1983a, b, c; Brush *et al*., 1987; Harrison, 1982; London *et al*., 1985; Nazzaro *et al*., 1985) as it offers a cheap, safe and usually effective way of controlling many moderate to average cases of PMS. On its own, it is unlikely to be sufficient to control the most severe cases and combination treatments may be needed in these circumstances (Brush, 1983a, b, c). Very recently, some doubts have been raised about the safety of vitamin B_6 when given in amounts of 200 mg day^{-1} upwards. This is discussed in detail later, but the present concensus is that up to 200 mg day^{-1} is quite safe.

Methods of Use   Originally, vitamin B_6 was used alone but more recently, combination of B_6 with other vitamins and minerals has become common.

1. Vitamin B_6 only. As a basis for the successful use of vitamin B_6, we would recommend the use of a well balanced diet with plenty of fruit and green vegetables as well as other vegetables, wholemeal bread, adequate but not excessive protein, and polyunsaturated margarine spreads. Use of sugar, salt, coffee and other caffeine-containing drinks should be kept to a minimum. Convenience foods and other foods containing preservatives and synthetic colourings should be avoided.

   The usual starting dose for adult women is 50 mg twice daily with meals, usually breakfast and evening meal, or one 100 mg long-acting tablet after breakfast. If this does not give enough help, the dose may be increased to 70 or 75 mg twice daily. In severe cases, 100 mg twice daily may be tried but this should not be exceeded as unpleasant gastric acidity may become a problem in a few cases. Treatment should be started three days before the expected start of any symptoms of PMS and continued until two days after the start of menstruation. If the menstrual cycle is very unpredictable, or after hysterectomy (with conservation of the ovaries), it may be better to take vitamin B_6 without a break.

   It is usually appropriate to try each dose level for two cycles before moving to a higher dose. Once treatment with vitamin B_6 is successful, it is usually continued for several cycles before any attempt is made to reduce or stop the treatment. If symptoms return on reducing the dose, the treatment can be restarted at the original level.

   For girls aged twelve to sixteen years and very mild adult cases, 20 mg twice or three times daily is suitable (see pp. 9–10 for further discussion of PMS in children).

   Vitamin B_6 can be taken in combination with medicines except the rarely used drug L-dopa and related compounds. However, it can be very unsafe to 'megadose' vitamin B_6, i.e. to take 500 mg day^{-1} or more on a regular basis, as this may lead in time to quite serious neuropathy (see p. 73 for details). Luckily, this type of megadosing is very rare in Britain though not uncommon among health enthusiasts in the USA. The doses recommended above are generally considered to be safe if taken as directed.

2. Vitamin B_6 combined with other vitamins and minerals. It is often stated, without adequate documentation, that vitamin B_6 should always be given in conjunction with supplements of other B vitamins, especially vitamins B_1, B_2 and niacin. Provided that a well balanced diet is being used, there is considerable doubt about the need for these additional supplements, but if there is any problem in keeping to a well balanced diet or if absorption is poor, then a good quality B complex supplement is certainly desirable. Those desiring the highest standards of physical fitness or having to cope with a particularly stressful lifestyle, may also benefit from an appropriate B complex supplement.

The separate intake of vitamin B_6 should be adjusted to allow for the B_6 content of the B complex taken, in order to ensure that the total daily B_6 intake does not exceed $150–200$ mg day^{-1}.

There are no experimental studies on combined treatment with various B vitamins since the pioneering studies of the Biskinds (Biskind, 1943; Biskind et al., 1944), who claimed deficiency of B vitamins in PMT, menorrhagia and cystic mastitis.

However, Abraham and colleagues have published several studies on a multivitamin and multimineral preparation (Optivite) which contains large amounts of all the B vitamins as well as other vitamins and various minerals, including zinc and magnesium (Goei and Abraham, 1983; Fuchs et al., 1985; Chakmakjian et al., 1985). Not altogether surprisingly, significant improvement over placebo was seen but the results are difficult to evaluate as no details of any previous treatments, nutritional or otherwise, are given. Before very complex and expensive nutritional supplements can be unreservedly recommended, it would be helpful if they could be compared on a double-blind basis with simpler nutritional regimes.

3. Vitamin B_6 combined with essential fatty acids and other nutrients. This will be discussed in the section on essential fatty acids.

4. Vitamin B_6 in combination with various hormones. Where some form of hormone treatment is indicated, e.g. for cycle regulation or preferred by clinician or patient, it may be desirable, especially in severe PMS, to give vitamin B_6 as well as the hormone treatment. Only brief reports on this type of combination are available.

Brush (1983a) reported on 26 cases studied in conjunction with various colleagues where the combination of dydrogesterone, 10 mg twice daily on days twelve to 26, with vitamin B_6, $100–150$ mg day^{-1} on days twelve to day two of the next cycle, was used. Good response was obtained in seventeen cases and partial response in seven cases. In all cases, either vitamin B_6 or dydrogesterone had been tried previously with no effect.

Varma (1983) and Williams (1983) also briefly mentioned the combination of dydrogesterone and vitamin B_6 with favourable results.

It may also be useful to add vitamin B_6 when natural progesterone suppositories are not well tolerated but treatment needs to be continued. Sometimes, unpleasant symptoms may occur after the progesterone is stopped on day 26, and vitamin B_6 continued to day three of the next cycle may be helpful in relieving this problem.

Toxicity of Very Large Doses of Vitamin B_6   Our experience, and that of many others in the UK, suggests that doses of vitamin B_6 up to 200 mg day^{-1} are well tolerated, apart from occasional complaints of nausea or indigestion at 150–200 mg day^{-1} (Kerr, 1977; Day, 1979; Taylor and James, 1979; Shangold, 1983; Barr, 1984; Williams *et al.*, 1985).

Although practice in the UK rarely, if ever, exceeds 200 mg day^{-1} vitamin B_6 in the treatment of PMS, there are reports of the use of 500 mg long-acting capsules used either continuously or for ten to fourteen days in each cycle (Abraham and Hargrove, 1980; Colin, 1982; London *et al.*, 1983) for treatment for PMS or benign breast disease, and no side-effects were noted.

Vitamin B_6 at 250–500 mg day^{-1} was used by Mitwalli *et al.* (1984) for one to six years in the successful treatment of kidney stones secondary to hyperoxaluria and no impairment of nerve conduction or other side-effects were detected. Ellis *et al.* (1982) and Del Tredici *et al.* (1985) treated carpal tunnel syndrome patients with vitamin B_6 100–300 mg day^{-1} with good results and no side-effects. Driskell *et al.* (1986) gave 100 mg vitamin B_6 or placebo daily to carpal tunnel syndrome patients for five to 58 weeks with vitamin B_6 showing substantial benefit as compared with placebo and no side-effects.

However, there are some health enthusiasts, mostly in the USA, who take much larger amounts than this, usually on a self-help basis but occasionally under medical direction.

Two recent studies in the USA have shown that very large doses of vitamin B_6 (0.5–6 g day^{-1}) may cause serious neuropathy (Schaumberg *et al.*, 1983; Parry and Bredesen, 1985). In the former report, seven patients were studied with dosages in the range 2–6 g day^{-1} and, in the latter study involving sixteen patients, the doses were 0.5–5 g day^{-1} with the exception of one case where neuropathy was noted on 200 mg day^{-1} taken continuously for three years. The patient details in this report were mostly very brief and, in some cases, were compiled on the telephone after press publicity. However, it is now clear that a risk of neuropathy may exist if 500 mg day^{-1} or more is taken continuously, especially for an extended period. With the exception of the one case mentioned above who took 200 mg day^{-1} continuously for three years, there are no other published cases of neuropathy in the dose range 100–200 mg day^{-1}, i.e. the common level for PMS treatment. There have been some alarmist, but unsubstantiated, reports in the popular media about dangers in the 100–200 mg day^{-1} dose range, but the overwhelming balance of experience from many sources continues to endorse the safety of this dose level. Nonetheless, professional and public awareness of this debate may serve to focus attention on any minor risks which could occur at low incidence levels. Some health professionals have advocated the regular use of other nutritional supplements in conjunction with vitamin B_6 to ensure that unphysiological vitamin balance is avoided. The use of other B vitamins, especially B_1 and B_2, is frequently suggested and magnesium and zinc are also recommended. Scientific evidence supporting these recommendations appears to be lacking at present, but our recent experience supports this approach, especially if the diet of the sufferer is in any way substandard. Dietary enquiry, followed by any necessary advice, should be an essential part of any PMS consultation.

If cases of excessive self-medication with vitamin B_6 are encountered, with or without symptoms, it is probably very unwise to stop vitamin B_6 intake abruptly. In the absence of symptoms, it may be possible to decrease the dose in a stepwise manner ending with a maintenance dose of 100–150 mg day^{-1}. If there are any signs indicating a possible neuropathy, the opinion of a consultant neurologist should be sought so that a full differential diagnosis can be made. Unfortunately, insufficient information is available on the absorption and metabolism of vitamin B_6 in abnormal states and, at present, blood and urine studies on vitamin B_6 and its metabolites cannot be recommended as a guide to clinical practice. In the future, blood levels of pyridoxal phosphate (PLP) and urinary excretion of 4-pyridoxic acid may be valuable in the assessment of PMS patients, especially those suspected of vitamin B_6 abuse. However, two preliminary reports (Ritchie and Singkamani, 1986; Van den Berg et al., 1986) have not shown a significant difference in plasma PLP values beteween controls and PMS sufferers. This suggests the possibility that vitamin B_6 therapy is either acting entirely at a pharmacological level or it is correcting a local deficiency of PLP in a specific organ or tissue.

The role of vitamin B_6 in the aetiology of PMS   Although the benefits of vitamin B_6 treatment in many cases of PMS have been known for over ten years, there is still considerable uncertainty as to the possible mechanism of action. There are several reasons for this, including the very large number of enzymatic processes which are known to depend on pyridoxal phosphate (PLP) as a co-factor and the inaccessibility of human organs, such as the hypothalmus and pituitary, which are thought to be involved. Furthermore, there are no known animal models for PMS and very little is known about the dynamics of the absorption of vitamin B_6 and its conversion to other pyridoxine derivatives, especially in varied physiological and pathological states.

Among the many important secretory activities of the hypothalamus is the production of two important neurotransmitter amines, dopamine and serotonin.

It has been known for some time that dopamine is inhibitory to the secretion of prolactin by the pituitary. PLP, the main active form of vitamin B_6, is a co-factor in the synthesis of dopamine from L-dopa. (Figure 1). Therefore, it is postulated (Brush, 1977, 1979) that any over-all deficiency of pyridoxine or local lack of PLP will reduce the synthesis of dopamine which, in turn, will lead to an imbalance in prolactin. Any abnormality in prolactin secretion is unlikely to be gross but sometimes quite small departures from normal may have adverse effects. Prolactin is known to have a role in regulating gonadotrophin activity at the ovarian level (McNatty *et al.*, 1974). Major increases in prolactin levels cause amenorrhoea (see Chapter 13) but minor increases may also have adverse effects on ovarian function. It is to be hoped that techniques will become available to allow the direct study of this chain of events, as it seems very likely that it plays an important but as yet not fully defined role in the aetiology of PMS.

Another important pathway in the hypothalamus leads from tryptophan to the neurotransmitter serotonin. The step from 5-hydroxytryptophan to serotonin is catalysed by 5-hydroxytryptophan decarboxylase, which is dependent on PLP as a co-factor (Figure 2). Thus, if there is a partial lack of PLP at the hypothalamic level, the conversion of 5-hydroxytryptophan to serotonin may be impaired. This may lead to depression and, possibly, other mood changes as there are known associations between low serotonin levels and depression (Ashcroft *et al.*, 1966; Adams *et al.*, 1973).

There are also complex and poorly understood inter-relationships between the hypothalamic pathways leading to serotonin, and dopamine synthesis. These interactions could be an important factor in mood regulation, but obviously much more information is required. The effects of the normal changes in ovarian function on these hypothalamic events also needs much

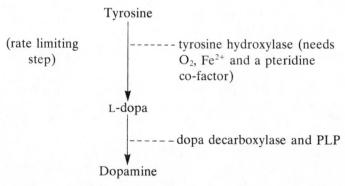

Figure 1. Biosynthesis of dopamine

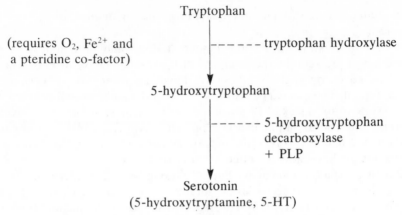

Figure 2. Biosynthesis of serotonin

further study. Despite the obvious difficulties in obtaining data on hypothalamic production of serotonin and dopamine in PMS sufferers the indirect evidence underlines the probable importance of this approach in the study of the aetiology of PMS.

Other factors may influence the metabolism of tryptophan and may, therefore, indirectly influence the biosynthesis of serotonin due to impaired availability of tryptophan. Several metabolic pathways from tryptophan have steps which are PLP-dependant and may therefore be impaired if partial deficiency of PLP exists in PMS sufferers.

Besides the formation of serotonin from 5-hydroxytryptophan, as mentioned earlier, the following steps shown in Figure 3 are PLP-dependent:

$$\text{Kynurenine} \xrightarrow[\text{PLP}]{\text{kynureninase}} \text{anthranilic acid}$$

$$\text{Kynurenine} \xrightarrow[\text{PLP}]{\text{aminotransferase}} \text{kynurenic acid}$$

$$\text{3-hydroxykynurenine} \xrightarrow[\text{PLP}]{\text{kynureninase}} \text{3-hydroxyanthranilic acid}$$

In vitamin B_6 deficiency, it is known that excretion of xanthurenic acid (XA) is increased, presumably due to partial block of the conversion of 3-hydroxykynurenine to 3-hydroxyanthranilic acid which relies on the PLP-dependant enzyme, kynureninase.

In women on oral contraceptive medication and oestrogen treatment for menopausal problems, there is increased activity via the kynurenine pathway with increased urinary excretion of various tryptophan metabolites, i.e.

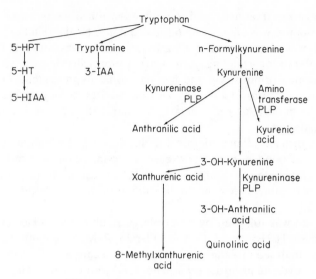

Figure 3. Metabolism of tryptophan

kynurenine, 3-hydroxykynurenine, 3-hydroxyanthranilic acid, xanthurenic acid and quinolinic acid (Rose, 1978; Wolff *et al.*, 1980). Similar studies in PMS sufferers would be valuable.

It is known that oestrogens will induce tryptophan oxidase and that this may be mediated by corticosteroids (Braidman and Rose, 1971). It was suggested by Mason *et al.* (1969) that oestrogens may compete with PLP for binding sites of apoenzymes. In addition, Bender and Wynick (1981) and Wolff *et al.* (1980) showed inhibition of kynureninase by oestrogens. As yet the possible significance of these findings as regards PMS is not known.

Essential Fatty Acids

Introduction

Over the last six years, there has been a very considerable increase in interest in the clinical uses of essential fatty acids (Horrobin, 1982). An accidental discovery by Horrobin, who was studying evening primrose oil (EPO) for other reasons, showed that this treatment helped some of his volunteers who had PMS. The effectiveness of EPO was thought to be due to its high content of γ-linolenic acid, an important essential fatty acid whose biochemical and clinical background is considered below. As a direct result of this finding, an open nutritional study was carried out at St Thomas's Hospital Medical School (Brush, 1982c) on 73 women with PMS who had failed at least one other recognized treatment, and sometimes two or three types of treatments. A good response was obtained in 62 per cent and partial relief in 22 per cent. No change was seen in the remaining 16 per cent. It was also noted that out of 36 women with longstanding premenstrual breast discomfort, 26 responded well to evening primrose oil and five had some improvement. Over several months, useful improvement may also be seen in fibrocystic breast disease (Brush, 1982c, 1983a,c) particularly if combined with abstinence from all forms of caffeine.

Open studies are often criticized as being confused by high rates of placebo effect but the good response of breast symptoms seen by Brush (1982c) is difficult to attribute to placebo effect. Also, the failure to respond to two or three other treatments lessens the likelihood of placebo response to evening primrose oil.

This study was followed by a very large double-blind placebo controlled study (Massil, H., Brush, M. G. and O'Brien, P. M. S., unpublished) which is now being analysed in detail. Initial results indicate a statistically significant response to evening primrose oil as compared with placebo. The dose used in this study was four 500 mg capsules twice daily without a break. Each treatment was given for four cycles before crossover. Open studies (Watson, J., Perry, M., Granger-Taylor, C. and Brush, M. G., unpublished) have also been continued with findings similar to the original open study of Brush (1982c).

Partial confirmation of these findings has come from Puolakka et al. (1985) and Ylikorkala et al. (1986) who studied 30 women with severe PMS who were treated with evening primrose oil or placebo from day fifteen until the start of menstruation. Although both agents gave improvement in PMS, evening primrose oil was more effective, especially as regards depression. The dose level and duration of treatment may have been insufficient to produce a more clear-cut effect.

A preliminary study from Sweden also confirms these findings (Ockerman et al., 1985).

Sources of γ-Linolenic Acid

At present, the most common source of γ-linolenic acid (GLA) is evening primrose oil (EPO) which contains 9 per cent GLA as well as 73 per cent linoleic acid, 12 per cent oleic acid and 5 per cent palmitic acid. EPO is derived from the seeds of the evening primrose and is available under several trade names (Efamol, Naudicelle, etc.). Nearly all the experimental work with GLA in the treatment of PMS has been carried out with EPO and the results are considered in this chapter.

GLA is also present in blackcurrant seeds and borage seeds. Blackcurrant seed oil contains 15–19 per cent GLA, 12–14 per cent α-linolenic acid,

45–60 per cent linoleic acid and 3–4 per cent stearidonic acid. Borage seed oil contains 25–27 per cent GLA and 35–36 per cent linoleic acid. As yet, they have not been extensively used in treatment of PMS but they appear to have considerable potential.

Methods of Use in Treatment of PMS

Several dose regimes hve been used for EPO treatment of PMS but, as yet, no formal comparison of these methods has been made.

In the original study of Brush (1982c), two 500 mg capsules of EPO twice daily were used from three days before the expected onset of PMS until the start of menstruation. If this did not give sufficient response, the dose was increased to three capsules twice daily. In very severe cases, vitamin B_6 50–75 mg twice daily, was added or a proprietary supplement containing vitamin B_6 100 mg day^{-1}, ascorbic acid 500 mg day^{-1}, zinc 10 mg day^{-1}, and niacin 30 mg day^{-1}, and results suggest that these combined regimes may give useful extra help.

Later experience in open studies (Watson, J., Perry, M., Granger-Taylor, C. and Brush, M. G., unpublished) has shown that it may be helpful in severe cases to give EPO continuously at the above dose levels. In a recent double-blind placebo-controlled study, four capsules of EPO twice daily were given continuously (Massil, H., Brush, M. G. and O'Brien, P. M. S., in preparation). Further studies may be needed to determined the range of dose levels of EPO needed to treat the different types of PMS of varying degrees of severity.

Biochemical and Clinical Aspects of GLA

The importance of GLA lies in two main factors. Firstly, it is a key intermediate in the n-6 series of essential fatty acids, which starts from *cis*-linoleic acid. Secondly, it is the precursor of prostaglandin E_1 (PGE_1) which is an important natural regulatory substance affecting a number of different body functions at the cellular level and is believed to be involved in the complex chain of events involved in PMS.

In normal circumstances, *cis*-linoleic acid derived from vegetable oils is converted to other EFAs and to PGE_1 as shown in Figure 4.

Although *cis*-linoleic acid is plentiful in most diets, it is used for a variety of functions in the body and its conversion to GLA is not always working at optimal efficiency. Several different factors may reduce the activity of the Δ_6-desaturase, including the presence of *trans*-linoleic acid, saturated fats, cholesterol, alcohol, diabetes mellitus, ageing and viral infections (Brenner and Peluffo, 1966; De Gomez Dumm *et al.*, 1976).

Low activity of the Δ_6-desaturase may also be present on a constitutional or

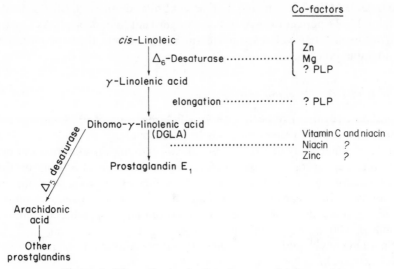

Figure 4. Biosynthesis of n-6 series essential fatty acids

genetic basis. Manku *et al.* (1984) and Wright (1985) showed significant reduction in Δ_6-desaturase in atopic eczema and atopic dermatitis respectively, and Brush *et al.* (1984) showed a similar reduction in 42 women with PMS as compared with normal controls.

The conversion of GLA to dihomo-γ-linolenic acid (DGLA) appears to be very efficient and is not rate-limiting. Little detailed information is available on the conversion of DGLA to PGE_1 or on its conversion to arachidonic acid via the Δ_5-desaturase pathway, although the latter is known to be rather inefficient in humans (Stone *et al.*, 1979).

Where there is a relative block of *cis*-linoleic to GLA for any reason, it is likely to be beneficial to give dietary supplements of GLA to by-pass the block and this has been shown to be the case (Manku *et al.*, 1984).

A further important factor is that Δ_6-desaturase requires several co-factors for its normal activity. These include zinc and magnesium (Horrobin *et al.*, 1979a,b; Horrobin and Cunnane, 1980), and it may be helpful to give supplements of these factors in some circumstances. The precise role of vitamine B_6 in the biosynthesis of the n-6 EFAs is still unclear. Witten and Holman (1952) showed that it is involved in the conversion of linoleic acid to arachidonic acid, but Kirschmann and Lepage (1979) suggest a more general role in EFA metabolism.

The conversion of DGLA to prostaglandin E_1 is thought to involve ascorbic acid at physiological concentrations (Manku *et al.*, 1979) and, in addition, zinc and niacin.

Despite the convincing evidence of the role played by the co-factors mentioned above in the biosynthesis of the n-6 series of EFAs and prostaglandin E_1, there is still some uncertainty about the need for the use of vitamin and mineral supplements to optimize the effectiveness of EPO in the treatment of PMS. Partly due to the need to complete formal studies of EPO alone to satisfy the needs of regulatory bodies such as the CSM, there have been no placebo-controlled double-blind studies of EPO plus vitamin B_6, ascorbic acid, niacin, zinc and magnesium. However, in our experience, the use of such supplements with standard doses of EPO can give a satisfactory response when EPO alone has not proved adequate. In some cases, the response to EPO plus vitamin B_6 together with diet improvement, is clearly better than EPO alone, but in other severe cases, full supplementation of EPO with vitamin B_6, ascorbic acid, zinc and magnesium is needed to obtain response. The need for niacin in such cases is unclear but some workers may wish to include it.

Minor defects in the absorption of zinc and magnesium are not uncommon and, therefore, trial of such supplements seems to be reasonable, especially as full assessment of zinc and magnesium status is not readily available in most centres.

As discussed above, there is now some evidence that blood PLP levels are not abnormal in PMS sufferers and that vitamin B_6 therapy in PMS may be acting at a purely pharmacological level. Despite the normal blood levels, there could still be problems at the tissue level in specific organs and, therefore, vitamin B_6 supplements seem to be fully justified in view of its known role in EFA metabolism and its importance in hypothalamic production of dopamine and serotonin (see pp. 75–76).

Specific practical evidence to support supplementation of EPO treatment with ascorbic acid and niacin is lacking, but in view of the safety and simplicity of this approach, it would appear reasonable to continue its use in the more difficult PMS cases.

Magnesium

There has been recent interest in the possible role of magnesium in the aetiology and treatment of PMS. Abraham and Lubran (1981) reported significantly reduced levels of magnesium in red blood cells in 26 women with well defined PMS. Serum magnesium levels were unchanged. A recent more detailed study with 105 women with PMS confirmed the previous report (Sherwood et al., 1986). The reason for the deficit in RBC magnesium is not known but possibly partial defects in absorption are most likely. Abraham et al. (1981) have reported that vitamin B_6 100 mg twice daily produces significant elevation of mean plasma and RBC magnesium levels. The RBC levels of magnesium were doubled after four weeks of vitamin B_6 therapy.

As mentioned above magnesium is also a co-factor which is important in the biosynthesis of essential fatty acids but further detailed information is required.

There have apparently been no formal studies on magnesium alone as a supplement in PMS but it is included in several commercially available vitamin–mineral supplements in amounts up to 250 mg day^{-1} elemental magnesium and in one case reports of beneficial results are available (Chakmakjian *et al.*, 1985; Fuchs *et al.*, 1985). Our own experience with a somewhat similar supplement which gives 145 mg day^{-1} magnesium is encouraging (Matthews, R., Lindfield, B., and Brush, M. G., unpublished). Clearly well designed scientific studies on the role of magnesium in the metabolism of vitamin B$_6$ and essential fatty acids in women with PMS would be very useful.

References

Abraham, G. E. and Hargrove, J. T. (1980). Effect of vitamin B$_6$ on premenstrual symptomatology in women with premenstrual tension syndrome. *Infertility*, **3**, 155–165.

Abraham, G. E. and Lubran, M. M. (1981). Serum and red cell magnesium levels in patients with premenstrual syndrome. *American Journal of Clinical Nutrition*, **34**, 2364–2366.

Abraham, G. E., Schwartz, U. D. and Lubran, M. M. (1981). Effect of vitamin B$_6$ on plasma and red blood cell magnesium levels in premenopausal women. *Annals of Clinical and Laboratory Science*, **11**, 333–336.

Adams, P. W., Rose, D. F., Folkard, J., Wynn, V., Seed, M. and Strong, R. (1973). Effect of pyridoxine hydrochloride (vitamin B$_6$) upon depression associated with oral contraception. *Lancet*, **i**, 897–904.

Ashcroft, G. W., Crawford, T. B. B., Eccleston, D., Sharman, D. F., MacDougall, E. J., Stanton, J. B. and Binns, J. K. (1966). 5-Hydroxyindole compounds in the cerebrospinal fluid of patients with psychiatric or neurologic diseases. *Lancet*, **ii**, 1049–1052.

Barr, W. (1984). Pyridoxine supplements in the premenstrual syndrome. *Practitioner*, **228**, 425–427.

Baumblatt, M. J. and Winston, F. (1970). Pyridoxine and the pill. *Lancet*, **i**, 832–833.

Bender, D. A. and Wynick, D. (1981). Inhibition of kynureninase by oestrone sulphate: an alternative explanation for abnormal results of tryptophan load tests in women receiving oestrogenic steroids. *British Journal of Nutrition*, **45**, 269–275.

Biskind, M. S. (1943). Nutritional deficiency on the etiology of menorrhagia, metrorrhagia, cystic mastitis and premenstrual tension: treatment with vitamin B complex. *Journal of Clinical Endocrinology and Metabolism*, **3**, 227–234.

Biskind, M. S., Biskind, G. R. and Biskind, I. H. (1944). Nutritional deficiency in the etiology of menorrhagia, metrorrhagia cystic mastitis and premenstrual syndrome. *Surgery, Gynecology and Obstetrics*, **78**, 49–57.

Braidman, I. P. and Rose, D. P. (1971). Effects of sex hormones on the glucocorticoid inducible enzymes concerned with amino acid metabolism in rat liver. *Endocrinology*, **89**, 1250–1255.

Brenner, R. R. and Peluffo, R. O. (1966). Regulation of unsaturated fatty acid biosynthesis, *Biochimica Biophysica Acta*, **176**, 471–479.

Brush, M. G. (1977). The possible mechanisms causing the premenstrual syndrome, *Current Medical Research and Opinion*, **4, Supplement 4**, 9–15.

Brush, M. G. (1979). Endocrine and other biochemical factors in the aetiology of the premenstrual syndrome, *Current Medical Research and Opinion*, **6, Supplement 5**, 19–27.

Brush, M. G. (1982a). Premenstrual syndrome: aetiology and treatment, *Pulse*, **42**, 62–63.

Brush, M. G. (1982b). The pill, pyridoxine and PMS symptoms, *MIMS Magazine*, **April 1 1982**, 18–24.

Brush, M. G. (1982c). Efamol (evening primrose oil) in the treatment of the premenstrual syndrome, in *Clinical Uses of Essential Fatty Acids*, (Ed. D. F. Horrobin) Eden Press, London, pp. 155–161.

Brush, M. G. (1983a). The significance of pyridoxine and gamma-linolenic acid in premenstrual syndrome, in *Premenstrual Syndrome*, (Ed. R. W. Taylor) Medical News Tribune, London, pp. 57–59.

Brush, M. G. (1983b). Pharmacological rationale for the management of PMS, *Journal of Psychosomatic Obstetrics and Gynaecology*, **2**, 35–39.

Brush, M. G. (1983c). Nutritional approaches to premenstrual tension, *Nutrition and Health*, **2**, 203–209.

Brush, M. G., Bennett, T. and Hansen, K. (1983). *A retrospective report on the use of pyridoxine in the treatment of premenstrual syndrome (PMS) at St Thomas's Hospital and Medical School*, 1976–1983. (Submitted for publication.)

Brush, M. G., Watson, J., Horrobin, D. F. and Manku, M. S. (1984). Abnormal essential fatty acid levels in plasma of women with premenstrual tension, *American Journal of Obstetrics and Gynecology*, **150**, 363–366.

Chakmakjian, Z. H., Higgins, C. E. and Abraham, G. E. (1985). The effect of a nutritional supplement, 'Optivite for Women', on premenstrual tension syndromes. II. Effect on symptomatology using a double-blind crossover design. *Journal of Applied Nutrition*, **37**, 12–17.

Colin, C. (1982). Etudes contrôlées de l'administration orale de progestagènes, d'un antioestrogènes et de vitamin B$_6$ dans le traitment des mastodynies. *Review Médical Bruxelles*, **3**, 605–609.

Day, J. B. (1979). Clinical trials in the premenstrual syndrome. *Current Medical Research and Opinion*, **6, Supplement 5**, 40–45.

De Gomez Dumm, I. N. T., De Alaniz, M. J. T. and Brenner, R. R. (1976). Comparative effects of glucagon, dibutyryl cAMP and epinephrine in the desaturation and elongation of linoleic acid by rat liver microsomes, *Lipids*, **11**, 833–836.

Del Tredici, A., Bernstein, A. and Chinn, K. (1985). Vitamin B$_6$ therapy for carpal tunnel syndrome (CTS). *Federation Proceedings*, **44**, 775.

Driskell, J. A., Wesley, R. L. and Hess, I. E. (1986). Effectiveness of pyridoxine hydrochloride treatment on carpal tunnel syndrome patients. *Nutrition Reports International*, **34**, 1031–1040.

Ellis, J., Folkers, K., Levy, M., Shizukuishi, S., Lewandowski, J., Nishii, S., Schubert, H. A. and Ulrich, R. (1982). Response of vitamin B$_6$ deficiency and the carpal tunnel syndrome to pyridoxine. *Proceedings of the National Academy of Sciences, USA*, **79**, 7494–7498.

Fuchs, N., Hakim, M. and Abraham, G. E. (1985). The effect of a nutritional supplement, Optivite for Women, on premenstrual tension syndromes. I. Effect on blood chemistry and serum steroid levels during the mid-luteal phase. *Journal of Applied Nutrition*, **37**, 1–11.

Goei, G. S. and Abraham, G. E. (1983). Effect of a nutritional supplement, Optivite, on symptoms of premenstrual tension. *Journal of Reproductive Medicine*, **28**, 527–531.

Harrison, M. (1982). *Self-help for Premenstrual Syndrome*, Random House, New York, pp. 103–104.

Horrobin, D. F. (Ed.) (1982). *Clinical Uses of Essential Fatty Acids*, Eden Press, London.

Horrobin, D. F., Oka, M. and Manku, M. S. (1979a). The regulation of prostaglandin E_1 formation: a candidate for one of the fundamental mechanisms involved in the action of vitamin C, *Medical Hypotheses*, **5**, 849–858.

Horrobin, D. F., Manku, M. S., Oka, M., Morgan, R. O., Cunnane, S. C., Ally, A. I., Ghayur, T., Schweitzer, M. and Karmali, R. A. (1979b). The nutritional regulation of T lymphocyte function, *Medical Hypotheses*, **5**, 969–985.

Horrobin, D. F. and Cunnane, S. C. (1980). Interactions between zinc, essential fatty acids and prostaglandins: relevance to acrodermatitis enteropathica, total parenteral nutrition, the glucagonoma syndrome, diabetes, anorexia nervosa and sickle cell anaemia, *Medical Hypotheses*, **6**, 277–296.

Kerr, G. D. (1977). The management of the premenstrual syndrome. *Current Medical Research and Opinion*, **4**, **Supplement 4**, 29–34.

London, R. S., Sundaram, G. S., Murphy, L. and Goldstein, P. J. (1983). Evaluation and treatment of breast symptoms in patients with the premenstrual syndrome. *Journal of Reproductive Medicine*, **28**, 503–508.

London, R. S., Murphy, L. and Kitlowski, K. E. (1985). Treatment of premenstrual syndrome with vitamin B_6: physicians' attitudes and perceptions, in *Vitamin B_6: Its Role in Health and Disease*, (Eds. R. D. Reynolds and J. E. Leklem) A R Liss, New York, pp. 469–477.

Manku, M. S., Oka, M. and Horrobin, D. F. (1979). Differential regulation of the formation of prostaglandins and related substances from arachidonic acid and from dihomogammalinolenic acid. II. Effects of vitamin C. *Prostaglandins and Medicine*, **3**, 129–137.

Manku, M. S., Horrobin, D. F., Morse, N. L., Wright, S. and Burton, J. L. (1984). Essential fatty acids in the plasma phospholipids of patients with atopic eczema, *British Journal of Dermatology*, **110**, 643–648.

Mason, M., Ford, J. and Wuh, H. L. C. (1969). Effects of steroid and non-steroid-binding metabolites on enzyme conformation and pyridoxal phosphate binding. *Annals of the New York Academy of Sciences*, **166**, 170–183.

Mattes, J. A. and Martin, D. (1982). Pyridoxine in premenstrual depression. *Human Nutrition: Applied Nutrition*, **36A**, 131–133.

McNatty, K. P., Sawers, R. S. and McNeilly, A. S. (1974). A possible role for prolactin in the control of steroid secretion by the human Graafian follicle *Nature*, **250**, 653–655.

Mitwalli, A., Blair, G. and Oreopoulos, D. G. (1984). Safety of intermediate doses of pyridoxine. *Canadian Medical Association Journal*, **131**, 14.

Nazzaro, A., Lombard, D. and Horrobin, D. (1985). *The PMT Solution*, Adamantine Press, London, pp. 99–100.

Ockerman, P. A., Glans, S., Rassner, S. and Bachrack, I. (1985). Essential fatty acids in the treatment of the premenstrual syndrome, in *2nd International Congress on Essential Fatty Acids, Prostaglandins and Leukotrienes, London, March 24–27, 1985*, Abstract 128.

Parry, G. J. and Bredesen, D. E. (1985). Sensory neuropathy with low dose pyridoxine. *Neurology*, **35**, 1466–1468.

Puolakka, J., Makarainen, L., Viinikka, L. and Ylikorkalo, O. (1985). Biochemical and clinical effects of treating the premenstrual syndrome with prostaglandin precursors. *Journal of Reproductive Medicine*, **30**, 149–153.

Ritchie, C. D. and Singkamani, R. (1986). Plasma pyridoxal 5'-phosphate in women with the premenstrual syndrome *Human Nutrition: Clinical Nutrition*, **40C**, 75–80.

Rose, D. P. (1978). The interactions between vitamin B_6 and hormones. *Vitamins and Hormones*, **36**, 53–99.

Schaumberg, H., Kaplan, J., Windebank, A., Vick, N., Rasmus, S., Pleasure, D. and Brown, M. J. (1983). Sensory neuropathy from pyridoxine abuse: a new megavitamin syndrome. *New England Journal of Medicine*, **309**, 445–448.

Shangold, M. M. (1983). Drug therapy for the premenstrual syndrome. *Journal of Reproductive Medicine*, **28**, 525–526.

Sherwood, R. A., Rocks, B. F., Stewart, A. and Saxton, R. S. (1986). Magnesium and the premenstrual syndrome. *Annals of Clinical Biochemistry*, **23**, 667–670.

Stone, K. J., Willis, A. L., Hart, M., Kirtland, S. J., Kernoff, P. B. A. and McNicol, G. P. (1979). The metabolism of dihomogammalinolenic acid in man, *Lipids*, **14**, 174–180.

Stokes, J. and Mendels, J. (1972). Pyridoxine and premenstrual tension. *Lancet*, **i**, 1177–1178.

Taylor, R. W. and James, C. E. (1979). The clinician's view of patients with premenstrual syndrome. *Current Medical Research and Opinion*, **6, Supplement 5**, 46–51.

Van den Berg, H., Louwerse, E. S., Bruinse, H. W. Thissen, J. T. N. M. and Schrijver, J. (1986). Vitamin B_6 status of women suffering from premenstrual syndrome. *Human Nutrition: Clinical Nutrition*, **40C**, 441–450.

Varma, T. R. (1983). Treatment of the premenstrual syndrome, in *Premenstrual Syndrome*, (Ed. R. W. Taylor) Medical News Tribune, London, pp. 63–65.

Williams, J. (1983). Experience in general practice, in *Premenstrual Syndrome*. (Ed. R. W. Taylor) Medical News Tribune, London, pp. 13–15.

Williams, M. J., Harris, R. I. and Dean, R. C. (1985). Controlled trial of pyridoxine in the premenstrual syndrome. *Journal of International Medical Research*, **13**, 174–179.

Winston, F. (1973). Oral contraceptives, pyridoxine and depression. *American Journal of Psychiatry*, **130**, 1217–1221.

Witten, P. W., and Holman, R. T. (1952). Effect of pyridoxine on essential fatty acid conversions. *Archives of Biochemistry and Biophysics*, **41**, 266.

Wolff, H., Walter, S., Brown, R. R. and Arend, R. A. (1980). Effect of natural oestrogens on tryptophan metabolism: evidence for interference of oestrogens with kyureninase. *Scandinavian Journal of Clinical Laboratory Investigation*, **40**, 15–22.

Wright, S. (1985). Atopic dermatitis and essential fatty acids: a biochemical basis for atopy? *Acta Dermatologica et Venereologia (Stockholm)*, **Supplement 114**, 143–145.

Ylikorkala, O., Puolakka, J., Makarainen, L. and Viinikka, L. (1986). Prostaglandins and premenstrual syndrome. *Progress in Lipid Research*, **25**, 433–435.

Functional Disorders of the Menstrual Cycle
Edited by M. G. Brush and E. M. Goudsmit
© 1988 John Wiley & Sons Ltd

CHAPTER 6

Endocrine factors in the aetiology of premenstrual syndrome

TORBJÖRN BÄCKSTRÖM

*Department of Obstetrics and Gynecology,
University of Umeå, S-901, 85 Umeå
Sweden*

The premenstrual syndrome (PMS) is a condition with cyclical mood and physical changes in relation to the menstrual cycle. The condition is common as about 30 per cent of women between 18 and 45 have moderate to severe complaints and about 10 per cent would like to have some treatment (Andersch *et al.*, 1986). There are, however, some disputes in the literature on diagnostic criteria and discrepancies in published results have often been ascribed to these differences. Patients seeking help for PMS usually give a similar case history but when they are investigated with daily prospective symptom ratings they are found to be a very heterogeneous group (Hammarbäck and Bäckström, 1985). It is therefore very important, when giving a treatment or investigating patients scientifically, that all differential diagnoses are cleared up especially regarding general psychological problems. The number of symptoms that change with the menstrual cycle varies between patients and over 100 symptoms are described to follow the menstrual cycle (Dalton, 1984), although a number of these are poorly defined or of uncertain relevance.

For the diagnosis of 'pure PMS' we apply the following criteria:

1. A cyclicity with significantly higher scores during the luteal phase compared to the follicular phase in at least three of the twelve most prominent symptoms.
2. A period free of symptoms during the preovulatory period, with not more than two days with symptoms in more than two of eight negative symptoms rated.
3. Symptoms must recur every premenstrual period for the last year. We accept variation between cycles in degree of severity of symptoms.
4. Moderate to severe mood change as defined by the severity rating.

The patients fulfilling criteria 1, 3 and 4 but not 2 we call premenstrual aggravation group and they seem to have psychological problems in addition to luteal phase provoked symptoms. The patients not fulfilling criteria 1 we do not consider to have PMS.

In our department we classify severity as follows:

1. Mild: The patient notices a change herself and this is also perceived by the family. There is no effect on social life and ability to work.
2. Moderate: The condition disturbs relations within the family. Social life is also affected, e.g., activities inhibited. Working capacity is affected but work can be done.
3. Severe: Relations within the family are disturbed. There is no social life. Housework or professional work is not done or markedly reduced. Need for treatment is clear.

Mild forms usually do not need medical treatment and it is often enough to discuss the phenomenon with the patient and her family. These patients with mild forms should not be included in research on aetiology or treatment of PMS, as environmental factors seem to greatly influence the presence or absence of symptoms.

Our experience is that it is necessary to do daily prospective symptom ratings in at least one menstrual cycle to achieve a clear picture of the symptom distribution during the menstrual cycle. We prefer to study at least two cycles as the degree of symptom change can vary between the cycles. We also measure plasma progesterone during the luteal phase to make sure that the cycle is ovulatory. The rating scale we use is a visual analogue scale (VAS) developed earlier (Sanders *et al.*, 1983).

Hormonally Linked Changes

PMS is characterized by cyclical mood changes. The exact relationship between symptom development and hormonal variations during the menstrual cycle was studied by asking women with a history of cyclical mood changes to rate their symptoms daily during one menstrual cycle and to give blood samples for plasma oestradiol and progesterone determinations during the same cycle (Bäckström *et al.*, 1983b). The results show that the maximum degree of symptoms occurred on the last five premenstrual days (Figure 1). When the menstrual period started, the symptom severity decreased quite rapidly, and the symptoms had disappeared three to four days after the onset of the menstrual period (Figure 1). This tallies well with the earlier clinical experience (Bäckström *et al.*, 1976, 1981; Dalton 1984; Sampson 1979; Steiner *et al.*, 1980). The severity of symptoms started to rise in parallel with the development of the corpus luteum. During the preovulatory oestradiol peak there were very few negative symptoms. Instead, there was a period of

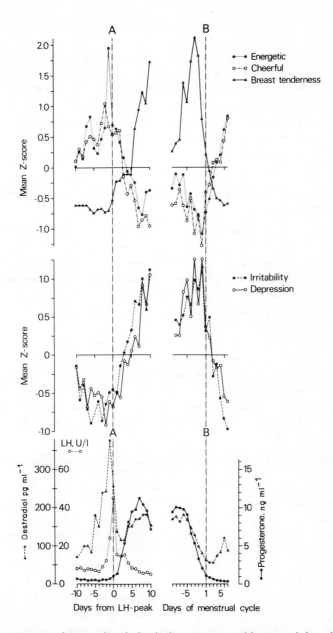

Figure 1. Mean Z-scores for mood and physical symptoms and hormonal data during the menstrual cycle in patients with PMT (n=12). (A) The data are synchronized around the day of LH surge. (B) The data are synchronized around the first day of menstrual bleeding. Day 1 = first day of menstrual bleeding. Reprinted with permission of Elsevier Science Publishing Co., Inc. from 'Mood, sexuality, hormones and the menstrual cycle. II. Hormone levels and their relationship to the premenstrual syndrome', by Bäckström *et al.*, *Psychosomatic Medicine* **45**, 503–507. © 1983 The American Psychosomatic Society Inc

well-being (Figure 1). These results indicate the possibility that one or more organic factors during the luteal phase provoke mental symptoms in these patients. The key issue thus becomes whether cyclical mood changes exist in anovulatory cycles or not. In anovulatory cycles induced by treatment LHRH analogues administered nasally or subcutaneously, the cyclical mood changes seem to disappear (Muse *et al.*, 1984; Bancroft 1986; Hammarbäck and Bäckström, unpublished).

Involvement of Oestradiol and Progesterone in the Development of Negative Mood Changes

Oestradiol and/or progesterone are the factors most often discussed in the aetiology of PMS. The reason for this is that these two hormones regulate the menstrual cycle and that the symptoms are so closely related to the different phases of the menstrual cycle. Both oestradiol and progesterone are accumulated in and have receptors in the brain as well as effects on the brain excitability (Bäckström *et al.*, 1984). They are also involved in the behaviour of animals (Leshner, 1978).

Oestradiol might have alerting effects on mood. There is an increased sense of well-being in relation to the preovulatory oestradiol peak (Figure 1). The general excitability of the brain seems to increase during oestrogen treatment (Bäckström *et al.*, 1984). Moreover, oestradiol has been shown to be effective in the treatment of general depression (Bowman and Bender, 1932; Klaiber *et al.*, 1979) although it has never been generally accepted as a treatment for depression.

Progesterone and especially some progesterone metabolites are also active in the brain, having sedative effects (Bäckström *et al.*, 1984). They might also have tranquillizing effects as many sedatives have, but this has not yet been investigated. However, progestagens, especially 19-nor-testosterone derivates, seem to be different as they have no sedative effects (Meyerson, 1967) but instead have been reported to provoke negative mood (Kane *et al.*, 1967). Medroxyprogesterone acetate and 17α-hydroxy-progesterone caproate do not seem to have negative mood provoking effects when given alone in high doses (Kohorn, 1978).

The combination of oestradiol and progesterone might have effects on mood other than those of the hormones separately. The combined situation occurs during the luteal phase when the symptoms are present (Figure 1, Bäckström *et al.*, 1983b). In postmenopausal women receiving sequential oestrogen–progestagen treatment the hormonal variations resemble the variations during an ovulatory cycle, while the treatment with only cyclical oestrogen resembles an anovulatory cycle. We have recruited eleven women with each treatment regime and followed them with daily prospective symptom ratings through the treatment cycle (Hammarbäck *et al.*, 1984). Women on the sequential

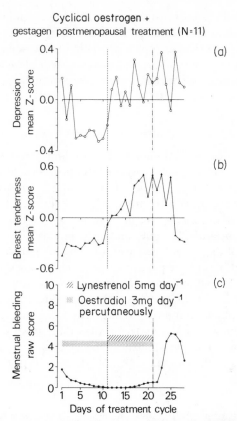

Figure 2. Mean depression, breast tender Z-scores and menstrual bleeding scores each day of treatment cycle in eleven postmenopausal women during sequential oestrogen/progestagen replacement therapy. Reproduced by permission of *Acta Obstetrica et Gynecologica Scandinavica* from Hammarbäck *et al.*, 1985

treatment developed negative mood soon after the progestagen was added to the treatment (Figure 2). Women on oestrogen only did not show any significant mood deterioration (Hammarbäck *et al.*, 1984). The results suggest that progesterone, perhaps in combination with oestradiol is involved in the provoking of negative mood.

In women taking oral contraceptives only patients with a previous history of PMS seem to react badly on the pill (Cullberg, 1972) and they reacted only on a combination with a low concentration of progestagen in the pill. The results suggest that an oral contraceptive pill with a low progestagen concentration is more symptom provocative than one with high concentration. This is in line with the findings of lower plasma progesterone concentrations in women with PMS (Bäckström and Carstensen 1974; Bäckström *et al.*, 1976; Munday *et al.*, 1981; Smith, 1975). However there are some studies not showing a significant decrease in plasma progesterone in patients compared to controls (Andersch *et al.*, 1979; Bäckström *et al.*, 1983b; O'Brien *et al.*, 1980). It is also clear that severe cyclical mood changes can occur in cycles with normal or high plasma progesterone concentrations (Bäckström *et al.*, 1983a).

Possible Difference Between Patients and Controls

Not all women have cyclical mood changes and those women with and without PMS must differ in some way is likely, as otherwise all or none should have cyclical mood changes. Cullberg (1972) noted in his oral contraceptive study that only the women who previously had suffered from PMS reacted badly on the pill. In our studies we have also noted that all women who tried the pill after the onset of PMS got mental changes as side-effects (Sanders *et al.*, 1983). Some of the women had also tried the pill before the onset of PMS and had no side-effects of the pill at that time. This suggests that women with PMS are more sensitive to hormonal provocation than women without. We also have some endocrine indications in the same direction. We have followed the first follicular phase after a corpus lute-ectomy with daily plasma hormone analysis in women with PMS and controls (Bäckström *et al.*, 1985). The results suggest that the hypothalamo–pituitary unit is more sensitive to ovarian hormones in the women with PMS compared to the controls.

Other Suggested Endocrine Factors

Aldosterone

Water retention has often been discussed as a possible aetiological factor (Janowsky *et al.*, 1973; O'Brien *et al.*, 1979) and as aldosterone participates in the water and sodium regulation it might be involved in PMS. Aldosterone levels change in parallel with the progesterone production via activation of the renin–angiotensive system (Sundsfjord and Aakvaag, 1970) and angiotensin II has been reported to have behavioural effects (Janowsky *et al.*, 1973). Plasma aldosterone has also been investigated in PMS women compared to controls but no difference has been found (O'Brien *et al.*, 1979; Munday *et al.*, 1981). A clinical trial with spironolactone, an aldosterone antagonist, has however shown beneficial effects over placebo on the mental symptoms (O'Brien *et al.*, 1979). This effect might, however, be due to effects separate from the anti-aldosterone effect. Spironolactone has been shown to inhibit the anaesthetic effects of progesterone and this might be of greater importance for the mental symptoms (Selye, 1969).

Testosterone

Testosterone treatment was suggested in some early studies (Rees, 1953). Patients also often report presence of acne during the luteal phase. So far no evidence of changed testosterone levels have been published (Bäckström and Aakvaag, 1981). The physiologically active part of the plasma testosterone concentration is the unbound concentration. Testosterone in plasma is bound to sex hormone binding globulin (SHBG) and albumin (Södergård *et al.*, 1982). A change in SHBG could result in changed androgen effect in the patients. Two studies have investigated SHBG in PMS patients and controls, with divergent results, thus giving no consistent picture (Dalton, 1981; Bäckström and Aakvaag, 1981). The total androgen picture has, however, not been studied in PMS patients.

Prolactin

Several authors have discussed prolactin as a possible aetiologic factor. This is mainly because it affects water and sodium regulation (Horrobin *et al.*, 1971) and the function of the corpus luteum (Robyn *et al.*, 1976). In animals prolactin has effects on behaviour and similar effects might exist in humans (Carrol and Steiner, 1978). Bromocriptine, an inhibitor of prolactin production, has been tried in PMS but the only consistent finding is a reduction of breast tenderness (Andersch *et al.*, 1978; Andersen *et al.*, 1977; Ghose and Coppen, 1977; Benedek-Jaszmann *et al.*, 1976; Elsner *et al.*, 1980). Plasma prolactin levels in PMS patients have been studied but were found to be similar to control levels (Andersch *et al.*, 1979; Bäckström and Aakvaag, 1981).

In conclusion, factors produced by the corpus luteum of the ovary seem to provoke a negative mood change in certain sensitive women. The factor or factors are not yet identified but the combination of oestradiol and progesterone is under suspicion.

Acknowledgements

These studies were supported by Swedish Medical Research Council (proj. 17x-6862), K. O. Hanssons foundation, University of Umeå foundation, Svenska Hoechst AB, Samverkansnämnden övre Norrland. M. Bergstén is acknowledged for secretarial assistance.

References

Andersch, B., Abrahamsson, L., Wendestam, C., Öhman, R. and Hahn, L. (1979). Hormone profile in premenstrual tension. Effects of bromocriptine and diuretics. *Clinical Endocrinology*, **11**, 657–664.

Andersch, B., Hahn, L., Andersson, M. and Isaksson, B. (1978). Body water and weight in patients with premenstrual tension. *British Journal of Obstetrics and Gynaecology*, **85**, 546–550.

Andersch, B., Wendestam, C., Hahn, L. and Öhman, R. (1986). Prevalence of premenstrual symptoms in a Swedish urban population. *Journal of Psychosomatic Obstetrics and Gynaecology*, **5**, 39–49.

Andersen, A. B., Larsen, J. F., Steenstrup, O. R., Svendstrup, B. and Nielsen, J. (1977). Effect of bromocriptine on the premenstrual syndrome. A double blind clinical trial. *British Journal of Obstetrics and Gynaecology*, **84**, 370–374.

Bäckström, T. and Aakvaag, A. (1981). Plasma prolactin and testosterone during the luteal phase in women with premenstrual tension syndrome. *Psychoneuroendocrinology*, **6**, 245–251.

Bäckström, T., Baird, D. T., Bancroft, J., Bixo, M., Hammarbäck, S., Sanders, D., Smith, S. and Zetterlund, B. (1983a). Endocrinological aspects of cyclical mood changes during the menstrual cycle or the premenstrual tension syndrome. *Journal of Psychosomatic Obstetrics and Gynaecology*, **2**, 8–20.

Bäckström, C. T., Boyle, H. and Baird, D. T. (1981). Persistence of symptoms of premenstrual tension in hysterectomised women. *British Journal of Obstetrics and Gynaecology*, **88**, 530–536.

Bäckström, T. and Carstensen, H. (1974). Estrogen and progesterone in plasma in relation to premenstrual tension. *Journal of Steroid Biochemistry*, **5**, 257–260.

Bäckström, T., Landgren, S., Zetterlund, B., Blom, S., Dubrovsky, B., Bixo, M. and Södergård, R. (1984). Effects of ovarian steroid hormones on brain excitability and their relation to epilepsy seizure variation during the menstrual cycle, in *Advances in Epileptology: XVth Epilepsy International Symposium*, (Ed. R. J. Porter) Raven Press, New York, pp. 269–277.

Bäckström, T., Sanders, D., Leask, R., Davidson, D., Warner, P. and Bancroft, J. (1983b). Mood, sexuality, hormones and the menstrual cycle II. Hormone levels and their relationship to the premenstrual syndrome. *Psychosomatic Medicine*, **45**, 503–507.

Bäckström, T., Smith, S., Lothian, H. and Baird, D. T. (1985). Prolonged follicular phase and depressed gonadotrophins following hysterectomy and corpus luteectomy in women with premenstrual syndrome. *Clinical Endocrinology*, **22**, 723–732.

Bäckström, T., Wide, L., Södergård, R. and Carstensen, H. (1976). FSH, LH, TeBG-capacity, estrogen and progesterone in women with premenstrual tension during the luteal phase. *Journal of Steroid Biochemistry*, **7**, 473–476.

Bancroft, J. (1986). The use of an LHRH-agonist in the investigation and treatment of premenstrual syndrome, in *Proceedings of 8th International Congress of Psychosomatic Obstetrics & Gynecology, Melbourne, 10–14 March 1986* International Congress Series, Elsevier, Amsterdam, p. 9.

Benedek-Jaszmann, L. J. and Hearn-Sturtevant, M. D. (1976). Premenstrual tension and functional infertility. *Lancet*, **i**, 1095–1098.

Bowman, K. M. and Bender, L. (1932). The treatment of involution melancholia with ovarian hormone. *American Journal of Psychiatry*, **11**, 867–872.

Carrol, B. J. and Steiner, M. (1978). The psychobiology of premenstrual dysphorea. The role of prolactin. *Psychoneuroendocrinology*, **3**, 171–180.

Cullberg, J. (1972). Mood changes and menstrual symptoms with different gestagen/ estrogen combinations. A double blind comparison with placebo. *Acta Psychiatrica Scandinavica*, **supplement 236**.

Dalton, K. (1984). *The Premenstrual Syndrome and Progesterone Therapy*. Heineman, London.

Dalton, M. E. (1981). Sex hormone binding globulin concentrations in women with severe premenstrual syndrome. *Postgraduate Medical Journal*, **57**, 560–561.

Elsner, C. W., Buster, J. E., Schindler, R. A., Nessim, S. A. and Abraham, G. E. (1980). Bromocriptine in the treatment of premenstrual tension syndrome. *Obstetrics and Gynecology*, **56**, 723–726.

Ghose, K. and Coppen, A. (1977). Bromocriptine and premenstrual syndrome: Controlled study. *British Medical Journal*, **1**, 147–148.

Hammarbäck, S., Bäckström, T., Holst, J., von Schoultz, B. and Lyrenäs, S. (1984). Cyclical mood changes as in the premenstrual syndrome during sequential estrogen-progestagen post-menopausal treatment. *Acta Obstetricia et Gynecologica Scandinavica*, **64**, 393–398.

Hammarbäck, S. and Bäckström, T. (1985). Premenstrual tension—diagnostical aspects and classification of patients. *Archives of Gynecology*, **237**, **Supplement**, p. 205.

Horrobin, D. F., Brustyn, P. G., Lloyd, I. J., Durkin, N., Lipton, A. and Muiruri, K. L. (1971). Actions of prolactin on human renal function. *Lancet*, **ii**, 352–353.

Janowsky, D. S., Berens, S. C. and Davis, J. M. (1973). Correlations between mood, weight and electrolytes during the menstrual cycle: A renin–angiotension–aldosterone hypothesis of premenstrual tension. *Psychosomatic Medicine*, **35**, 143–158.

Kane, F. J., Daly, R. J., Ewing, J. A. and Keeler, M. H. (1967). Mood and behavioural changes with progestational agents. *British Journal of Psychiatry*, **113**, 265–268.

Klaiber, E. L., Broverman, D. M., Vogel, W. and Kobayashi, Y. (1979). Estrogen therapy for severe persistent depression in women. *Archives of General Psychiatry*, **36**, 550–559.

Kohorn, E. I. (1978). Current Status of progestogens in the management of endometrial cancer, in *Endometrial Cancer*, (Eds. M. G. Brush, R. J. B. King, and R. W. Taylor) Baillière Tindall, London, pp. 179–187.

Leshner, A. I. (1978). *An Introduction to Behavioural Endocrinology*, Oxford University Press, New York.

Meyerson, B. (1967). Relationship between the anesthetic and gestagenic action and estrus behaviour-inducing activity of different progestins. *Endocrinology*, **81**, 369–374.

Munday, M., Brush, M. G. and Taylor, R. W. (1981). Correlations between progesterone, oestradiol and aldosterone levels in the premenstrual syndrome. *Clinical Endocrinology*, **14**, 1–19.

Muse, K. N., Cetel, N. S., Futterman, L. A. and Yen, S. S. C. (1984). Premenstrual syndrome-effects of 'Medical Ovariectomy'. *New England Journal of Medicine*, **311**, 1345–1349.

O'Brien, P. M. S., Craven, D., Selby, C. and Symonds, E. M. (1979). Treatment of premenstrual syndrome by spironolactone. *British Journal of Obstetrics and Gynaecology*, **86**, 142–174.

O'Brien, P. M. S., Selby, C. and Symonds, E. M. (1980). Progesterone, fluid and electrolytes in premenstrual syndrome. *British Medical Journal*, **1**, 1161–1163.

Rees, L. (1953). The premenstrual tension syndrome and its treatment. *British Medical Journal*, **1**, 1014–1016.

Robyn, C., Vekermans, M., Cautriez, A. and L'Hermite, M. (1976). Effects of sulpiride-induced hyperprolactinemia on circulating gonadotrophins and sex steroids during the menstrual cycle. *International Research Communication Systems*, **4**, 14.

Sanders, D., Warner, P., Bäckström, T. and Bancroft, J. (1983). Mood, sexuality, hormones and the menstrual cycle I. Changes in mood and physical state: description of subjects and methods. *Psychosomatic Medicine*, **45**, 487–501.

Sampson, G. A. (1979). Premenstrual syndrome. A double-blind controlled trial of progesterone and placebo. *British Journal of Psychiatry*, **135**, 209–15.

Selye, H. (1969). Spironolactone actions, independent of mineralocorticoid blockade. *Steroids*, **13**, 803–807.

Smith, S. L. (1975). Mood and the menstrual cycle, in *Topics in psychoneuroendocrinology*, (Ed. E. J. Sachar) Grune and Stratton, New York, pp. 19–58.

Södergård, R., Bäckström, T., Shanbhag, V. and Carstensen, H. (1982). Calculation of free and bound fractions of testosterone and estradiol-17β to human plasma proteins at body temperature. *Journal of Steroid Biochemistry*, **16**, 801–810.

Steiner, M., Haskett, R. F. and Carrol, B. J. (1980). Premenstrual tension syndrome: the development of research diagnostic criteria and new rating scales. *Acta Psychiatrica Scandinavica*, **62**, 177–190.

Sundsfjord, J. A. and Aakvaag, A. (1970). Plasma angiotensin II and aldosterone excretion during the menstrual cycle. *Acta Endocrinologica*, **64**, 452–456.

Functional Disorders of the Menstrual Cycle
Edited by M. G. Brush and E. M. Goudsmit
© 1988 John Wiley & Sons Ltd

CHAPTER 7

Endocrine treatments for premenstrual syndrome: principles and clinical evaluation

GWYNETH A. SAMPSON
Department of Psychiatry,
Whiteley Wood Clinic,
Woofindin Road,
Sheffield S10 3TL

Although premenstrual symptoms have been described for many years it is only as the ability to measure hormones has developed that links between the two have been postulated and developed.

In 1931 Frank who measured 'female sex hormone' in 'mouse units' wrote:

'It would thus appear that the continued circulation of an excessive amount of female sex hormones in the blood may in labile persons produce serious symptoms, some cardiovascular, but the most striking definitely psychic and nervous (autonomic). These periodic attacks are incapacitating and lead occasionally to extreme unhappiness and family discord. They can be directly ascribed to the excessive hormonal stimulus' (Frank, 1931).

One major problem in assessing endocrine abnormality is knowing what to consider as a 'normal' endocrine pattern. Lenton and Landgren (1985) point to the philosophical difficulties associated with 'normal' subject selection. They suggest that 'the normal cycle' does not exist but that cycles should be described as normal with respect to ovulation, or to fertility or to prolactin concentrations, etc.; they have demonstrated that there are many versions of the normal cycle. They comment:

'. . . that there are marked qualitative and quantitative differences in endocrine function between women but not within a woman where cycles will generally be very reproducible with respect to endocrine features, although less so when follicular growth dynamics are considered'.

97

The debate as to whether it is normal or abnormal to have some physical and psychological symptoms in relation to menstruation highlights a further philosophical question: 'is the cycle without any symptoms in relation to menstruation abnormal or normal?'.

Possible Endocrine Aetiological Models for Premenstrual Syndrome

There have been many different aetiological models for the condition now known as premenstrual syndrome (PMS) whose definitions are discussed in Chapter 3. With the rapid development in assay techniques it is likely that old models will continue to be discarded and new ones hypothesized.

Ovarian Hormones

Frank (1931) suggested oestrogen excess as the cause of PMS and Israel (1938) considered that change in the oestrogen–progesterone ratio was a principal factor. Morton (1950) gave oestrogen to women following oophorectomy and produced bloatedness and irritability whilst Gillman (1942) reported that he could produce similar symptoms in the follicular phase by injecting 10–30 mg progesterone. Zondek and Bromberg (1947) postulated that premenstrual symptoms resulted from hyper-sensitivity to progesterone or its metabolites at multiple gonadal steroid sites but unfortunately very little work has been carried out to investigate this interesting hypothesis.

As hormonal assays became more feasible these early hypotheses were tested in several studies in which ovarian hormones were directly measured during the menstrual cycles of women with PMS (see Chapters 6 and 8). However, a variety of queries have been raised about the design of most of these studies and there is therefore some debate as to their validity. In particular earlier studies have been criticized regarding frequency of sampling and lack of standardized collection times both during the day and during the cycle. Of equal concern is that there has often been inadequate recording of symptoms. There is rarely any attempt to correlate actual symptoms with endocrine values although in many cases this would present complex statistical problems. There is also the problem of defining the 'subject'—in some studies subjects were not primarily premenstrual symptom complainers but women attending general gynaecology or infertility clinics (Benedek-Jaszmann and Hearn-Sturtevant, 1976; Hargrove and Abraham, 1983).

Several studies have measured oestrogen and progesterone levels and although some report modest abnormalities (Bäckström et al., 1976; Munday et al., 1981) others do not find abnormal levels or an abnormal oestrogen–progesterone ratio (Taylor, 1979; Bäckström et al., 1983). Unfortunately the patients in the various studies are not directly comparable due to differences in mean age, symptom definitions and groupings and the number of subjects included e.g. the median age of the subjects of Taylor (1979) was 23 years which was much younger than in other studies and the symptomatology criteria were wide enough to include 'menstrual distress' subjects (see p. 5). However, there is no evidence to support the hypothesis that there is a major progesterone deficiency in the second half of the cycle. Although nearly all studies on premenstrual symptomatology relate to the luteal phase, there is some evidence that a PMS-like condition can occur in anovulatory cycles (Adamopoulos et al., 1972; E. A. Lenton and G. A. Sampson, unpublished data). Patient inclusion criteria used by Adamopoulos et al. (1972) were not well defined and 'menstrual distress' subjects may have been included. The early theory of Gillman (1942), has gained support from a study in a group of postmenopausal women who received progestogen in addition to their oestradiol and developed negative mood changes one to three days after the onset of the progestogen administration which ceased two to three days after the hormones were stopped (Hammarback et al., 1985).

Other investigators have argued that it is not the difference in total hormonal levels which is important but the free hormone levels (Dalton, 1984) although others do not find abnormal SHBG levels (Bäckström et al., 1976).

From the above evidence it now seems rather unlikely that abnormal levels of ovarian hormones play a critical role in the aetiology of PMS although the normal changes in oestrogen and progesterone levels from ovulation onwards may play a key part in the triggering of premenstrual symptoms. It is possible that central brain mechanisms controlling both mood and endocrine cycles represent an important area for future research in the aetiology of PMS with changes in ovarian hormones being relegated to a secondary role (see also Chapters 5 and 8).

Gonadotrophins

It is known that PMS symptoms may be relieved when ovulation is suppressed by drug induced reduction in gonadotrophin levels. However, no abnormalities in FSH and LH levels were found in their PMS subjects by O'Brien (1979) and Andersch et al. (1979). Bäckström et al. (1976) found significant increases in FSH levels on days nine, eight, seven and six before menstruation and suggested that this may lead to increased activity from newly formed ovarian follicles. Watts et al. (1985) did not find changes in FSH levels but did see small increases in LH immediately prior to menstruation. Thus, it seems that further research is needed in order to clarify the possible role of gonadotrophins in PMS.

Prolactin

Although Horrobin (1973) hypothesized that prolactin plays an important role in the aetiology of PMS, levels have been measured in several studies and no consistent abnormalities have been shown (Andersch *et al.*, 1979; O'Brien and Symonds, 1982).

Testosterone

A possible role for testosterone has been considered but no abnormal levels reported (Bäckström and Aakvaag, 1981).

Vasopressin

Vasopressin is an effective uterine stimulant in the non-pregnant human uterus especially around the onset of menstruation. It has been hypothesized that it could well contribute to the onset of premenstrual pain and also, because of its effect on water balance, to the fluid retention symptoms. Vasopressin levels were found to be increased in a group with premenstrual pain compared with a control group (Strömberg *et al.*, 1984).

Adrenal Hormones

Three studies have measured aldosterone levels—in two an increase in levels was found; in one study this increase was also in the control group but the control group did develop cyclical mood changes in treated cycles and could be described as having premenstrual changes (Perrini and Pilego, 1959; O'Brien *et al.*, 1979). Munday *et al.* (1981) found no significant difference betwen PMS subjects and controls. Studies on manic-depressive patients have suggested a correlation between mood and aldosterone levels (Jenner *et al.*, 1967).

Pancreatic Hormones

Several authors consider hypoglycaemia to be a contributory mechanism in PMS; however, there is conflicting evidence as to variations in glucose tolerance during the menstrual cycle and there is no study reporting differences in glucose tolerance between women with PMS and women who are symptom-free.

Melatonin

This pineal hormone varies with the menstrual cycle and is at its highest during the premenstrual and menstrual phases—it has also been reported to exacerbate dysphoria in depressed patients (Kashiwagi *et al.*, 1976). However, it has not been measured in women with PMS.

TRH and Thyroid Hormones

Several reports suggest the hypothalamic–pituitary axis is disturbed in PMS, and one study reports significantly higher cortisol levels in response to TRH stimulation in PMS patients compared with controls (Chiodera *et al.*, 1982). A preliminary report assessing thyroid dysfunction in women reporting PMS symptoms suggested that 94 per cent of 54 patients studied had one or more indicators of thyroid dysfunction compared with none of twelve patients without PMS symptoms (Brayshaw and Brayshaw, 1986).

Growth Hormone

Two studies have assessed growth hormone in PMS. Chiodera *et al.* (1982) found that although basal growth hormone concentrations were in the normal range there was a significant response to TRH in six out of seven patients. Steiner *et al.* (1984) measured circadian secretory profiles and found no relationship with PMS.

Conclusions

Although there are many reported studies it is difficult to state that there is a consistently detectable hormonal abnormality differentiating women with PMS from other women.

In terms of proven endocrine theories we have no more consistent data than Frank in 1931, except that our increased endocrine knowledge suggests that the answer will not be a simplistic one.

Endocrine therapy for PMS continues to be largely empirical though based in part on various aetiological theories none of which have at present been proven or disproven. The many varied results available allow almost any theory to be supported by a reported study and emphasize the need for further well-designed endocrine studies.

In order to evaluate the current hormonal treatments for PMS the various treatment models may be arbitarily divided into subgroups:

1. Hormone replacement: these theories suggest that a hormone deficiency causes PMS symptoms either by itself or by altering a hormonal ratio and imply that suitable hormone therapy will rectify the deficiency.
2. A direct pharmacological effect: these theories suggest that a direct action or loss of action of the hormone produces symptoms and imply that by using hormones in pharmacological rather than physiological dosage the symptoms will be abated.

Table 1. Possible rationale for current endocrine therapies for premenstrual syndrome

	Hormone replacement	Pharmaco-logical	Subtle cycle manipulation (still menstruating)	Cycle ablation (not menstruating)
Oral Contraceptive		×	×	
Progesterone	×	×	×	×
Progestogens	×	×	×	×
Oestrogen		×	×	×
Bromocriptine			×	
Danazol				×
GnRH agonist				×

3. A 'subtle manipulation' of the menstrual cycle to be more like a non-PMS cycle is in keeping with those theories of complex endocrinological change being the cause of PMS.
4. Ablation of the menstrual cycle removes the cyclical hormonal fluctuations which are hypothesized as being the key to PMS.

In reality 3 and 4 are arbitary points on a spectrum of disruption of the menstrual cycle, in 3 menstruation as a marker still occurs whilst it is ablated in 4. However, the endocrine change which ablates bleeding in one woman may not consistently do so in another.

Table 1 indicates which endocrine therapies could be used for each of these four categories.

Clinical Evaluation of Endocrine Therapy

In any study of PMS there must be a clear definition of the condition; the problems in defining this have been discussed (Chapters 1 and 3). In a clinical study of the effects of endocrine therapy there should be a fully documented diagnosis based upon daily prospective rating of symptoms.

The subjects in whom the therapy is being assessed should be patients with severe symptoms interfering with home, work or social life with demonstrable PMS over several cycles, some of which could be placebo treated cycles (Metcalf and Hudson, 1985). Evaluations required include detailed history taking, appropriate rating scales, e.g. to measure neuroticism, self-esteem etc., and appropriate physical examination. The history, pattern and timing of symptoms may allow separation into subgroups which might respond differently to medication. Any trial should have clear inclusion and exclusion criteria, enough patients should be recruited and complete the trial to allow for adequate statistical interpretation of results. Ideally at least 100 subjects should start the trial as this will allow for the inevitable drop-outs.

As techniques of endocrine assay improve and are extended to saliva as well as blood, it is more feasible to measure endocrine parameters during a treatment study although the length of such studies (six months minimum) means this will be an expensive and time-consuming operation. It could even be argued that there is no point in endocrine studies if a treatment is used which is still to be proven as consistently effective, and that endocrine studies should only be undertaken for 'proven' therapies. Our limited knowledge of the detailed endocrine profile of 'normal' and 'PMS' cycles suggests that a simplistic evaluation of a hormonal profile is inappropriate.

However, there are several benefits to be obtained from endocrine studies of women receiving endocrine therapy:

1. By assessing the untreated cycle one has a baseline from which to compare treated cycles; it is possible that endocrine 'sub-groups' in terms of abnormalities in different hormonal profiles or length of luteal phase can be identified which might respond differently to treatment regimes.
2. By assessing the endocrine changes in treated cycles compared with untreated, to assess if symptom alterations (improvements or deteriorations) correlate with endocrine changes. In fact, for many endocrine treatments there is a paucity of knowledge on their 'usual' effects on the endocrine profile of the menstrual cycle when they are given in differing dosage regimes. It would be beneficial to PMS research if there was an increase in the knowledge of the effect of endocrine therapies on 'normal' cycles.
3. By comparing endocrine responses to treated cycles which produce a total amelioration of symptoms with cycles in which symptoms are reduced in intensity or time and cycles where symptoms do not respond to treatment it may be feasible to identify specific changes in dosage or its timing which alter symptom profiles.
4. With varying aetiological models it would be interesting to correlate endocrine levels with, for example, amines, essential fatty acids or other substances suggested as being involved in the aetiology of PMS.
5. If one suggests a direct pharmacological action of the endocrine agent it would be important to measure levels of the therapeutic agent and also record any endocrine response to the agent. Again there is a paucity of knowledge of the 'pharmacological' effect of endocrine treatments in humans and an expansion of knowledge in this field would benefit PMS research.

If one does undertake endocrine studies it seems appropriate to measure as many hormones as is feasible, (both in terms of the reality of collecting samples and of analysing them); in an ideal world this would include ovarian, pituitary, adrenal and perhaps thyroid, pancreatic, pineal and parathyroid hormones! Many authors point to the need for at least daily sampling and Steiner *et al.* (1984) comments:

> '. . . it is clear from our data that measurement of circadian profiles is superior to plasma level estimation in single samples. The pulsatile secretion pattern of these hormones clearly demonstrates the difficulties of interpreting values obtained from single samples.'

A realistic endocrine study is clearly a compromise.

It is now accepted that there is a high placebo response in many controlled treatment studies of PMS. This is not surprising in view of the affective nature of many of the symptoms and the high response to placebo in trials of psychotropic drugs (Jenner, 1977). Figure 1 and Table 2 demonstrate the placebo response obtained during a double-blind cross-over study of progesterone and placebo (Sampson, 1979). Metcalf and Hudson (1985) in a study of placebo given for three cycles following three untreated cycles found

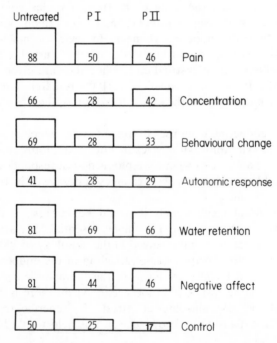

Figure 1. The percentage of total cycles which showed a significant increase in symptoms premenstrually ('A') for each of the symptom clusters of Moos Menstrual Distress Questionnaire during untreated and placebo treated (PI, PII) months

Table 2. Significant differences between untreated and placebo treated (PI, PII) cycles in terms of the percentage of cycles having a significant increase in symptoms premenstrually ('A'). Differences are shown for each of the separate symptom clusters of the Moos Menstrual Distress Questionnaire

Symptom cluster	Untreated/PI	Untreated/PII
Pain	× ×	×
Concentration	× ×	
Behavioural change	× ×	× ×
Autonomic response		
Water retention		
Negative affect	× ×	× ×
Control	×	× ×

× $p < 0.05$ × × $p < 0.01$

placebo administration was associated with an over-all reduction in the incidence of 'premenstrual tension', mood-related symptoms were diminished but there was no reduction of physical symptoms. Placebo administration was associated with a reduction of symptom severity. There were marked variations in the response of the individual to placebo. They analysed their data to quantify factors which related to the consistent presence of 'premenstrual tension', and they conclude that treatment studies should only be done on women with consistent forms of the disorder who, (a) perceive their PMS to be severe or moderately severe, and (b) continue to experience premenstrual symptoms when a placebo is given.

Some studies find a more marked placebo reponse to mood rather than physical symptoms (Metcalf and Hudson, 1985) whilst others find both physical and mental symptoms respond to placebo (Sampson et al., 1987). There are no long term studies (over one year) of treatment response to any PMS medication including placebo; many treatment studies compare responses in consecutively treated cycles and find a large placebo and treatment response in the first cycle. In some studies this response continues and in others it appears to diminish with increasing duration of treatment (Magos et al., 1986).

In a placebo controlled endocrine treatment study it would seem appropriate to estimate endocrine profiles during placebo as well as active treated cycles in order to, (a) keep the trial 'blind', (b) to observe if placebo alters endocrine profiles and (c) observe if improvements or deteriorations in symptoms are related to endocrine changes.

In the clinical evaluation of an endocrine treatment for PMS it is important not only to define the 'treatment' but also to propose a rationale for the treatment, for example, if devising a trial of progesterone therapy it would be appropriate to suggest that the therapy is presumed to replace a 'hormone deficiency', act as a pharmacological agent, or disrupt or ablate the endocrine cycle.

Endocrine measures should be made throughout the study, using at least daily assessment but for some patients might involve more frequent sampling; symptoms should be recorded in detail to allow correlation with endocrine status.

The treatment study should be double-blind cross-over (which poses practical problems when the rationale for the therapy is cycle ablation); it would seem appropriate to have short-term (six months) and longer term treatment (over one year) studies as although some patients request short-term therapy many require and request medication over a period of several years. The analysis of data should include ways of assessing carry-over effects of treatment from one cycle to the next (Sampson and Prescott, 1981); data from all or most of the cycle should be used rather than just from the premenstrual week. There seems now good evidence that the different symptoms of PMS respond differently to varying treatment regimes, therefore, it would seem important to analyse several symptoms or symptom groups independently.

The presence of side-effects should be fully recorded with both the placebo and active treatments. Women with severe PMS may require long-term therapy and it is therefore important to select the treatment known to show the least side-effects in long-term clinical studies.

Current Endocrine Treatments for PMS

Although most endocrine treatment currently used has been assessed in a clinical trial, the value of the reported trial data varies considerably.

Combined Oral Contraception

Several studies (Herzberg and Coppen, 1970; Royal College of General Practitioners, 1974) suggest oral contraceptives help premenstrual symptoms; it has been suggested that the more progestogenic formulations are more effective (Cullberg, 1972). Further discussion of oral contraception in relation to PMS is given in Chapter 4. As most oral contraceptives suppress ovulation and modify the normal endogenous hormonal pattern it can be hypothesized that their action is by manipulation or ablation of the endocrine cycle; however, this may be simplistic as there is also a direct pharmacological effect of the constituents of the various oral contraceptives.

Oestradiol Implants

Magos et al. (1986) advanced the hypothesis:

'The corollary of considering cyclical ovarian activity as fundamental in the aetiology of premenstrual syndrome is that suppression of ovulation should abolish symptoms . . .'

as the rationale for a parallel, but not cross-over study comparing oestradiol implants with placebo implants. Progestogen was added for seven days each month to ensure that menstruation occurred. Analysis of prospective ratings showed a significant superiority of oestrogen over placebo, although there appear to be pharmacological effects of the progestogen. An initial placebo response of 94 per cent was a noticeable feature of this study.

Progesterone

The initial rationale for using progesterone appears to have been to correct supposed abnormal hormone levels or ratios, treatment being given between ovulation and the onset of bleeding. Several double-blind studies of progesterone and placebo have been reported; there were double-blind cross-over studies which report that although progesterone was beneficial it was no more so than placebo (Maddocks *et al.*, 1986; Sampson, 1979; Van der Meer *et al.*, 1983). Maddocks *et al.* (1986) used 200 mg twice daily by the vaginal route and Sampson (1979) used both 200 and 400 mg twice daily doses usually by vaginal administration. A double-blind cross-over study of oral micronized progesterone given for ten days of each menstrual cycle starting roughly three days after ovulation is reported by Dennerstein *et al.* (1985). The results found progesterone more effective than placebo for some symptoms, but it is difficult, because of the data analysis, to assess if this is a direct effect on premenstrual symptoms or a global improvement throughout the cycle. A further study (Smith, 1975) on women with premenstrual depression only was placebo controlled using intramuscular progesterone 50 mg on alternate days from day nineteen and no consistent improvement attributable to progesterone therapy was reported.

The above studies using modest amounts of progesterone to correct a hypothetical deficiency suggest it is often no more effective than placebo. However, some of the benefits attributed to the use of larger amounts of progesterone in open studies (Dalton, 1977) may be due to pharmacological effects related directly to its effect on cerebral functioning. It is known that progesterone affects brain amines (Shaw, 1983) and Bancroft and Bäckström (1985) suggest there is now a *prima facie* case for considering the direct effects of oestradiol and progesterone on central nervous system activity. Several women using progesterone develop a dependence syndrome, with a need to increase the dosage in frequency and time and experience withdrawal effects when it is stopped. In humans intravenous administration of 250–500 mg progesterone induces sleep (Merryman *et al.*, 1954). The current United Kingdom Data Sheet for progesterone lists euphoria as a side-effect from 'overdosage'.

Table 3. The number of days of symptoms and bleeding per calendar month in one woman using differing therapeutic progesterone regimes

Treatment	Number of days of symptoms per calendar month	Number of days bleeding per calendar month	Number of days interval between first day of bleeding
Untreated	10	6	31
Progesterone 400 mg vaginally twice daily day twelve to 26	11	7	27
Progesterone 400 mg vaginally twice daily day five to onset of bleeding	6	14	14
Progesterone 400 mg vaginally twice daily continuously	2	0	—

After surveying the dosage regimes described by Dalton and reviewing clinical case studies Sampson (1981) comments that only when the menstrual cycle is disrupted is there usually, but not always, an improvement in symptoms. One example is shown in Table 3, which describes the effects of varying progesterone regimes in the management of a 35 year-old woman with ten days of psychological and physical symptoms which were relieved on the first day of bleeding. Her initial regime could be perceived as an attempt to correct a deficiency of progesterone and this was unhelpful. Using the same dosage but commencing on day five, the incidence of symptoms was halved but her bleeding pattern unacceptably disrupted. She has had her cycle ablated by continuous progesterone 400 mg twice daily given vaginally for nine years with total suppression of PMS, although she continues to have 'off' days which are randomly distributed.

As methods of collecting daily endocrine samples improve it will allow an assessment of the varying endocrine profiles produced by these different regimes.

Dalton (1977) reports several cases treated continuously with intramuscular progesterone 100 mg daily. Such a dose will ablate the cycle but will also have a direct pharmacological action.

Progestogens

Although several progestogens have been used for the treatment of PMS only dydrogesterone has been widely evaluated in controlled clinical trials as well as in uncontrolled studies. It was originally advocated in a dosage regime (10 mg twice daily on days twelve to 26) which could be regarded as correcting an endocrine deficiency and uncontrolled and single-blind studies using this regime reported therapeutic success (Taylor, 1977; Kerr *et al.*, 1980). A multi-centre general practice double-blind placebo controlled study, using a dosage regime of 10 mg twice daily from day twelve until the onset of bleeding (Williams *et al.*, 1983) with physician rating forms completed retrospectively found that both placebo and dydrogesterone gave significant improvement in twelve of fourteen symptoms studied, but in the third treatment month a retrospective global evaluation by physician and patient indicated a significant preference for dydrogesterone over placebo. A double-blind cross-over study in a hospital clinic and self-referring clinic (Sampson *et al.*, 1987) found on daily prospective rating analysis that dydrogesterone and placebo were effective in relieving symptoms but there was no significant difference; the treatment regime was dydrogesterone 10 mg twice daily from day twelve to 26 of a standardized 28 day cycle.

As with progesterone it seems unlikely that progestogens correct an underlying endocrine deficiency; they may have a direct pharmacological effect on brain and breast, for example, Sampson *et al.* (1987) found a significant increase in breast tenderness as a side-effect in dydrogesterone compared with placebo treated cycles.

There is now good evidence that the same dosage of dydrogesterone given at differing times in the cycle will produce different endocrine profiles (Lenton, 1984). Figures 2 and 3 are profiles of symptoms and progesterone levels from a pilot study assessing the response of premenstrual symptoms to

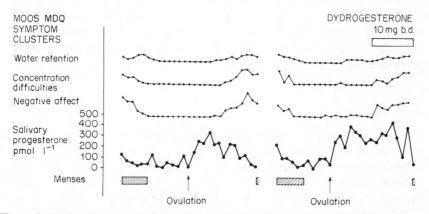

Figure 2. Daily symptom profiles (Moos Menstrual Distress Questionnaire symptom clusters) and progesterone levels in a subject with PMS receiving treatment with dydrogesterone 10 mg twice daily from day nineteen to the onset of bleeding

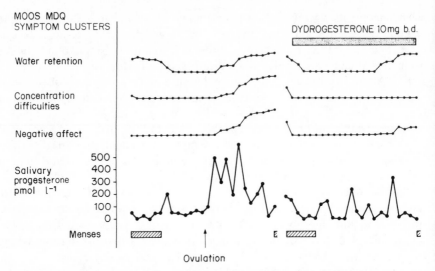

Figure 3. Daily symptom profiles (Moos Menstrual Distress Questionnaire symptom clusters) and progesterone levels in a subject with PMS receiving treatment with dydrogesterone 10 mg twice daily from day five to day 26 of her menstrual cycle

different dosage regimes of dydrogesterone. In Figure 2 the dosage regime (day nineteen to onset of bleeding) is compatible with a 'replacement' aetiological model, in Figure 3 the dosage regime (day five to day 26) with a manipulation of the endocrine cycle model.

Some progestogens have been used to ablate the menstrual cycle. Keye (1985) reported a pilot study of depo-medroxy progesterone acetate (150 mg every one to three months) with useful improvements in fifteen out of 20 subjects, and there are clinical reports of cycle ablation by continuous oral progestogens.

Bromocriptine

Bromocriptine is a dopamine agonist and inhibits prolactin secretion. The rationale for use is that there is excess prolactin secretion in PMS which is rectified by the use of bromocriptine. There are several double-blind studies of bromocriptine and placebo although the dosage regime varies. The majority of studies (Mansel *et al.*, 1978; Anderson *et al.*, 1977; Andersch *et al.*, 1978) report on improvement in breast but not mood symptoms—suggesting physical and psychological symptoms could have a different aetiology.

Danazol

Danazol could be effective in PMS by cycle ablation. Two preliminary reports of placebo controlled double-blind studies have been reported which show a higher percentage response to danazol than placebo. However, in both studies adverse side-effects caused those patients on active medication rather than placebo to withdraw (Watts *et al.*, 1985; Gilmore *et al.*, 1985). Watts *et al.* (1987) report that danazol helps symptoms of breast pain, lethargy, anxiety and increased appetite.

Gonadotrophin Releasing Hormone (GnRH) Agonists

GnRH agonists cause anovulation and amenorrhoea by down-regulating pituitary gonadotrophin secretion; their effectiveness in PMS could relate to cycle ablation. Two studies have been reported. Muse *et al.* (1984) in a double-blind cross-over study of GnRH agonist against placebo in eight patients report both physical and behaviour symptoms were improved compared with placebo. Bancroft *et al.* (1985) report preliminary work with the LH-RH agonist Buserelin, where the most convincing results were in women who showed follicular suppression. These data confirm that the area of cycle manipulation/cycle ablation is a complex one.

Conclusions

As methods of hormonal collection and analysis improve, our awareness of the complexity of the endocrinology of the menstrual cycle grows; similarly as our information-gathering on PMS improves our awareness of its complexity increases. Correlating the two is a fascinating but intricate task. It may be more appropriate in the future to concentrate research on studies involving a more thorough assessment of relatively small numbers of patients rather than large-scale treatment studies of a heterogenous group of women.

It is clearly simplistic to say an endocrine treatment helps or does not help PMS; we need to identify the endocrine agent, its correct dosage and timing of dosage in relation to the cycle as well as the endocrine and symptom factors it changes and the side-effects it produces.

Acknowledgements

I am grateful to Dr E. A. Lenton for endocrine assays, Gillian Gill for library help and Elsa Forsythe for typing assistance.

References

Adamopoulos, D. A., Loraine, J. A., Lunn, S. F., Coppen, A. J. and Daly, R. J. (1972). Endocrine profiles in premenstrual tension. *Clinical Endocrinology*, 1, 283–292.

Andersch, B., Hahn, L., Wendestam, C. and Abrahamsson, L. (1978). Treatment of premenstrual syndrome with bromocriptine. *Acta Endocrinologica*, 88, Supplement 216, 165–174.

Andersch, B., Abrahamsson, L., Wendestam, C., Ohman, R. and Hahn, L. (1979). Hormonal profiles in premenstrual tension—effects of bromocriptine and diuretics. *Clinical Endocrinology*, 11, 657–664.

Anderson, A. N., Larsen, J. F., Steenstrup, O. R., Svendstrup, B. and Nielson, J. (1977). Effect of bromocriptine on the premenstrual syndrome: a double blind clinical trial. *British Journal of Obstetrics and Gynaecology*, 84, 370–374.

Bäckström, T. and Aakvaag, A. (1981). Serum prolactin and testosterone during the luteal phase in women with premenstrual tension syndrome. *Psychoneuroendocrinology*, 6, 245–251.

Bäckström, T., Sanders, D., Leask, R., Davidson, D., Warner, P. and Bancroft, J. (1983). Mood, sexuality, hormones and the menstrual cycle. II. Hormone levels and their relationship to the premenstrual syndrome, *Psychosomatic Medicine*, 45, 503–507.

Bäckström, T., Wide, L., Södegard, R. and Carstensen, H. (1976). FSH, LH, TeBG-capacity, estrogen and progesterone in women with premenstrual tension during the luteal phase. *Journal of Steroid Biochemistry*, 7, 473–476.

Bancroft, J. and Bäckström, T. (1985). Premenstrual syndrome, *Clinical Endocrinology*, 22, 313–316.

Bancroft, J., Boyle, H., Davidson, D. W., Gray, J. and Fraser, H. M. (1985). The effects of an LH-RH agonist on the premenstrual syndrome: a preliminary report, in *LH-RH and its analogues, Fertility and Anti-Fertility Aspects*, (Ed. M. Schmidt-Gollwitzer) Walter de Gruyter, Berlin, pp. 307–319.

Benedek-Jaszmann, L. J. and Hearn-Sturtevant, M. D. (1976). Premenstrual tension and functional infertility. Aetiology and treatment. *Lancet*, i, 1095–1098.

Brayshaw, N. D. and Brayshaw, D. D. (1986). Thyroid hypofunction in premenstrual syndrome. *New England Journal of Medicine*, 315, 1486–1487.

Chiodera, P., Coiro, V. and Butturini, A. (1982). High based cortisol levels and growth hormone response to thyrotropin releasing hormone in patients with premenstrual syndrome. *Journal of Obstetrics and Gynaecology*, 2, 252–254.

Cullberg, J. (1972). Mood changes and menstrual symptoms with different gestogen/oestrogen combinations. *Acta Psychiatrica Scandinavica*, Suppl. 236, 1–86.

Dalton, K. (1977). *The Premenstrual Syndrome and Progesterone Therapy*, Heinemann, London.

Dalton, M. E. (1984). The effect of progesterone administration on sex hormone binding globulin capacity in women with severe premenstrual syndrome. *Journal of Steroid Biochemistry*, 20, 437–439.

Dennerstein, L., Spencer-Gardner, C., Gotts, G., Brown, J. B., Smith, M. A. and Burrows, G. D. (1985). Progesterone and the premenstrual syndrome: a double-blind cross-over trial. *British Medical Journal*, 290, 1617–1621.

Frank, R. T. (1931). The hormonal causes of premenstrual tension. *Archives of Neurology and Psychiatry*, 26, 1053–1057.

Gillman, J. (1942). The nature of subjective reactions evoked in women by progesterone with special reference to the problem of premenstrual tension. *Journal of Clinical Endocrinology and Metabolism*, 2, 157–160.

Gilmore, D. H., Hawthorn, R. J. S. and McKay-Hart, J. (1985). Danol for premenstrual syndrome: A preliminary report of a placebo controlled double-blind study. *Journal of International Medical Research*, **13**, 129–130.

Hammarback, S., Bäckström, T., Holst, J., von Schoultz, B. and Lyrens, S. (1985). Clinical mood changes as in the premenstrual tension syndrome during sequential oestrogen–progestogen post-menopausal replacement therapy. *Acta Obstetrica et Gynecologica Scandinavica*, **64**, 393–397.

Hargrove, J. T. and Abraham, G. E. (1983). The ubiquitousness of premenstrual tension in gynaecologic practice. *Journal of Reproductive Medicine*, **28**, 435–442.

Herzberg, B. and Coppen, A. (1970). Changes in psychological symptoms in women taking oral contraceptives. *British Journal of Psychiatry*, **116**, 161–164.

Horrobin, D. F. (1973). *Prolactin. Physiology and Clinical Significance*, MTP Press, Lancaster.

Israel, S. L. (1983). Premenstrual tension. *Journal of the American Medical Association*, **110**, 1721–1723.

Jenner, F. A. (1977). Some of the problems and difficulties associated with clinical studies of antidepressant agents. *British Journal of Clinical Pharmacology*, **4**, 199s–208s.

Jenner, F. A., Gjessing, L. R., Cox, J. R., Davies-Jones, A., Hullin, E. J. and Hanna, S. M. (1967). A manic-depressive psychotic with a persistent 48-hour cycle. *British Journal of Psychiatry*, **113**, 895–910.

Kashiwagi, T., McClure, J. N. and Wetzel, K. D. (1976). Premenstrual affective syndrome and Psychiatric Disorder, *Diseases of the Nervous System*, **37**, 116–119.

Kerr, G. D., Day, J. B., Munday, M. R., Brush, M. G., Watson, M. and Taylor, R. W. (1980). Dydrogesterone in the treatment of the premenstrual syndrome. *Practitioner*, **224**, 852–855.

Keye, W. R. (1985). Medical management of premenstrual syndrome. *Canadian Journal of Psychiatry*, **30**, 483–488.

Lenton, E. A. (1984). The effect of dydrogesterone on the mid-cycle gonadotrophin surge in regularly cycling women. *Clinical Endocrinology*, **20**, 129–135.

Lenton, E. A. and Landgren, B. M. (1985). The normal menstrual cycle, in *Clinical Reproductive Endocrinology*, (Ed. R. P. Shearman) Churchill Livingstone, Edinburgh, pp. 81–108.

Maddocks, S., Hahn, P., Moller, F. and Reid, R. (1986). A double-blind placebo controlled trial of progesterone vaginal suppositories in the treatment of premenstrual syndrome. *American Journal of Obstetrics and Gynecology*, **154**, 573–581.

Magos, A. L., Brincat, M. and Studd, J. W. W. (1986). Treatment of the premenstrual syndrome by subcutaneous oestradiol implants and cyclical oral norethisterone: placebo controlled study. *British Medical Journal*, **292**, 1629–1633.

Mansel, R. E., Preece, P. E. and Hughes, L. E. (1978). A double-blind trial of the prolactin inhibitor bromocriptine in painful benign breast disease. *British Journal of Surgery*, **65**, 724–727.

Merryman, W., Boiman, R., Barnes, L. and Rothchild, I. (1954). Progesterone 'anaesthesia' in human subjects. *Journal of Clinical Endocrinology and Metabolism*, **14**, 1567–1569.

Metcalf, M. G. and Hudson, S. M. (1985). The premenstrual syndrome. Selection of women for treatment trials. *Journal of Psychosomatic Research*, **29**, 631–638.

Morton, J. H. (1950). Premenstrual tension. *American Journal of Obstetrics and Gynecology*, **60**, 343–352.

Munday, M. R., Brush, M. G. and Taylor, R. W. (1981). Correlations between progesterone, oestradiol and aldosterone levels in the premenstrual syndrome. *Clinical Endocrinology*, **14**, 1–9.

Muse, K. N., Catel, N. S., Futterman, L. A. and Yen, S. S. C. (1984). The premenstrual syndrome. Effects of medical ovariectomy. *New England Journal of Medicine*, **311**, 1345–1349.

O'Brien, P. M. S. (1979). M. D. Thesis, University of Wales.

O'Brien, P. M. S., Craven, D., Selby, C. and Symonds, E. M. (1979). Treatment of premenstrual syndrome by spironolactone. *British Journal of Obstetrics and Gynaecology*, **86**, 142–147.

O'Brien, P. M. S. and Symonds, E. M. (1982). Prolactin levels in the premenstrual syndrome. *British Journal of Obstetrics and Gynaecology*, **89**, 306–308.

Perrini, A. and Pilego, N. (1959). The increases in aldosterone in premenstrual tension. *Minerva Medicine*, **50**, 2897–2899.

Royal College of General Practitioners (1974). *Oral Contraceptives and Health*, Pitman Medical, London.

Sampson, G. A. (1979). Premenstrual syndrome. A double-blind controlled trial of progesterone and placebo. *British Journal of Psychiatry*, **135**, 209–215.

Sampson, G. A. (1981). An appraisal of the role of progesterone in the therapy of premenstrual syndrome, in *The Premenstrual Syndrome*, (Ed. P. A. Van Keep and W. H. Utian), MTP Press, Lancaster, pp. 51–69.

Sampson, G. A., Heathcote, P. R. M., Wordsworth, J., Prescott, P. and Hodgson, A. (1987). Premenstrual syndrome. A double-blind cross-over study of treatment with dydrogesterone and placebo (in press).

Sampson, G. A. and Prescott, P. (1981). The assessment of the symptoms of premenstrual syndrome and their response to therapy. *British Journal of Psychiatry*, **138**, 399–405.

Shaw, D. M. (1983). Hormones, amines and mood, in *Premenstrual Syndrome*, (Ed. R. W. Taylor) Medical News-Tribune, London, pp. 33–35.

Smith, S. L. (1975). Mood and the menstrual cycle, in *Topics in Psychoendocrinology*, (Ed. E. J. Sacher) Grune & Stratton, New York, pp. 19–58.

Steiner, M., Haskett, E. F., Carrol, B. J., Hays, S. E. and Rubin, R. T. (1984). Circadian hormone secretory profiles in women with severe premenstrual tension syndrome. *British Journal of Obstetrics and Gynaecology*, **91**, 466–471.

Strömberg, P., Akerlund, M., Forsling, M. L., Granstrom, E. and Kindahl, H. (1984). Vasopressin and prostaglandins in premenstrual pain and primary dysmenorrhoea. *Acta Obstetrica et Gynecologica Scandinavica*, **63**, 533–538.

Taylor, J. W. (1979). Plasma progesterone, oestradiol 17β and premenstrual symptoms. *Acta Psychiatrica Scandinavica*, **60**, 76–86.

Taylor, R. W. (1977). The treatment of premenstrual syndrome with dydrogesterone (Duphaston). *Current Medical Research and Opinion*, **4**, Supplement 4, 35–40.

Van der Meer, Y. G., Benedek-Jaszmann, L. J. and Van Loenen, A. V. (1983). Effect of high dose progesterone on the premenstrual syndrome: a double-blind cross-over study. *Journal of Psychosomatic Obstetrics and Gynaecology*, **2**, 220–222.

Watts, J. F., Butt, W. R., Edwards, R. L. and Holder, G. (1985). Hormonal studies in women with premenstrual tension. *British Journal of Obstetrics and Gynaecology*, **92**, 247–255.

Watts, J. F., Butt, W. R. and Edwards, R. L. (1987). A clinical trial using danazol for the treatment of premenstrual tension. *British Journal of Obstetrics and Gynaecology*, **94**, 30–34.

Watts, J. F., Edwards, R. L. and Butt, W. R. (1985). Treatment of premenstrual syndrome using danazol: Preliminary report of a placebo controlled double-blind dose ranging study. *Journal of International Medical Research*, **13**, 127–128.

Williams, J. G. C., Martin, A. J. and Hulkensberg-Tromp, T. E. M. L. (1983). PMS in

four European countries, Part 2, A double-blind placebo controlled study of dydrogesterone. *British Journal of Sexual Medicine*, **10**, 8–18.
Zondek, B., and Bromberg, Y. M. (1947). Clinical reactions of allergy to endogenous hormones and their treatment. *Journal of Obstetrics and Gynaecology of the British Empire*, **54**, 1–9.

Functional Disorders of the Menstrual Cycle
Edited by M. G. Brush and E. M. Goudsmit
© 1988 John Wiley & Sons Ltd

CHAPTER 8

New concepts in the endocrinology of premenstrual syndrome

W. R. BUTT

Department of Clinical Endocrinology,
Birmingham and Midland Hospital for Women,
Showell Green Lane, Sparkhill,
Birmingham B11 4HL

In spite of many theories and treatments the aetiology of the premenstrual syndrome (PMS) remains obscure. The cyclical nature of the symptoms suggests that the basic problem is related to a hormone, or other agent, which varies in a cyclical manner. What has become clear is that there is no known hormone which is grossly abnormal in this condition. If there is a basic endocrine cause it must be a subtle abnormality in a hormone or group of hormones which is not recognized in the weekly or daily samples of serum that have been employed in most investigations.

Interest in the syndrome is illustrated by the number of reviews published and meetings held on the subject in recent years. Early observations were restricted to the types of assays which were available at the time and many of these would not be regarded very favourably nowadays, so in discussing new concepts much of the early work will be ignored. The major cyclical changes in the normal menstrual cycle and in the syndrome will be dealt with first and then the possible influence of other hormones and related substances.

Symptoms and Hormonal Disorders

The condition is diagnosed by the use of diary charts on which the patient herself enters the degree and number of symptoms. There are symptoms which can be classified as psychological and others as physical, so that it is possible that the same endocrine abnormality would not occur in all patients. Usually however, both psychological and physical symptoms occur together.

One of the most common complaints is abdominal bloating. Here it might be expected that there is some abnormality of factors controlling salt and water metabolism (see pp. 119–120). Breast pain is also common and here prolactin may be implicated (see also p. 124). Unfortunately it does not appear that anything so clear cut has emerged relating hormonal abnormality to symptom and at present there is no hormone assay which can be claimed to be diagnostic for PMS.

The Normal Menstrual Cycle

Although many observations have been made on hormonal changes in the menstrual cycle very few authors have made clear whether or not their subjects suffered from any premenstrual symptoms. In fact, can some symptoms be classified as normal? One of the characteristics of the syndrome is that symptoms tend to persist for several days together in the last week or ten days of the cycle with almost complete freedom from complaints in the second week of the cycle. In the patients considered to be symptom-free any that do occur tend to be present for only a day or two at a time. In the control subjects included in the study of Watts *et al*. (1985) diary charts indicated considerable freedom from symptoms. Five of twelve subjects complained of a mild degree of lethargy, abdominal bloating, breast discomfort or increased appetite for a day or two premenstrually. Most women to a greater or lesser degree show some fluid retention with ankles swelling in hot weather and on prolonged standing which is rarely seen in men. Physiological fluid retention occurs in pregnancy, lactation and menstruation and the point at which the normal becomes pathological is not sharply defined. A woman can be considered to suffer from PMS when the premenstrual symptoms become so severe that they interfere with her daily life.

So-called normal ranges for hormones measured during the menstrual cycle probably show such large ranges because of the difficulty of defining what is truly normal, symptoms of premenstrual tension being only one set of examples of many possible situations affecting hormone production. Clearly, in trying to define any abnormal hormonal patterns in PMS it is essential to obtain control subjects for comparison who have been extremely well documented.

Hormone Changes in PMS

The day to day variation in some hormones is considerable so that frequent sampling is required. There may also be diurnal and other rhythms and some studies suggest there may even be seasonal variations, although these do not appear to have been investigated in PMS. In addition to these factors most of the reproductive hormones are released episodically, an essential requirement for normal responsiveness at the target cells but nothing has been reported on this important mechanism in PMS.

The severity of symptoms is greatest in the last week of the cycle and therefore many investigators have confined their studies to this time although in some cases PMS may be present throughout the luteal phase. It has been considered that the syndrome involves some factor or factors produced from the corpus luteum. This may be so, but the events of the luteal phase are dependent on those of the follicular phase and on the process of ovulation and it is therefore necessary to investigate hormonal changes throughout the cycle. Defects in the luteal phase may be associated with abnormalities in the development of the pre-ovulatory follicle following inappropriate priming with gonadotrophins in the follicular phase. On the other hand a follicle may develop normally and produce oestrogen but the positive oestrogen feedback on LH release might fail so that the follicle does not rupture, or there may be luteinization without ovulation. Progesterone production will then be deficient in the luteal phase. When ovulation does occur, however, oestrogen and progesterone are produced and the development of large antral follicles is suppressed and only recommences when the secretion of FSH and LH rises following regression of the corpus luteum. If the corpus luteum is enucleated at any stage of the luteal phase, follicular development recommences (Bäckström et al., 1985).

Hormones Showing Cyclical Variations

Hypotheses to explain the endocrinology of PMS have usually implicated the steroid hormones progesterone and oestrogens. Besides arising from the corpus luteum and exerting their well known actions on the endometrium etc., they have effects on salt and water metabolism. Since bloating is a common symptom it was early suggested that this may result from salt and water retention induced by oestrogen. However, there is no clear relationship between the symptom and salt and water retention. O'Brien et al. (1980) studied eighteen patients and ten controls and found that sodium excretion was lowest immediately before ovulation and highest just after ovulation with intermediate values premenstrually in both groups. There were no significant differences between the results of patients and controls in the sodium excretion or the sodium–potassium ratios. Varma (1983) also found no differences in serum concentrations of sodium or potassium in either the follicular or luteal phases of the cycle in 25 patients compared with ten asymptomatic controls.

The theory has been that oestrogens among their many actions, cause retention of sodium and water, whereas progesterone tends to have the reverse effect. A deficiency of progesterone in the luteal phase would therefore favour water retention. In two studies (Bäckström and Carstensen, 1974; Munday, 1977) progesterone concentrations lower than normal were found in some patients but not in all. Others, however, (O'Brien et al., 1979, 1980;

Watts *et al.*, 1985) found higher than normal values for progesterone during the early part of the luteal phase in some patients with PMS. Bäckström and Mattson (1975) attributed more significance to oestrogens. Bäckström *et al.* (1976) and Munday *et al.* (1981) found higher than normal levels of oestrogen in the luteal phase but again others (Andersch *et al.*, 1979; Watts *et al.*, 1985) found no significant differences. However, these steroids cannot be the sole factors as there are patients with severe PMS and relatively high or high-normal progesterone and normal oestrogen levels in the same cycle (Bäckström *et al.*, 1983).

The sodium and water retaining effects of oestrogens are slight and transitory in normal women. They have been summarized by Reid and Yen, (1981). Oestrogens increase the levels of plasma renin substrate (PRS), possibly through enhanced synthesis in the liver and this leads to elevation of plasma renin activity (PRA) and angiotensin II. Increased secretion and excretion of aldosterone results from this, but there is evidence that the sodium retaining effect of oestrogen is independent of its ability to increase aldosterone production. In contrast, progesterone does not increase PRS but it can induce an increase in PRA and aldosterone secretion and excretion. It has been postulated that the sodium excreting effect of progesterone is a blocking effect of aldosterone at the renal tubules, an effect which appears to be independent of changes in the renin–angiotensin–aldosterone axis.

In the normal cycle there appears to be no change in the luteal phase levels of PRS, but there is an increase in renin and aldosterone. As the rise in aldosterone occurs in the absence of a rise in PRS it is likely that progesterone may be involved. In PMS patients however, neither O'Brien *et al.* (1979) nor Munday *et al.* (1981) were able to show any abnormality in aldosterone concentrations.

According to Dunnigan (1983) the commonest factor associated with the onset of fluid retention is weight gain. There is also an association with psychosocial problems and fluid retaining symptoms may follow stress independently of weight gain. This clearly may be relevant to PMS but there is little evidence of true fluid retention in the syndrome. Morning and evening weights were recorded in the study of Watts *et al.* (1985) and although there was a raised level in the evening in some patients compared with controls it was only a small increase averaging about 1.2 lb and the change in weight from the late follicular to the late luteal phase was only 1.5 lb. Faratian *et al.* (1984) likewise found no consistent increase in premenstrual weight, but found that the patients' own perception of body size increased and the discrepancy between perceived and actual body size was significant. The suggestion has been made therefore that bloatedness recorded by nearly all patients might be related to redistribution of fluid into different body compartments in response to an alteration of vascular permeability, resulting in distension without weight increase. Although this may result from a change in angiotensin, experimental work to confirm this is lacking. It is likely that in many patients the feeling of bloatedness is related to the gaseous distension of the bowel and the constipation which they experience.

Watts *et al.* (1985) were able to divide their patients into two groups, A and B. Women in group A (seventeen patients) appeared to ovulate fourteen days or less before the next period, similar to ten out of twelve control subjects without symptoms. The time of ovulation was judged by the LH surge and by ultrasonic scanning of the follicles. Women in group B (eighteen patients) ovulated more than fourteen days before the next period. The gonadal and pituitary hormones attained the same peak levels in both groups (Table 1) but oestradiol reached maximum levels in group B patients two to three days earlier than in group A patients and progesterone began to rise two days earlier. Follicular growth as judged by ultrasound, gave results consistent with these and it was interesting to note that on average the maximum follicular diameter in the patients, whether group A or B, was 2 mm less than in control subjects, tending to suggest that ovulation was premature. Ovulation would be related to the release of LH triggered by the oestrogen positive feedback and it may be therefore that the syndrome is related to some modulation of this feedback sensitivity. In the last week of the cycle Watts *et al.* (1985) found that patients with PMS had significantly higher levels of LH than control subjects and this again suggests some change in feedback sensitivity as

Table 1. Peak values of pituitary and ovarian hormones in PMS patients and control subjects. Although eighteen of the 35 patients ovulated earlier in the cycle than ten of the twelve control subjects there were no differences in these hormone levels. (Data from Watts *et al.*, 1985)

	Peak values (mean and S.E.M.)		
	Oestradiol (pmol l^{-1})	LH (u l^{-1})	Progesterone (nmol l^{-1})
PMS patients			
Group A (n = 17) Ovulation fourteen days or less before next period	896 (77)	46.4 (8.5)	48.4 (3.5)
Group B (n = 18) Ovulation more than fourteen days before next period	964 (73)	38.8 (6.8)	55.8 (2.4)
Control subjects (n = 10) Ovulation fourteen days or less before next period	1023 (87)	48.1 (9.7)	48.8 (3.6)

122   FUNCTIONAL DISORDERS OF THE MENSTRUAL CYCLE

Table 2. LH and oestradiol concentrations in 35 PMS patients and twelve control subjects on days six and two before menstruation. Although the LH values were significantly higher in the PMS patients than in controls the oestradiol values were the same in each group (Data from Watts *et al.*, 1985)

	LH (u l⁻¹) (mean and S.E.M.)		Oestradiol (pmol l⁻¹) (mean and S.E.M.)	
Days before menstruation	6	2	6	2
PMS patients	5.6 (0.5)	5.9 (0.5)	580 (37)	327 (43)
Control subjects	3.5 (0.8)	3.8 (0.6)	583 (49)	363 (38)
Significance (P) of difference PMS vs controls (unpaired t-test)	<0.05	<0.01	NS	NS

NS = not significant.

at this time there were no differences in oestrogen concentrations (Table 2). Added to this Bäckström *et al.* (1976) reported that FSH levels were raised for part of the luteal phase.

There has been considerable discussion as to whether the symptoms would develop in the absence of ovulation but there is not a great deal of firm evidence to provide an answer (see also pp. 57 and 90). In some early publications claims that patients ovulated or did not ovulate were not well supported by satisfactory experimental evidence. Bäckström *et al.* (1983) however, reported three women with anovular cycles in a group of 22 with severe symptoms. In the anovulatory cycles the women complained of some breast tenderness and bloating premenstrually, but there was no cyclical change in mood. Some methods of treatment for this condition inhibit ovulation while relieving symptoms but whether this relief is related to the anovulation or to another effect of the drugs used is difficult to assess. Thus the anti-gonadotrophic drug danazol is of some benefit but at effective doses it usually inhibits ovulation. Long-acting analogues of gonadotrophin releasing hormone (GnRH) also alleviate the symptoms of PMS while inhibiting ovulation. Muse *et al.* (1984) found that by one month of treatment with such an analogue, ovulation was inhibited and symptom scores were reduced considerably to the low levels associated with the follicular phase. Bancroft and Bäckström (1985) reported that in the initial phase of treatment when the analogue is stimulatory the symptoms may be aggravated if given in the luteal phase and produce the symptoms if given in the follicular. This offers an example therefore of symptoms occurring without ovulation.

Hammarbäck *et al*. (1983) noted premenstrual symptoms of mood changes and some physical changes in postmenopausal women given cyclical oestrogen–progestogen treatment. The symptoms appeared only when a progestogen was added to oestrogen giving evidence that hormonal changes without ovulation may lead to symptoms.

Consideration of the steroid patterns in PMS itself and in the various treatment cycles leads to the conclusion that symptoms occur when oestrogen concentrations are changing rapidly, progesterone augmenting this effect. When oestrogen concentrations are stabilized by suppression with danazol or GnRH analogue, or as Magos and Studd (1985) have reported, by giving oestradiol implants with cyclical progestogen, symptoms are controlled.

Another important property of the gonadal steroids is their influence on mood, affective state and behaviour related to reproduction mediated through nerve cells, particularly in the hypothalamus (Pfaff and McEwen, 1983). There are specific receptor-like macromolecules in the soluble fraction of the target tissue which bind the steroid and carry it to the cell nucleus. Oestrogens and progesterone interact with receptors and trigger messenger RNA formation and in turn the synthesis of specific proteins. Oestrogens increase the number of progesterone receptors in the ventromedial nuclei and this could be the reason for the synergistic action between these two steroids affecting several endocrine and behavioural phenomena. In this way the steroids alter nerve cell electrical activity shown by alterations in discharge rates of hypothalamic neurones which has been demonstrated to occur in the oestrous cycle of rats. Elevation of electrical activity of arcuate nucleus neurones in the hypothalamus has been found to correlate with ovulation.

Follicular Fluid Factors

Several interesting materials have been recognized in follicular fluid, one of the most important being the glycoprotein, inhibin (Tsonis *et al*., 1986). As follicles grow, production of inhibin increases in parallel with oestrogen and it has also been recognized in lower concentrations in fluid taken from follicles in the luteal phase of the cycle (Tanabe *et al*., 1983). Progesterone tends to suppress the secretion of inhibin and Marrs *et al*. (1984) while finding a positive correlation between inhibin and oestrogens or androgens found a negative correlation with progesterone. The biological effect of inhibin is a specific suppression of FSH secretion and it is therefore one of the factors preventing the growth of multiple follicles in the human. There are no observations of inhibin concentrations in PMS yet available: as there is no evidence that women with PMS have an increased incidence of multiple pregnancies it seems unlikely that secretion of inhibin or other follicular fluid factors is abnormal in the follicular phase. Changes in progesterone secretion premenstrually, however, may lead to recognizable changes in inhibin secretion which would be worth investigating.

Other Hormones

Prolactin

There has been interest in the possibility that prolactin is involved in PMS. It would not be surprising to find somewhat elevated levels of prolactin in patients undergoing the stress of PMS and it might also help to explain the common symptom of breast discomfort. However, most up to date studies have failed to detect any gross abnormalities (O'Brien and Symonds, 1982; Steiner et al., 1984; Watts et al., 1985). True hyperprolactinaemia would lead to amenorrhoea as the prolactin interferes with the positive feedback of oestrogens on gonadotrophin release (Glass et al., 1976) and by definition, amenorrhoea could not be associated with the syndrome. Prolactin itself cannot be considered to be the direct cause since hyperprolactinaemic women are not noted for having any of the symptoms associated with PMS.

Horrobin (1979) has suggested that an alternative explanation may be that in PMS there is an excessive sensitivity to normal levels of prolactin and possibly other hormones. This may result from a deficiency of essential fatty acids, including prostaglandin precursors, leading to low levels of prostaglandin E_1, a suggestion that has been followed up in the work of Brush et al. (1984). Levels of linoleic acid, the main dietary n-6 essential fatty acid, were above normal, indicating no deficit of intake or absorption. Concentrations of metabolites of linoleic acid however were reduced, possibly because of a defect in the conversion of linoleic to γ-linolenic acid. Since this abnormality was present in both follicular and luteal phases, it cannot be the direct cause of the luteal phase symptoms, but it may still be a mechanism whereby tissues are sensitized so that they respond abnormally to normal levels of reproductive hormones probably through an effect of a prostaglandin.

Cortisol

Cortisol is another hormone which may be affected by the stress of PMS. There seems to be little information available on the levels in this syndrome however. There is no cyclical variation and corticosteroids do not play an important part in treatment. Watts et al. (1985) measured cortisol concentrations in 35 patients and found that results were within the normal range but were uniformly higher than in twelve control subjects without symptoms. Interestingly the observations were made from a time in the cycle before symptoms had developed and prolactin measurements at the same time showed no significant changes. These observations were extended to include measurements of cortisol in saliva. Because of diurnal variations samples were collected several times during the day and throughout the cycle. Significant differences between patients with symptoms and control subjects were noted only in the evening samples premenstrually when symptoms were most severe and then the levels were higher in the patients. The most obvious explanation for these results is that in serum the slightly elevated levels in patients were related to the stress of travelling to the hospital and having venepunctures, whereas the control subjects were hospital staff already at their place of duty for some time before venepuncture. When patients were able to collect saliva at home this stress was avoided and changes occurred only when related to the stress of the symptoms. This suggests that any changes in cortisol are most likely to be the results of the syndrome rather than a cause.

Androgens

No abnormalities of androgenic steroids have been recorded in PMS. It has generally been considered that elevated levels of androgen affect the normal menstrual cycle. In polycystic ovarian disease where hirsutism frequently occurs, anovulation is a common feature. Dewis *et al*. (1986) have recently investigated this point by measuring hormone changes in six women given 100 mg implants of testosterone. Five of the subjects chosen suffered from PMS with symptoms including loss of libido, and they had failed to respond to other therapy. Elevated levels of testosterone were achieved but in two months' trial there were no significant changes in FSH, LH, prolactin, oestradiol or progesterone and no alteration in cycle length. This study did not support the view that elevated testosterone led to menstrual disturbances but the patients reported some relief of symptoms and a further trial is planned.

Increased levels of testosterone reduce sex hormone binding globulin (SHBG) binding capacity and such a change has been implicated in PMS and would be important as oestrogens bind to the same protein. With a fall in SHBG it would be expected that the biologically active free oestrogen fraction would increase and disturb the balance between oestrogen and progesterone, particularly at the end of the cycle. There is one study in which low SHBG capacity was reported in PMS (Dalton, 1981) and a similar trend has emerged in a study of the direct measurement of SHBG by radioimmuno-assay (Payne *et al*., 1987).

Prostaglandins

Increased synthesis and release of prostaglandins occurs in the luteal phase and during menstruation. These compounds have diverse actions and many of the symptoms of PMS could be attributed to the effects of prostaglandins (Craig, 1980). They have a depressive action on behaviour and affect motor function and body temperature and modulate the release of neurotransmitters. Prostaglandins of the E series facilitate pain induced by various stimuli by sensitizing pain receptors, and these may be involved in premenstrual pain and headache. Aspirin-like compounds achieve their analgesic effect by inhibiting prostaglandin synthesis and some encouraging preliminary results were obtained in the treatment of PMS using the prostaglandin synthetase inhibitor mefenamic acid (Jakubowitz, 1983). On the other hand some therapeutic value of evening primrose oil (Efamol), a source of γ-linolenic acid and a prostaglandin precursor, has been reported (Brush, 1983). Synthesis of γ-linolenic acid from dietary *cis*-linoleic acid is rather inefficient so that in some situations γ-linolenic acid and therefore prostaglandin E_1 may be deficient.

Prostaglandin $F_{2\alpha}$ has convulsant properties at pharmacological doses so that indirectly the sex steroids may be involved in the cyclical exacerbations of epilepsy which has been observed in some patients. Peaks in the concentrations of this prostaglandin have been found to occur premenstrually secondary to endometrial synthesis.

In general the determination of prostaglandins in blood is not entirely satisfactory because of rapid metabolism and the production of artefacts. Reliable results therefore are few. In the study of Jakubowitz *et al.* (1984) there was some evidence that concentrations of prostaglandins E_2, F_2 and FM were low in PMS. There was no direct evidence for raised PGE_1 to account for the beneficial effects of mefenamic acid. Furthermore Abraham (1983) postulated that some symptoms were caused by PGE_1 deficiency providing a reason for the use of a precursor such as evening primrose oil.

Endogenous Opioids

The hypothesis that endogenous opioids and related compounds may be involved at some stage in the aetiology of PMS seems reasonable (Halbreich and Endicott, 1981; Reid and Yen, 1981). The endogenous opioids are known to arise from three precursors which are produced in separate neural systems: all three are found in the hypothalamus. They are pro-opiomelanocortin producing β-endorphin, pro-enkephalin producing methionine- and leucine-enkephalins and pro-dynorphin which gives dynorphin and neo-dynorphins. The pro-opiomelanocortin neurones are localized in the arcuate nucleus and tuberal regions with extensive processes to other hypothalamic and extra-hypothalamic sites, pro-enkephalin neurones are widely distributed in the brain and pro-dynorphin neurones in several brain areas, in the hypothalamus being restricted to the supra optic, paraventricular and accessory hypothalamoneurophysial cell groups.

Each family of opioid shows some selectively for binding to various receptors, thus enkephalins may act as endogenous ligands for δ receptors, dynorphin and α-neo-endorphin for the κ receptor and β-endorphin for μ and also δ receptors. Direct experimental evidence that the endogenous opioids are in any way abnormal in the syndrome is lacking and the hypothesis rests on the known consequences of their under- or over-secretion and on the withdrawal of opioids.

The effects of gonadal steroids on opioids are now well established. Wardlaw *et al.* (1982) examined the effects on β-endorphin in hypophysial portal blood of female monkeys. In ovariectomized animals β-endorphin was undetectable even after the administration of 2 μg oestradiol. After oestrogen replacement for two to three weeks however, β-endorphin was detectable in portal blood in two of four animals. When the animals received oestradiol and progesterone replacement to mimic the normal cycle however, high levels of β-endorphin were detected in each of the four animals, the mean concentration being more than ten times higher than before replacement. Ovarian steroids are thought to affect not only opioids but oxytocin, vasopressin, serotonin and noradrenaline and these are involved in modulating mood behaviour and motor co-ordination.

Some of the reasons why it has been considered that endogenous opioids may be involved in the aetiology of PMS are:

1. It is known that β-endorphin secretion increases in pregnancy as does oestrogen. After delivery oestrogen concentrations fall dramatically and some of the symptoms of post partum depression resemble those of PMS. These include depressed mood, lethargy, anxiety and tearfulness.
2. Halbreich and Endicott (1981) produced some evidence, although on small numbers of experiments, that administration of β-endorphin affects mood and pain perception. Much research has centred on the relation of endogenous opioids to pain: pain relief induced through electro-acupuncture may be mediated through the release of endogenous opioids and other compounds such as serotonin and the analgesia is readily blocked by the opiate antagonist naloxone. Elevated levels of endogenous opioids may lead to increased agitation and anxiety and pain perception may be altered.
3. Opioids affect certain neuronal activities such as an interaction with dopamine pathways. Met-enkephalin has been reported to elevate the rate of synthesis and turnover of dopamine and its metabolites and other neurotransmitters including noradrenaline and serotonin may also be affected. Decreased serotonin levels have been related to increased depression, irritability, pain sensitivity and changes in libido. It has been noted that pyridoxine, in the form of pyridoxal-5-phosphate is a co-factor in two key pathways leading to the production of dopamine and serotonin

(Brush, 1979). Pyridoxine is widely used to relieve PMS and depression in some women taking oral contraceptives may be related to a lack of pyridoxine: Adams *et al*. (1973) showed that pyridoxine was beneficial in comparison with placebo in relieving this condition. Deficient synthesis of dopamine however, would be associated with increased secretion of prolactin and most women with PMS have normal prolactin secretion. Likewise, although serotonin levels are affected by oestrogen and progesterone (Janowsky and Rausch, 1985) any effects produced would be similar to those in the normal cycle.

4. Opioids affect glucose metabolism and it is known that morphine can cause hyperglycaemia. These compounds therefore influence appetite and thirst.

5. Immunocytochemical studies have been used to show that oxytocin neurones and secretory terminals contain immunoreactive enkephalins whilst vasopressin neurones and terminals contain immunoreactive dynorphin. In contrast to the indirect action of opioids on gonadotrophin secretion, the inhibition of release of vasopressin and oxytocin by opioids is directly on the neurohypophysial neurones. The effect of opiates such as morphine on the inhibition of oxytocin secretion and subsequent milk ejection is well known. The physiological roles of oxytocin outside of lactation or parturition are not clear, however. The modulation of the release of vasopressin, however, may not only be important with regard to fluid balance, but may also modulate anterior pituitary function and affect memory processes.

The withdrawal effects of opiates may be important. Activation of presynaptic receptors by opiates decreases cell firing rate producing a 'disuse hypersensitivity' and tolerance develops. When opiates are withdrawn resumed sensitivity leads to temporary overactivity resulting in the withdrawal symptoms. The decreased neurotransmission of biogenic amines has been implicated in the pathogenesis of depression, while excessive activity has been linked to irritability and aggression. These features are common in acute opiate withdrawal and vary in intensity depending on the duration of exposure and the rapidity of withdrawal. Halbreich and Endicott (1981) have hypothesized that premenstrual decrease of opioids, presumably related to falling oestrogen levels, may be involved in the pathophysiology of 'atypical depressive' PMS, i.e. depressed mood, loss of interest, increased appetite and libido change, while the disordered regulation of opioids may be involved in anxiety and agitation. Likewise Reid and Yen (1981) consider that disordered release of, or sensitivity to, β-endorphin and maybe other peptides such as α-MSH during the luteal phase may be the central event which triggers a series of neuroendocrine changes leading to the symptoms. Opioid-induced inhibition of central biogenic amine systems may produce mood changes, increased appetite and thirst. Breast pain, fluid retention and bloating could possibly be related to opioid induced changes in prolactin and vasopressin and they may also inhibit prostaglandin E in the bowel. Withdrawal would afford some relief but may trigger other symptoms such as irritability and aggression.

Bancroft and Bäckström (1985) have considered these theories and drew attention to the complicated interactions between the various factors. They outlined a so-called 'system model' considering that symptoms such as mood changes are centrally determined, whereas others such as breast pain and bloating result from differing sensitivities to ovarian feedbacks.

In the absence of direct evidence to support these hypotheses it seems likely that different sensitivity at receptor levels is involved as presumably endorphin and related compounds exhibit similar changes in symptomless cycles. Direct measurements in the peripheral circulation of endogenous opioids is difficult and is unlikely to be of much help in assessing activities at the hypothalamic or other levels. Chuong et al. (1985) however, have recently attempted to measure β-endorphin serum levels in 20 women with PMS and the results appeared to be lower premenstrually than in controls. Another approach is to observe any of the established effects of endorphins on the release of pituitary hormones, notably the negative influence of opioids on LH release. Opioids do not act directly on the pituitary to affect the secretion of gonadotrophins and this gland contains very few opioid receptors. Instead they act at the level of the hypothalamus preventing secretion of GnRH from the median eminence. Effects on GnRH are probably indirect and mediated through opioid interaction with monoaminergic neurones. Bicknell (1985) has proposed that the activity of GnRH cell bodies in the pre-optic-anterior hypothalamic region is excited or facilitated by noradrenaline or adrenaline released from neuroterminals of the ventral noradrenergic tract. Secretory output from these terminals is inhibited by opioid peptides. There may also be inhibition of GnRH released directly in the median eminence or through inhibition of dopamine. Furthermore gonadal steroids may regulate GnRH output by acting on both monoamine and opioid neurones. Most clinical evidence for the effect of opioids on LH secretion has come from the use of the opioid antagonist naloxone. This drug stimulates LH release if given during the late follicular or luteal phases of the cycle, the effect being modulated by oestrogen levels.

Thus it seems likely that endogenous opioids are involved in the regulation of LH secretion during the phases of the menstrual cycle when oestrogen or oestrogen and progesterone are raised (Quigley and Yen, 1980). The premature release of LH in some patients with PMS demonstrated by Watts et al. (1985) may reflect therefore deficient opioid levels, or changes in feedback sensitivity. In the last six days of the luteal phase in this series of patients there was also a slightly increased release of LH compared to control subjects, again fitting in with the theory of decreased opioid activity. If this is so it must be

Table 3. Major endocrine changes and controlling mechanisms in the menstrual cycle and observations on these in PMS

Major hormones	Controlling mechanisms	Observations in PMS
Follicular phase Episodic release of gonadotrophins	Pulsatile release of GnRH from hypothalamus influenced by oestrogen and other hormones including catecholamines, vasopressin, endogenous opioids and related compounds.	FSH, LH, prolactin and androgens normal. No observations on opioids, catecholamines, inhibin.
Follicular fluid factors including Inhibin Oestrogens	Inhibition of FSH secretion by inhibin. Negative feedback of oestrogens on gonadotrophin secretion.	
Ovulation phase Surge of LH and FSH	Oestrogen (with progesterone) positive feedback at hypothalamus and pituitary. Effect modulated by prolactin, endogenous opioids, dopamine, serotonin, catecholamines, prostaglandins.	Tendency for early release of gonadotrophins. (? Altered feedback sensitivity. ? Lack of opioids). Slight decrease in conversion of linoleic acid to γ-linolenic acid possibly leading to prostaglandin defect.
Luteal phase Progesterone and oestrogen production	Tonic secretion of LH at low pulse rate to maintain corpus luteum. Oestrogen and progesterone control of gonadotrophin secretion so that large antral follicles do not develop. Inhibin secretion affected by oestrogen (positive effect) and progesterone (negative effect). Regression of corpus luteum accompanied by decreasing oestrogen and progesterone and opioid secretion leading to release of gonadotrophin which stimulates follicles for the next cycle.	Slightly raised gonadotrophin secretion in last week of cycle. (? Lack of opioids. ? Altered feedback sensitivity). No observations reported on opioids, inhibin etc.

assumed that endogenous opioids are low at a time in the cycle well before symptoms develop as well as premenstrually, and it must be supposed that other factors are involved to explain why symptoms should appear only in the second half of the cycle.

From all the evidence it is clear that no one mechanism explains all the manifestations of the syndrome. Further research into the relationships between endogenous opioids and other compounds with neurotransmitters and the bearing on symptoms will hopefully lead to a better understanding of the different forms of the syndrome.

Conclusions

There appear to be no gross hormonal abnormalities in women with PMS. Hormone concentrations in serum are within the range found in women without symptoms and probably the falling concentrations of oestrogens which occur premenstrually are more important as many other biologically interesting substances are affected. Some of the major hormones involved in the menstrual cycle are listed in Table 3 with comments on the various mechanisms by which these hormones are controlled. These relationships are sometimes complicated and finely adjusted and in addition variable sensitivity at target sites may be involved in the syndrome. The regression of the corpus luteum in the last week of the cycle and the falling concentrations of progesterone and oestrogen are accompanied by altered secretion of endogenous opioids, inhibin and prostaglandins. Although there are as yet no direct biochemical observations on many of these compounds, the possibility that some are involved in the syndrome, particularly those like the opioids which have biological effects which relate to the symptoms of PMS, is an attractive concept.

References

Abraham, G. E. (1983). Nutritional factors in the etiology of the premenstrual tension syndromes. *Journal of Reproductive Medicine*, **28**, 446–464.

Adams, P. W., Rose, D. P., Folkard, J., Wynn, V., Seed, M. and Strong, R. (1973). Effect of pyridoxine hydrochloride (vitamin B_6) upon depression associated with oral contraception. *Lancet*, **2**, 897–904.

Andersch, B., Abrahamsson, L., Wenderstam, C., Ohman, R. and Kahn, L. (1979). Hormone profile in premenstrual tension: effects of bromocriptine and diuretics. *Clinical Endocrinology*, **11**, 657–664.

Bäckström, T. and Carstensen, H. (1974). Estrogen and progesterone in plasma in relation to premenstrual tension. *Journal of Steroid Biochemistry*, **5**, 257–260.

Bäckström, T. and Mattson, B. (1975). Correlation of symptoms in premenstrual tension to oestrogen and progesterone concentrations in blood plasma: a preliminary study. *Neuropsychobiology*, **1**, 80–86.

Bäckström, T., Sanders, D., Leask, R., Davidson, D., Warner, P. and Bancroft, J.

(1983). Mood, sexuality, hormones and the menstrual cycle II. Hormone levels and their relationship to premenstrual syndrome. *Psychosomatic Medicine*, 45, 503–507.

Bäckström, T., Smith, S., Lothian, H. and Baird, D. T. (1985). Prolonged follicular phase and depressed gonadotrophins following hysterectomy and corpus lutectomy in women with premenstrual tension syndrome. *Clinical Endocrinology*, 22, 723–732.

Bäckström, T., Wide, L., Södergard, R. and Carstensen, H. (1976). FSH, LH, TeBG-capacity, estrogen and progesterone in women with premenstrual tension during the luteal phase. *Journal of Steroid Biochemistry*, 7, 473–476.

Bancroft, J. and Bäckström, T. (1985). Premenstrual syndrome. *Clinical Endocrinology*, 22, 313–336.

Bicknell, R. J. (1985). Endogenous opioid peptides and hypothalamic neuroendocrine neurones. *Journal of Endocrinology*, 107, 437–446.

Brush, M. G. (1979). Endocrine and other biochemical factors in the aetiology of the premenstrual syndrome. *Current Medical Research and Opinion*, 6 (Supplement 5), 19–27.

Brush, M. G. (1983). The significance of pyridoxine and gamma-linolenic acid to premenstrual syndrome, in *Premenstrual Syndrome*, (Ed. R. W. Taylor) Medical News-Tribune Ltd, London, pp. 57–59.

Brush, M. G., Watson, S. J., Horrobin, D. F. and Manku, M. S. (1984). Abnormal essential fatty acid levels in plasma of women with premenstrual tension. *American Journal of Obstetrics and Gynecology*, 150, 363–366.

Chuong, C. J., Coulam, C. B., Kao, P. C., Bergstralh, E. J. and Go, V. L. W. (1985). Neuropeptide levels in premenstrual syndrome. *Fertility and Sterility*, 44, 760–765.

Craig, G. M. (1980). The premenstrual syndrome and prostaglandin metabolism. *British Journal of Family Planning*, 6, 74–77.

Dalton, M. E. (1981). Sex hormone-binding globulin concentrations in women with severe premenstrual syndrome. *Postgraduate Medical Journal*, 57, 560–561.

Dewis, P., Newman, M., Ratcliffe, W. A. and Anderson, D. C. (1986). Does testosterone affect the normal menstrual cycle? *Clinical Endocrinology*, 24, 515–521.

Dunnigan, M. G. (1983). The recognition and management of the fluid retention syndrome of women, in *Premenstrual Syndrome* (Ed. R. W. Taylor) Medical News-Tribune Ltd, London, pp. 25–32.

Feratian, B., Gaspar, A., O'Brien, P. M. S., Johnson, I. R., Filshie, G. M. and Prescott, P. (1984). Premenstrual syndrome: weight, abdominal swelling and perceived body image. *American Journal of Obstetrics and Gynecology*, 150, 200–204.

Glass, M. R., Shaw, R. W., Williams, J. W., Butt, W. R., Logan Edwards, R. and London, D. R. (1976). The control of gonadotrophin release in women with hyperprolactinaemic amenorrhoea: effect of oestrogen and progesterone on the LH and FSH response to LHRH. *Clinical Endocrinology*, 5, 521–530.

Halbreich, U. and Endicott, J. (1981). Possible involvement of endorphin withdrawal or imbalance in specific premenstrual syndromes and post-partum depression. *Medical Hypotheses*, 7, 1045–1058.

Hammarbäck, S., Bäckström, T., Holst, J. and von Schoultz, B. (1983). PMS mood changes in menopause. *Acta Obstetrica et Gynecologica Scandinavica*, Supplement 116, Abstract 104.

Horrobin, D. F. (1979). Cellular basis of prolactin action: involvement of cyclic nucleotides, polyamines, prostaglandins, steroids, thyroid hormones, Na/KATPases and calcium: relevance to breast cancer and the menstrual cycle. *Medical Hypotheses*, 5, 599–620.

Jakubowitz, D. L. (1983). The significance of prostaglandins in the premenstrual syndrome, in *Premenstrual Syndrome*, (Ed. R. W. Taylor) Medical News-Tribune Ltd, London, pp. 50–56.

Jakubowitz, D. L., Godard, E. and Dewhurst, J. (1984). The treatment of premenstrual tension with mefenamic acid: analysis of prostaglandin concentration. *British Journal of Obstetrics and Gynaecology*, **91**, 78–87.

Janowsky, D. S. and Rausch, J. (1985). Biochemical hypotheses of premenstrual tension syndrome. *Psychological Medicine*, **15**, 3–8.

Magos, A. and Studd, J. (1985). Effects of the menstrual cycle on medical disorders. *British Journal of Hospital Medicine*, 68–77.

Marrs, R. P., Lobo, R., Campeau, J. D., Nakamura, R. M., Brown, J., Ujita, E. L. and DiZerega, G. S. (1984). Correlation of human follicular fluid inhibin activity with spontaneous and induced follicle maturation. *Journal of Clinical Endocrinology and Metabolism*, **58**, 704–709.

Munday, M. (1977). Hormone levels in severe premenstrual tension. *Current Medical Research and Opinion*, 4, **Supplement 4**, 16–22.

Munday, M. R., Brush, M. G. and Taylor, R. W. (1981). Correlation between progesterone, oestradiol and aldosterone levels in the premenstrual syndrome. *Clinical Endocrinology*, **14**, 1–9.

Muse, K. N., Cetel, N. S., Futterman, L. A. and Yen, S. S. C. (1984). The premenstrual syndrome. Effects of 'medical ovariectomy'. *New England Journal of Medicine*, **311**, 1345–1349.

O'Brien, P. M. S., Craven, D., Selby, C. and Symonds, E. M. (1979). Treatment of premenstrual syndrome by spironolactone. *British Journal of Obstetrics and Gynaecology*, **86**, 142–147.

O'Brien, P. M. S., Selby, C. and Symonds, E. M. (1980). Progesterone, fluid and electrolytes in premenstrual syndrome. *British Medical Journal*, **280**, 1161–1163.

O'Brien, P. M. S. and Symonds, E. M. (1982). Prolactin levels in the premenstrual syndrome. *British Journal of Obstetrics and Gynaecology*, **89**, 306–308.

Payne, E., Thomas, P. and Rudd, B. (1987). Effect of danazol on SHBG and hormonal profiles in women with premenstrual syndrome, (in preparation).

Pfaff, D. W. and McEwen, B. S. (1983). Actions of estrogens and progestins on nerve cells. *Science*, **219**, 808–814.

Quigley, M. E. and Yen, S. S. C. (1980). The role of endogenous opiates on LH secretion during the menstrual cycle. *Journal of Clinical Endocrinology and Metabolism*, **51**, 179–181.

Reid, R. L. and Yen, S. S. C. (1981). Premenstrual syndrome. *American Journal of Obstetrics and Gynecology*, **139**, 85–104.

Steiner, M., Haskett, R. F., Carroll, B. J., Hays, S. E. and Rubin, R. T. (1984). Circadian hormone secretory profiles in women with severe PMT syndrome. *British Journal of Obstetrics and Gynaecology*, **91**, 466–471.

Tanabe, K., Gagliano, P., Channing, C. P., Nakamura, Y., Yoshimura, Y., Iizuka, R., Fortuny, A., Sulewski, J. and Rezai, N. (1983). Levels of inhibin-F activity and steroids in human follicular fluid from normal women and women with PCO-disease. *Journal of Clinical Endocrinology and Metabolism*, **57**, 24–31.

Tsonis, C. G., McNeilly, A. S. and Baird, D. T. (1986). Measurement of exogenous and endogenous inhibin in sheep serum using a new and extremely sensitive bioassay for inhibin based on inhibition of ovine pituitary FSH secretion *in vitro*. *Journal of Endocrinology*, **110**, 341–352.

Varma, T. R. (1983). Hormones and electrolytes in premenstrual syndrome, in

Premenstrual Syndrome, (Ed. R. W. Taylor) Medical News-Tribune Ltd, London, pp. 60–63.

Wardlaw, S. L., Wehrenberg, W. B., Ferin, M., Antunes, J. L. and Frantz, A. G. (1982). Effect of sex steroids on β-endorphin in hypophyseal portal blood. *Journal of Clinical Endocrinology and Metabolism*, **55**, 877–881.

Watts, J. Ff., Butt, W. R., Logan Edwards, R. and Holder, G. (1985). Hormonal studies in women with premenstrual tension. *British Journal of Obstetrics and Gynaecology*, **92**, 247–255.

Functional Disorders of the Menstrual Cycle
Edited by M. G. Brush and E. M. Goudsmit
© 1988 John Wiley & Sons Ltd

CHAPTER 9

Inter-relationships between the environment and premenstrual syndrome

WILLIAM J. REA

Environmental Health Center,
8345 Walnut Hill Lane,
Suite 205
Dallas, Texas 75231,
USA

Introduction

The suggestion that there could be environmental aspects of premenstrual syndrome (PMS) occurred during observations of hundreds of patients with environmentally triggered vascular disease studied in an ultra-controlled environment. It became clear that many women had a history and subsequent course which included PMS.

The PMS symptoms in many of these patients responded favourably to dietary and environmental manipulation including removal of incitants found as a result of inhaled challenge reactions to ambient doses of <0.50 ppm phenol, <0.002 ppm formaldehyde, <0.33 ppm chlorine, <0.5 ppm petroleum alcohol, and <0.0034 ppm pesticide (2-4-DNP). These same patients were found to have numerous organochlorine pesticides and volatile organic hydrocarbons in their blood. (See Figure 1 and Table 1.)

In addition animal studies have shown alterations of hormones on exposure to similar toxic chemicals (Rattner *et al.*, 1984). For example monkeys fed a diet with pesticide levels similar to those in the average human diet had abnormal variations in their oestrogen and progesterone levels with irregularities in their menstrual cycles (Hinsdill and Thomas, 1978). These were the first symptoms along with periorbital oedema.

A programme was then devised to systematically evaluate PMS patients on an out-patient basis to see if manipulation of specific environmental incitants could trigger the syndrome. From there a practical approach with subsequent

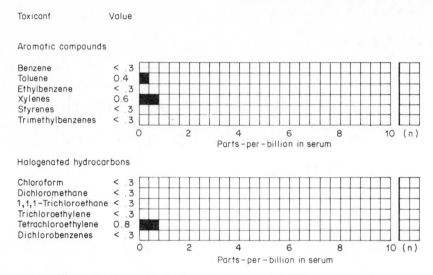

Figure 1. General volatile screening test (GVST)—an example

removal of incitants was developed thus allowing relief. This involved the development and intake of less polluted air, water, vitamins, minerals, and hormones. The over-all approach will be discussed in this chapter by considering various aspects:

1. Principles.
2. Pollution data with scientific basis of studies in Environmental Control Unit.
3. Applicability to PMS.
4. Ways the environment including nutrition could be manipulated in order to help patients with PMS.

Principles

In order to effectively diagnose and treat the environmental aspects of different disease including PMS, it is necessary to understand the following basic principles.

Total Body Burden

Total body load or burden can be defined as the total of all the pollutants that the body takes in and has to handle in order to maintain homeostasis (see Rea, 1980). The pollutants may be biological (pollens, dusts, parasites,

Table 1. Chlorinated pesticide screening test (CPST)—an example

Compound	Results (ng ml^{-1} ppb)	Frequency per 100	Arithmetic mean
Aldrin	<0.1	5.0	<0.1
Dieldrin	<0.1	61.9	0.2
α-BHC	<0.1	9.8	<0.1
β-BHC	<0.1	67.9	0.8
γ-BHC	<0.1	2.2	<0.1
δ-BHC	<0.1	0.3	<0.1
DDT	<0.1	46.3	0.2
DDE	<0.1	98.2	4.2
DDD	<0.1	1.7	<0.1
α-Chlordane	<0.1	0.7	<0.1
γ-Chlordane	<0.1	1.1	<0.1
Heptachlor	<0.1	0.5	<0.1
Heptachlor epoxide	<0.1	80.8	0.6
trans-Nonachlor	<0.1	83.3	0.2
Endosulphan I	<0.1	6.3	<0.1
Endosulphan II	<0.1	0.7	<0.1
HCB	<0.1	94.9	0.5
Endrin	<0.1	2.3	<0.1

Variability factor ± 19.86 per cent calculated from a control level of 0.02 ppb.
Note: Any level other than zero is abnormal. These compounds are foreign and serve no beneficial function to the body. In certain medical or legal instances serial testing may be advisable.

viruses, bacteria), chemical (organic or inorganic), or physical pollutants (heat, cold, electromagnetic radiation, radon, positive and negative ions, noise, light, weather changes) (see Rea and Brown, 1986 for more detailed discussion). In order to prevent disease, the body must deal with this burden by either utilization or elimination. If the load is excessive, premenstrual symptoms may occur and not be cleared until the load is reduced.

This principle has been well documented and commonly understood in relation to bacteria and body function. The case of infectious agents of childbed fever is an excellent example of increased total bacterial load. Institution of sterile techniques reduced the total bacterial load resulting in a decrease in maternal mortality. Reduction of bacterial load is practised in nearly every facet of modern civilization. Attempts are made to free most indoor environments of agents which are known to foster infectious diseases including dust, garbage, vermin, human and animal excrement.

No physician today would consider treating a wound with antibiotics alone. He would first eliminate the overload of bacteria present by vigorously cleansing the wound, and applying a sterile bandage thus reducing the total body burden. In fact, zealous attempts to eliminate infectious agents have inadvertently increased exposure to toxic chemical agents through the use of phenol, chlorine, formaldehyde, and various organic solvents for cleaning purposes.

The control of non-infectious pollutants has not been as successful as control of infectious agents. Overall levels of inhalation of sulphur dioxide from car exhausts or refineries, formaldehyde fumes from new clothes, and exposures to radon or electromagnetic fields increase markedly though individual variation due to personal and geographical factors is considerable. As accumulations of pollutants increase, total body burden increases. The accumulation of total body load encompasses two phenomena: (a) sudden massive exposures and (b) gradual toxic build-up of commonly occurring biological, chemical, and/or physical incitants. An acute exposure can be due to a physical trauma such as a car accident or to a toxic injury such as an acute pesticide exposure, or to a massive viral or bacterial exposure. Subtoxic doses of substances may be involved including such common things as pollens, dusts, moulds, water contaminants, food, food contaminants, inhaled ambient doses of chemicals (Rinkel, et al., 1951; Randolph, 1962; Miller, 1972; Dickey, 1976; Speer, 1977), electromagnetic radiation, and positive air ions, or electrical field changes (Becker and Marino, 1982). Additionally, subtoxic doses of multiple different agents acting in synergism or additive fashion can cause insults producing injury resulting in increased sensitivity to small doses of the aforementioned agents.

The total body load or burden tends to disturb many of the body's mechanisms, often becoming too great for persons with hereditary or acquired limitation to handle. Consequently, an individual susceptibility occurs with resulting generalized inflammatory disease or a change in one end-organ as Nadal and Lee (1977), Matsumura et al. (1972) and Lee et al. (1977) showed with nitrogen dioxide, sulphur dioxide or ozone over-exposure resulting in damage to the bronchial mucosa. This was also shown to occur with oral ingestion of foods containing pesticides with resultant disturbances of oestrogen and progesterone levels (Hinsdill and Thomas, 1978).

Masking or Adaptation or Acute Toxicological Tolerance

Masking (Rinkel *et al.*, 1951) or adaptation (Selye, 1946) or acute toxicological tolerance (Stokinger, 1965; Mustafa and Tierney, 1978) is a change in the homeostasis induced by the internal or external environment followed by accommodation of body function to a new set point. Adaptation is an acute survival mechanism in which the individual apparently 'gets used to' a constant acute toxic exposure in order to initially survive while paying the price of a long term decrease in efficient functioning and perhaps longevity. Because of this phenomenon, the total body load may increase unknown to an individual. At this point, the toxic substance then appears to no longer bother her. Even though there are no apparent correlated symptoms, repeated exposures continue to damage her immune and enzyme detoxification systems. The eventual result often is end-organ failure. This may account for the 20–30 year delay of the onset of vascular and pulmonary diseases before end-organ failure manifests itself. The hormone disturbance of PMS will occur with much less delay. Specific avoidance of the inciting substances for four days, will unmask symptoms and allows for their scientific reproduction. After the unmasking, re-exposure will result in an immediate and clearly definable reaction; cause and effect are now easily distinguishable. Failure to unmask for at least four days often results in negative challenge reactions.

The effects of this process can be readily observed in daily practice. Sensitivities are often missed because offending foods are eaten or harmful substances are breathed daily resulting in masking. In the masked state, challenge tests are frequently negative due to the increased activity of the already induced immune and enzyme detoxification systems. Because of the masking of symptoms, a person can no longer perceive the harmful effects of a substance and she believes herself to be 'healthy' until the next stage of disease occurs. The initial signs and symptoms of vascular and gynaecological disease are often obscured due to these masking effects. The acute survival mechanisms involved in bringing the body back to a steady state certainly sustain life, but only on a shortened and less efficient functioning basis. The dysfunction associated with PMS certainly falls into the latter category. Adaptation has been characterized in three stages: alarm, adaptation, and exhaustion (Selye, 1946). The alarm stage triggers an acute response to initial exposure while the adaptation stage is the 'getting used to' response. The exhaustion stage encompasses end-organ failure.

The process of adaptation (stage 2) has two phases. The first is a physiological adjustment to an incitant. This phase is probably defined by narrow limits depending on the quantity of enzymes and other immunodetoxification systems available for induction and response. There is minimal strain on the system with no chronic inflammation or severe metabolic depletion. Development of the second phase of stage 2 signals more severe difficulties. A series of metabolic events occur which strains the availability of ATP and the metabolism of minerals, glucose, carbohydrates, and fats. Enzyme systems, such as the glucose-6-phosphate dehydrogenase, glutathione peroxidase, superoxide dismutase, monoamine oxidase, aryl hydrocarbon hydroxylase, mixed function oxidase, and cytochrome P-450 systems are stimulated. Gradually they are over extended by continuing stress which increases body load by virtue of gradual inability to detoxify substances, therefore the gradual depletion of essential nutritional elements occurs. Finally, end-organ failure or stage 3 maladaptation occurs resulting in heart (Rea, 1978), lung (Mustafa and Tierney, 1978), blood vessel (Rea, 1977), gastro-intestinal (Ward, 1985), or genito-urinary (Eroschenko and Osman, 1986) disease. One can see that PMS clearly falls into the 2 B phase.

Studies with common inorganic pollutants such as nitrogen dioxide and ozone soundly support this masking concept (McGrath and Smith, 1984; Menzel, 1976; Crapo *et al.*, 1978). Stokinger and Coffin (1968), Bennett (1962), and the National Research Council (1962) pointed out that although daily exposures to pollutants may initially decrease pulmonary function from 15 per cent to 20 per cent, by the fourth day the pulmonary function returns to control levels, thus demonstrating masking. Rinkel *et al.* (1951) showed the same phenomenon after repeated ingestion of offending foods. Cellular and metabolic changes then occur. Variations in metabolic changes are dependent on the concentration and virulence of pollutants as well as the volume of offending substances, time, nutritional state of the organism and the presence of other disease (Kon, 1978; Horrobin *et al.*, 1977). Since people get 'used to' a toxic substance they will continue to increase body burden inadvertently. This phenomenon can occur in any smooth muscle organ and is apparent in the environmentally sensitive PMS patient.

Bipolarity

Bipolarity is another factor which contributes to the total body burden. When exposed to a toxic substance, the body initially develops a bipolar response with a stimulatory phase followed by a depressive phase. Initially, induction of the immune and enzyme detoxifiction system occurs. If the incitant is sufficiently virulent, substantial in amount, or the duration of exposure is extended, the biological enzyme and immune detoxification systems are then depleted (depressed) by overstimulation. Parallel to this pathological phenomenon, an individual may experience the stimulatory reaction in the brain and perceive the inciting substance as not being harmful to her initially, but actually making her feel better or 'high'. Therefore she continues to acquire more exposures either to maintain the 'high' or inadvertently from accidental exposure. After a period of time, however, be it minutes, months or years her body's defences break down from over use and she develops disabling depression–exhaustion symptoms. These stimulation and depression–exhaustion phenomena have been observed with many pollutant exposures including ozone (National Research Council, 1962; Bennett, 1962; Stokinger, 1965; Stokinger and Coffin, 1968; Mustafa and Tierney, 1978).

Due to initially sufficient immune and enzyme inductivity, the body appears to be tricked into initially tolerating a toxic substance or even liking it, again probably for acute survival, although it is adding to the damaging long-term load due to over-utilization of the nutrient fuel of the induction process and direct toxic damage. The depressive phase occurs when the various metabolic systems become depleted or sustain sufficient toxic damage to the point that they can no longer respond as well to the stimuli. Fixed pathological cellular changes then occur with abnormal healing or scar formation. During the stimulation phase, enzyme and immune induction had occurred initially with increases in energy production (adenosine triphosphate, glucose, protein, lipid metabolism, and enzyme response). When an incitant is acutely removed, a symptomatic withdrawal period may be experienced. This is not to be confused with the depression phase which occurs with continued excessive stimulation. The symptomatic withdrawal period is probably due to a sudden removal of an incitant with a slow three to four day turn off of response systems. A prime example of withdrawal is seen in people drinking alcohol on a Saturday night in order to get high. The withdrawal period is expressed as a 'hang over' on Sunday morning while the depressive phase comes years later with eventual brain and liver deterioration. A second example involves workers who get hang-over-like symptoms on Saturday morning at home following exposures to toxic substances in the workplace during the week. They feel well during the work week, but they experience headaches, muscle aches, shakiness, and impaired ability to function on Saturday through early Sunday. By Sunday afternoon, as their systems rid themselves of the toxic substances and induced systems return to prestimulatory levels, the workers are again able to function well and feel fit to work on Monday. This cycle may be repeated weekly for months or years before the person develops end-stage disease. During this time, the PMS patient continues to accentuate her symptoms. It can easily be seen how this occurrence can lead to an addictive phenomenon (constant withdrawal and re-exposure) as seen in many PMS patients. Cycle observations under controlled conditions have suggested that this stimulatory–addictive withdrawal phenomenon can spill over into cross-reactivity, i.e. an individual working in a plastic factory may develop severe thirst or hunger. She then drinks carbonated beverages or eats 'junk foods' until she sets up more addictive patterns taking more harmful substances into the body including medications and drugs in order to maintain her precarious balance. She develops a spreading phenomenon becoming sensitive to more chemicals as she adds to the body burden. As her load or burden increases, she becomes more and more sensitive to new foods and chemicals (Symington *et al.*, 1981) which further derange body metabolism predisposing to severe PMS.

Biochemical Individuality

The final principle necessary to the understanding of the environmental aspects of gynaecological health and disease is that of individuality. Biochemical individuality is our uniqueness accounting for individual susceptibility. We have individually differing quantities of carbohydrates, fats, proteins, enzymes, vitamins, minerals, and immune parameters with which to respond to environmental factors. This individuality allows us to clear the body of noxious substances or to contribute to our own body burden. Biochemical individuality is dependent on at least three factors: genetics, state of fetus's nutritional health and toxic body burden during pregnancy, and the individual's present toxic body burden in relation to her present nutritional state at the time of exposure, e.g. some individuals are born with significantly less quantities of a specific enzyme (may be 25 per cent, 50 per cent or even 75 per cent). While she may be able to respond to an environmental stimulant, her response is often considerably less than that of the individual who was born with 100 per cent of the expected detoxifying enzyme and immune parameters. The over 2000 genetic metabolic defects already described in the literature appear to be 'time bombs' awaiting environmental triggers to elicit their expression. It is likely that any given individual may have one or more genetic defects. A common example, of the 'time bomb' effect is the children with phenylketonuria who do well as long as they do not take in phenylalanines although they have a genetic enzyme defect. Smith (1986) has shown that a group of individuals exist in the general population (approximately 25 per cent) who are slow sulphoxidisors. When they are exposed to a substance such as succinyl cysteine they will slowly metabolize it and become ill during the process. He also found another group (about 10 per cent) of the general population, who had genetic deficiency through the cytochrome P-450 system, who could not tolerate debrisoquine compounds. Monro (1986) studying a select group of chemically sensitive people showed as many as 60 per cent of the patients to have defects in these systems. It should be emphasized that many different toxic chemicals, additives, preservatives, pesticides, and chlorinated hydrocarbons may cause vitamin, amino acid, lipid, enzyme, and mineral depletion resulting in a selectively depleted individual. This may be due to in-utero depletion in the fetus which is due to bioconcentration of toxic chemicals, direct toxic effects of chemicals on nutrients, competitive inhibition; (e.g. some drugs like hydralazine are selectively absorbed in preference to vitamin B_6), over utilization of the detoxification systems with depletion of their fuel sources (vitamins, etc.), or selective nutrient malabsorption due to toxic damage to intestinal walls or flora. An individual whose immune and enzyme detoxification systems are depleted is unable to respond as well to more toxic environmental exposures which are normally received in routine living. This cycle appears to occur in the PMS patient.

Pollution Facts

Food

Food can influence the PMS process in many ways. This can be due to the nutritive quality, toxic effects of the food itself, sensitivity to the food, and sensitivity to its additives and preservatives. Many women on monotonous diets tend to get nutrient deficiencies because of limited variety of intake or poor nutritional quality.

Nutritive Quality

There appears to be a decrease in the quality of foods raised on soils which have been regularly treated with pesticides and herbicides, and also soils that are naturally depleted of minerals (Pottigener, 1936; Hill, 1983). In addition processing is known to destroy nutrients, e.g. vitamin D is lost in the pasteurization of milk. Individuals who eat the so-called ultra-processed and preserved 'junk food' will tend to have more vitamin and mineral depletion. Vitamin B_6 and magnesium depletion especially seem to occur with this type of diet. Also, selenium, zinc, and calcium intake may not be appropriate. Vitamins such as the other B vitamins, C, A and E may also be deficient in some diets. Fatty acids may also be deficient especially if there is a lack of fish and non-heated polyunsaturated oils or high amounts of animal protein. Diets high in simple rather than complex carbohydrates, or high in refined sugars increase the need for the B-complex vitamins. Also, excessive total carbohydrate intake seems to be a problem in many PMS patients.

Toxic Effects of Foods

Many foods contain their own toxins. If these are ingested in large quantities or repetitively problems can arise. Toxins involved in food processing and storage include carcinogens such as nitrosamines, bleaching agents such as methionine sulphoximine, solvent extraction by trichloroethylene and fumigation with ethylene oxide. Natural toxins from plants may be both endogenous and exogenous. Cabbage and related vegetables contain glucosinolates which have goitrogenic activity although clinical symptoms are unlikely. Sweet potatoes or legumes may produce cyanogens thus producing neuropathy and mental confusion. *Datura stramonium* may produce atropine with resultant hallucinations. Bananas may produce pressor amines thus causing headache and hypertension. Solanine may be found in potatoes, especially when badly stored, which may result in headaches, incoherence, hallucination and dizziness. Exogenous sources include peanuts and grains which may contain aflatoxins if contaminated with certain moulds. Aflatoxins can cause encephalopathy, hallucinations, and hepatic disease. Nitrites originating from endogenous nitrates may be present in some green vegetables including spinach with potential risk of headache, hepatic disease and methaemoglobinaemia. Conversion to nitrosamines results in potential risk of carcinogenic activity. Naturally occurring toxins from animals occur. Endogenous examples include fish which contain certain lipoproteins which may result in symptoms of vomiting, headache, and dizziness. Other examples include cheese which contains tyramine which can give headache and elevated blood pressure in susceptible individuals. Saxitoxin originating from dinoflagellates may be found in fish or shellfish possibly giving symptoms of dyspnoea, paralysis, or haemorrhage.

Food Sensitivities

These have been shown to cause mild to severe problems causing abnormal smooth muscle reactions. This occurs more in the uterus, tubes, and ovaries than previously thought and reactions occur especially in the blood vessels. This means that the ovaries, tubes and uterus could be a double target organ with the vessels contained in them and the intrinsic muscles themselves becoming sensitized. The mechanism of these sensitivities can be through IgE, but probably more often occurs via Type II, III, and IV mechanisms or even from direct non-immune triggering (Rea and Brown, 1986). Avoidance for four days with rechallenge usually allows the diagnosis of food sensitivity. The most common offenders for the tubes, ovaries, and uterus are coffee, tea, cane sugar, wheat, corn, milk, beef, eggs, chicken, and pork. Many of the accessory signs and symptoms such as headache, depression, and agitation of the PMS patient occur or may be accentuated as a result of sensitivity to these and other foods.

Food Additives

These consist of preservatives, colourings, pesticides, herbicides, and flavourings (Rea and Brown, 1986). All commercial foods in the USA now have pesticides and herbicides in them. This is probably so in the UK also. Reactivity in the PMS patient can occur from these and may well be one of the major reasons that menstrual cycles become disordered. Aldehydes are used in some foods as flavouring and when coupled with formaldehyde used as preservatives in others can trigger reactions of the gynaecological system. Sulphites, monosodium glutamate, benzoic acids, and tartrazine dyes can also trigger reactions. Many heavy metals like lead, cadmium and mercury may be found in foods and may trigger severe metabolic reactions especially through the glutathione pathway with resultant gynaecological dysfunction. All of the food parameters tend to increase total body burdens in the PMS patient.

Water Contamination

Water contains minerals, toxic organic and inorganic chemicals, particulates, and radiation. Mineral content has an effect on the vascular and other smooth muscles. Water with high calcium and magnesium content tends to have a soothing effect on the smooth muscle of blood vessels and probably the gynaecological organs. We have seen the immediate cessation of severe premenstrual cramps with the administration of magnesium intravenously. Those waters with a high sodium content tend to accentuate the frequent oedema problems of PMS. Most public water supplies are not only contaminated by the chlorination process, but also at the source of the water. Drinking and bathing water sources are from lakes, wells, and ponds. Most of this water comes from:

1. Rain (contaminated with hydrocarbons, sulphuric acid, nitric acid, or radioactivity).
2. Agricultural run off (contaminated with pesticides, herbicides, nitrates).
3. Factory effluent (containing a wide variety of organic and inorganic chemicals including formaldehyde, PBC, PBB, lead, mercury, cadmium etc.)
4. Public sewage treatment (more of the above metals, household products with detergents, solvents, etc.).

Contamination with particulate material may be organic decay from leaves, faeces, carcasses, etc., which combine with chlorine in the chlorination process to form the most toxic materials, the trihalomethanes. These can be absorbed through the GI tract, lungs, and/or skin to cause gynaecological problems by altering the integrity of blood vessel walls triggering oedema.

Radiation occurs naturally in some water due to the emission from the earth. The content varies depending on where and which type of stone the water comes from. External radiation can come from rain run-off from nuclear plants as seen dramatically in the Chernobyl accident.

In 1965, a serious drinking water problem existed in one in 25 patients hospitalized in the Environmental Control Unit. Today it is up to 80 per cent. Patients susceptible to water contaminants usually exhibit multiple sensitivities with advanced chemical susceptibility problems especially to airborne chemicals; 50 per cent of these menstruating females admitted to the Environmental Control Unit have severe PMS problems. They often experience some PMS symptoms which are triggered by water contaminant problems and cannot clear until this aspect is eliminated by using one of the less contaminated waters such as spring, distilled, or charcoal filtered. The water also must be contained in glass or steel rather than plastic in order to avoid recontamination.

Air Pollution

Air pollution has long been known to enhance disease processes. There are basically two types, outdoor and indoor.

Outdoor Air Pollution

According to Environmental Protection Agency studies (Gilpin, 1978), there has been no fresh air in the USA in 20 years. This probably holds true for the UK and Europe as well. Air pollution can arise from natural sources such as volcanoes, forest fires, marshes, and animal emanations which account for 55 per cent of the world air pollution. However, 45 per cent comes from man-made sources such as factory, automobile, heating and electrical generating plant emissions. Of course, around urban areas major sources are man-made far exceeding the natural sources. Smog, the combination of fog and man-made pollution can be devastating as was seen in London earlier in the century and Los Angeles at the present. Weather conditions and terrain can markedly change air pollution, while cities now generate their own autogenous heat islands and local weather. Worse case situations occur due to subsidence and radiation inversions where there is a cap of stable pollution topping the city to accentuate more pollution from a layer coming from the lower levels. This is the worst of all possible conditions and can increase the pollutant gradient thousands of times. Inversions will make living more hazardous and often accentuates the PMS in already susceptible people. The major outdoor air pollutants include sulphur dioxide, nitrous oxide, carbon monoxide, ozone, particulates (pollens, moulds, hydrocarbons), lead with other heavy metals and chlorinated compounds and cyanides. Most of these pollutants have been shown to trigger various detoxification systems by the generation of free radicals. Many PMS patients find that when they go to areas of less polluted air their syndrome disappears only to return when they get back to areas of higher air pollution.

Indoor Air Pollution

Indoor air is now the most polluted place in our environment. This is due to the sealing of buildings to prevent heat and cold loss, and the stocking of homes with rapidly disintegrating synthetics. The most common cause of problems in the new homes less than three years of age are the stains, dyes, solvents, paints, and formaldehyde-impregnated plywood, pressboard, and gypsum board. Alkanes, alkabenzenes, and terpenes are also present. In addition older homes contain petroleum alcohols and moulds. Gas, oil or coal stoves and heaters are the most common offenders that increase total body burden in the home environment. These are followed by routine use of pesticide. Other significant contaminants are foam stuffed furniture and mattresses, synthetic fabrics, termite proofing, Scotch gard finishes, dry cleaned clothes, washing detergents, chlorinated compounds, and other solvents.

Blood levels of pesticides and volatile organic hydrocarbons in patients with environmentally influenced PMS usually contain numerous pollutants found all around us in the air, water, and food (Figure 1 and Table 1). These and their relatives apparently are a significant part of total body load disturbing both the immune and enzyme detoxification systems. Then disturbed metabolism occurs with the resultant PMS.

EHC-Dallas has seen 200 patients with severe PMS, who had to radically alter their home environments in removing pollutants just described in order to decrease their syndrome, e.g. they often reported that after the heating came on or spraying was done that they had a severe increase in their PMS and removal of these pollutants decreased their problems.

Applicability of Environmental Precepts to PMS

A less polluted environment in an isolated wing of the hospital was created. Other areas were sealed from all inlets. Double doors with air locks were used in order to prevent entry of contaminants. Air depollution devices were installed and no smoking, perfumes, or synthetics were allowed in order to decrease pollutants. Floors and walls were all ceramic. All food was grown in a less chemically contaminated environment in the relative absence of pesticides and herbicides. Less contaminated water includes spring, distilled, or charcoal filtered, all bottled in glass. Air analysis by particulate counters, gas chromatography, and mass spectroscopy was done daily inside and outside the unit revealing 80–100 per cent reduction of pollutants in the unit. The unit is free of formaldehyde and pesticides. Reports on several series of patients suffering from arthritis (Kroker *et al.*, 1984), phlebitis (Rea *et al.*, 1981), vasculitis (Rea, 1977), cardiac arrhythmias (Rea, 1980), asthma and recurrent sinusitis (Rea and Mitchell, 1982) have shown clearing with manipulation of environmental incitants without use of medication. Improvement of numerous laboratory parameters were seen including eosinophils, C-reactive protein, total and fractions of serum complements, T and B lymphocytes and immunoglobulins other than IgE, pesticide levels, volatile organic hydrocarbon levels, and brain functions in over 2000 environmentally sensitive patients. The patient can be taken off medications and not fed for two to seven days until she is deadapted in this less polluted environment. Challenge with (oral) water contaminants, food, food contaminants, and (inhaled) air can be carried out. The above principles, facts, and procedures were used as a scientific basis for evaluating the PMS patient.

Several characteristics seen in some PMS patients suggest environmental

Rate symptoms for level of severity: 1, 2, 3, 4 or 5

Month _____

Days of month

SYMPTOMS	1	2	3	4	5	6	7	8	9	10	11	12	13	14	15	16	17	18	19	20	21	22	23	24	25	26	27	28	29	30	31
Anxious																															
Blackouts																															
Breasts swelling and tenderness																															
Hallucination																															
Tense																															
Withdrawn feelings																															
Ovulating																															
Menstruating																															
Seizures																															
Tremor / Convulsions																															
Nipples sensitive																															
Cramping																															
Abdominal bloating																															
Diarrhoea																															
Allergic reactions																															
Rashes / skin eruptions																															
Lowered motor co-ordination																															
Depressed																															
Irritable																															
Difficulty concentrating																															
Nauseated																															
Suicidal																															
Angry outbursts																															
Hot flashes																															
Water retention																															
Listless																															
Headache																															
Food cravings																															
Mental confusion																															
Undue confusion																															
Undue fatigue																															
Change in sex ↑ ↓																															
Want to be left alone																															
Crying spells																															
Negative attitude																															
Clumsy																															
Fainting spells																															
Difficulty controlling behaviour																															

Figure 2. Symptom score sheet

triggers; e.g. headache, cyclic oedema, drug sensitivity, inability to tolerate oral contraception, bloating, periorbital oedema, increased sinus congestion, post nasal drip, asthma, flare of skin problems, worse after each pregnancy, spontaneous bruising, petechiae, purpura, cold sensitivity, history of threatened abortion, inability to tolerate most medications, weather sensitivity, anaesthestic sensitivity, decreased tolerance for alcohol, food or alcohol craves, history of hypertension or pre-eclampsia. Severe odour sensitivity to perfumes, hairsprays, deodorants, gasoline, car exhaust fumes, pesticides, or formaldehyde is almost pathognomonic of environmental overload and is often seen in PMS patients.

Once a PMS patient is suspected of having environmental triggers, a symptom score sheet is done (Figure 2). Tracking of symptoms throughout a cycle is then easily accomplished. Patients are then evaluated to see if they

Table 2. Intradermal symptom neutralization

Hormone	Concentrate			
Oestrone	2 mg ml^{-1}			
Progesterone	50 mg ml^{-1}			
Luteinizing	20 000 USP units vial^{-1} (10 ml vial)			
	Dilution	Dose (mg)	Symptoms	Wheal
No. 1	0.25 ml^3 1/5	2.5	Provoked	11 × 11
No. 2	0.05 ml^3 1/25	0.5	Same	9 × 9
No. 3	0.05 ml^3 1/25	0.1	Relieved	7 × 7
No. 4	0.05 ml^3 1/625	0.02		
No. 5	0.05 ml^3 1/3125	0.004		

Examples of intradermal injection for method of determining correct dose by the Lee–Miller method for hormonal treatment for relief of PMS symptoms. If no symptoms provoked the first dose that gives a 7 × 7 wheal will usually be the neutralizing dose.

have hormone sensitivity. Sensitivity to the hormones (luteinizing hormone, progesterone, and oestrogen) is assessed by the provocation neutralization technique either sublingually or intradermally. This is done by using 1:5 progressive serial dilution of each hormone individually, provoking and then relieving the symptoms and/or the wheal. One can frequently find a dose that will immediately stop symptoms. The first report of endocrine susceptibility demonstrated with skin testing was by Zondek and Bromberg in 1947. Heckel in 1953 treated by injection and cleared numerous patients. G. Fricke (personal communication) using the Lee–Miller method found immediate results with the intradermal provocation neutralization technique in PMS. Mabray et al. (1982) studied a large series of women with progesterone related symptoms (Table 2).

His technique of managing sensitivities by optimum-dose (provocative neutralization) testing and treatment using aqueous progesterone has been studied in 132 women having progesterone-related symptoms due to the menstrual cycle, pregnancy, or exogenous hormone administration. When extremely small doses of progesterone (0.0016 mg or below, up to a maximum of 2.5 mg) were administered following determination of specific dose requirement by skin testing, rapid and effective clearing of symptoms was observed (Table 3). With these individualized doses, symptoms cleared completely or almost completely within 30 min in the majority of patients. A single-blind technique was employed to rule out placebo effect (Mabray et al., 1982). Some common problems found to respond well to the procedure were

Table 3. Presenting symptoms and response to initial minidose progesterone administration

	Base study group (N = 100)			Blind study group (N = 32)			Total (N = 132)		
	No.	Marked or complete relief	%	No.	Marked or complete relief	%	No.	Marked or complete relief	%
Dysmenorrhoea	37	32	86	6	4	67	43	36	84
Headache	29	26	90	10	10	100	39	36	92
Backache	14	13	93	11	10	91	25	23	92
Abdominal pain	11	10	91	9	8	89	20	18	90
Abdominal pressure, bloating	2	2	100	4	4	100	6	6	100
Neck, leg, and hip pain	4	3	75	6	5	83	10	8	80
Breast pain	2	2	100	5	5	100	7	7	100
Nausea	18	16	89	2	2	100	20	18	90
Nervousness, irritability, depression	26	25	96	18	17	94	44	42	95
Vertigo, dizziness	6	6	100				6	6	100
Fatigue, weakness	3	3	100	7	6	86	10	9	90
Flushing, hot flashes	1	1	100	3	2	67	4	3	75
Urticaria of pregnancy	1	1	100				1	1	100
Tinnitus	1	1	100				1	1	100

Many patients presented with more than one complaint. Mabray *et al.*, 1982.

nausea and vomiting during pregnancy (100 per cent), PMS (96 per cent), and dysmenorrhoea (84 per cent) (Table 3). Hormone sensitivities are then treated with the optimum dose therapy 0.05 ml of the appropriate dose which will either control the sensitivity and/or balance the hormonal dysfunction. The following schedule is used once this symptom neutralizing dose is found.

1. Oestrone: the prescribed dose, usually 0.05 ml of appropriate dilution (injection or sublingual), is taken every fourth day and as needed for symptoms throughout the cycle. Dosage may be repeated up to four times a day.
2. Progesterone: the prescribed dose, usually 0.05 ml of appropriate dilution (injection or sublingual), is taken daily with onset of premenstrual symptoms. Dosage may be taken up to four times a day to relieve symptoms. The dose on the day menstruation is expected should be held until onset of menses occurs. Then progesterone may be resumed if needed to control menstrual symptoms.
3. Luteinizing hormone: the prescribed dose, usually 0.05 ml of appropriate dilution (injection or sublingual), is taken daily one to two weeks prior to

Table 4. Protocol for optimum dose hormonal injection treatment of PMS determining neutralizing dose by the Lee–Miller method

Oestrone	0.05 cm^3 of appropriate dilution	Every four days as required by symptoms. May repeat up to four times a day.
Progesterone	0.05 cm^3 of appropriate dilution (sublingual or injection)	Daily with onset of premenstrual symptoms. May repeat up to four times a day. Hold day that menstruation is due until onset of menses then may be resumed if needed to control menstrual symptoms.
Luteinizing hormone	0.05 cm^3 of appropriate dilution (sublingual or injection)	Daily one to two weeks prior to onset of menses. When symptoms occur and are not neutralized by oestrone or progesterone. May repeat up to four times a day.

onset of menses when symptoms occur and are not neutralized by oestrogen and progesterone. Dosage may be repeated up to four times a day.

This schedule may be used for ovulatory symptoms. This regimen will clear
75–85 per cent of the patients (Mabray *et al.*, 1982; G. Fricke, personal
communication). Some patients who are more environmentally sensitive also
require supplementation with more oestrogen and progesterone. Here vaginal
suppositories, composed of a naturally occurring hormone in a fatty acid
base which avoids the use of petrochemicals or plastic derived base, are used.
Complicating factors are myriad for the environmentally sensitive PMS
patient. Some patients have specific food sensitivities or are addicted to 'junk
foods'. Often patients are placed on a fresh, raw, whole food diet avoiding
foods that are processed, canned, packed, etc. Sometimes patients do very
well with cessation of many of their symptoms. Others are sensitive to specific
foods. These food sensitivities can be proven by their elimination for four
days then rechallenged by eating. Therapy can be devised by using the
intradermal provocation neutralization technique and the administration of
food injections or sublingual drops every four days. Other patients are
extremely sensitive to water contaminants and have to drink less polluted
(charcoal filtered, distilled or spring) glass bottled water. Also, some patients
have to eat foods free from pesticides and herbicides. Finally, some patients are
exquisitely sensitive to odours of synthetics, formaldehyde, phenol, pesticides,
chlorine, petroleum-derived products, and many need an environmental oasis

within their homes. This oasis is designed to decrease pollution and thus total body load by being relatively free of particulates, dust, moulds, pollens, and toxic organic and inorganic materials. No gas, oil, or coal heat and no pesticides are mandatory in some patients. Occasionally a patient needs desensitization for pollens, dust, or moulds in order to control seasonal variations of PMS. In addition any other unsatisfactory nutritional factors must be corrected.

Many PMS patients have symptoms related to an overgrowth of the vaginal and/or gastro-intestinal tracts with yeast (especially *Candida albicans*) and other fungi. In these cases yeast and high sugar containing foods such as cheese, vinegar, alcohol, sweets, and breads are discouraged. Also local and systemic anti-fungal therapy are applied. Nystatin 500 000 units twice daily for two to three months may be needed. Ketoconazole 200 mg daily for one to two weeks can be used or oral amphotericin-B 250 mg, three times a day, for two weeks may be used. Oral douches of chlotrimazole may be used up to four times a day for one month plus vaginal douches daily.

Nutritional Deficiencies

Correction of nutritional deficits is important when trying to correct vascular or other smooth muscle pollutant damage.

Vitamin A

β-Carotene and vitamin A are used as potent antioxidants, being shown to affect free radicals, adversely. They also fight bacteria and other infections, maintain healthy epithelial tissue, and are essential for a normal menstrual cycle in the female. Up to 5000 i.u. daily for one to two months has been used in our centre without side effects. β-Carotene is preferable because it is less prone to rancidity and thus will trigger fewer free radicals. The patients with vascular acne-like lesions sometimes will respond to vitamin A-*cis*-retenoic acid. Care has to be taken here due to the multiple potential side effects (Pfeiffer, 1975). Careful monitoring of vitamin A compounds should be carried out to avoid liver damage. Vitamin A has been shown to blunt the effects of radiation probably through its free radical scavenger effect. It should not be taken for a long period of time without attempting to find the triggering agents. Vitamin A toxicity is rare but is characterized by irritability, headaches, skin desquamation, vomiting and loss of appetite.

Vitamin B

PABA (*para*-aminobenzoic acid) will decrease the toxicity of ozone by neutralizing the free radical formation of lipid peroxidation (Goldstein *et al.*, 1972). Deficiencies in thiamine, riboflavin, niacin, and pyridoxine enhance the toxicity of PCBs. Pyridoxine is a cofactor in many reactions in intermediary metabolism and has been shown to be of value in relieving the symptoms of PMS. Doses of up to 100 mg daily may be given. Care should be taken to be sure that adequate absorption occurs since some pollutant sensitive patients have selective malabsorption. Pyridoxine also helps to maintain the sodium balance. Many of the PMS patients can also have their central nervous system symptoms improved by the administration of thiamine, riboflavin and niacin in addition to vitamin B_{12}. Vitamin B_5 (pantothenic acid) is a component of co-enzyme A which serves in metabolic reactions involving transfer of acetyl groups. Symptoms of deficiency are headache, nausea, occasional vomiting and abdominal cramps.

Vitamin C

Vitamin C can be depleted with chemical exposures particularly to substances like benzene (Forsman and Frykholm 1947), carbon monoxide (Zaffiri et al., 1971), ethanol (Yunice and Lindeman, 1979), smoking (Pelletier, 1975), nitrous compounds (Varghese et al., 1978), vinyl chloride (Gedigk et al., 1975), heavy metals (Samitz et al., 1968) and pesticides (Chakraborty et al., 1978). Amorphous ground substance of the vessel wall is somewhat dependent on vitamin C. Vitamin C supplements can be used to not only strengthen the blood vessel wall but also used as a free radical scavenger and antioxidant. Usually a range of $1-10$ g day^{-1} of powdered vitamin C has been used in patients with vascular and PMS dysfunction. One must be careful of the source of carbohydrate excipients in vitamin C tablets since many individuals become intolerant of the food of origin, such as corn, sago palm, potato, and carrot, as well as the excipients of talc, silica, etc. The powder is much safer. Excessive use of vitamin C may cause gas and diarrhoea.

Vitamin D

Vitamin D is needed to help regulate calcium metabolism. Those who live in northern climates have more difficulty generating vitamin D due to less exposure time to the sun. It has been shown that those persons living where the oxidant pollutant levels are high may have a concommitant decrease in vitamin D accumulations by as much as 15 per cent over a 25 year period. Pasturization also eliminates vitamin D. Supplementation must be carefully monitored in order to avoid toxicity. Excess leads to hypercalcaemia. The safest therapy is exposure to sunlight.

Vitamin E

Vitamin E has been used in some vascular and PMS patients. It is particularly important in maintenance of lipid membrane integrity and the preservation of tissue polyunsaturated fatty acid content. Deficiency results in more inflammation in animals while oral Vitamin E has been shown to stop lipid peroxidation (Menzel, 1976). Clearly vitamin E is not only a free radical scavenger but also a stabilizer of the cellular membranes. It has been shown to be an effective anti-pollutant. From 400 to 1400 units per day have been used.

Calcium

Calcium is clearly a mineral that is necessary for membrane stability and thus vascular wall tone. It also is a co-factor in many metabolic steps. Calcium has been found to be inversely proportional to radiostrontium thus it would be of use in protecting a patient against this pollutant (Nordin *et al.*, 1967). Doses of 1–3 g of calcium have been given daily to patients with vascular disease and PMS and have been found to stabilize cell membranes. It has reduced the damage caused by carbon tetrachloride ingestion in animals.

Magnesium

Magnesium is a membrane stabilizer. It is complexed with ATP and ADP and therefore is a mandatory co-factor for all kinases and other enzymes containing magnesium. The daily dose is 500 to 1000 mg.

Surgery on the PMS Patient

EHC-Dallas has eight patients who were severely incapacitated with their PMS after all of the aforementioned modalities. They were all in their late 30s and wished to have no more children. Oophorectomy was preferred with satisfactory results in this highly selected group. Each was able to tolerate hormone supplementation where she previously could not. Follow-up from one to eight years has shown continued improvement.

Stress Management

Stress management may be needed in many of these patients including the family. This lifestyle change may be accomplished in many ways. Biofeedback, relaxation therapy, imagery, and tension awareness as well as individual and group psychotherapy are used in our centre.

In conclusion it may be said that there are some new methods which have promise for the effective treatment of PMS. Today, however, the best mode of treatment and prevention of most PMS symptoms is avoidance of incitants, replacement of nutrients, and hormone neutralization and replacement.

References

Becker, R. O. and Marino, A. A. (1982). *Electromagnetism and Life*, New York Press, Albany.

Bennett, G. (1962). Ozone contamination of high altitude aircraft cabins. *Aerospace Medicine*, 33, 969–973.

Crapo, J. D., Sjestiom, K., and Drew, R. T. (1978). Tolerance and cross-tolerance using NO_2 and O_2. I. Toxicology and biochemistry. *Journal of Applied Physiology*, 4, 364–369.

Chakraborty, D., Bhattacharyza, A., Majumdar, K., Chatteyee, K., Chatteyee, S., Sen, A. and Chatteryee, G. C. (1978). Studies on L-ascorbic acid metabolism in rats under chronic toxicity due to organophosphorus insecticides and effects of supplementation of L-ascorbic acid in high doses. *Journal of Nutrition*, 108, 973–980.

Dickey, L. D. (Ed.) (1976). *Clinical Ecology*, Thomas, Springfield.

Eroschenko, V. P. and Osman, F. (1986). Scanning electron microscopic changes in vaginal epithelium of suckling neonatal mice in response to oestradiol or insecticide chlordecone (Kepone) passage in milk. *Toxicology*, 38, 175–185.

Forsman, S., and Frykholm, K. O. (1947). Benzene poisoning. II. Examination of workers exposed to benzene with reference to the presence of extersulfate, muconic acid, urochrome A and polychenols in the urine together with vitamin C deficiency. Prophylactic measures. *Acta Medica Scandinavica*, 128, 256–280.

Gedigk, P., Muller, R. and Bechtelsheimer, H. (1975). Morphology of liver damage among polyvinyl chloride production workers: A report of 51 cases. *Annals of the New York Academy of Sciences*, 246, 278–285.

Gilpin, A. (1978). *Air Pollution*, (2nd edition), University of Queensland Press, St Lucia, Queensland.

Goldstein, B. D., Levine, M. R., Cuzzi-Spada, R., Cardenas, R., Buckley, R. D. and Balcham, O. J. (1972). p-Aminobenzoic acid as a protective agent in ozone toxicity. *Archives of Environmental Health*, 24, 243–247.

Heckel, G. P. (1953). Endocrine allergy and the therapeutic use of pregnanediol. *American Journal Obstetrics and Gynecology*, 66, 1297–1312.

Hill, L. (1983). *Vegetable Pest and Disease Control the Organic Way* Henry Doubleday Research Association, Braintree, Essex.

Horrobin, D. F., Karmali, R. A., Ally, A. I., Manku, M. S., and Morgan, R. D. (1977). Immunological deficiency, cancer, and prostaglandins. *British Medical Journal*, 2, 1086–1087.

Hinsdill, R. D. and Thomas, P. T. (1978). Effect of polychlorinated biphenyls on the immune responses of rhesus monkeys and mice. *Toxicology and Applied Pharmacology*, 44, 41–51.

Kon, S. H. (1978). Underestimation of chronic toxicities of food additives and chemicals: the bias of a phantom rule. *Medical Hypotheses*, 4, 324–339.

Kroker, G. F., Stroud, R. M., Marshall, R., Bullock, T., Carroll, F. M., Greenberg, M., Randolph, T. G., Rea, W. J. and Smiley, R. E. (1984). Fasting and rheumatoid arthritis: a multi-centre study, *Clinical Ecology*, 2, 137–144.

Lee, L. Y., Bleecker, E. R., and Nadel, J. (1977). Effects of ozone on bronchomotor response to inhaled histamine aerosol in dogs. *Journal of Applied Physiology*, 434, 626–631.

Mabray, C. R., Burditt, M. L., Martin, T. L., Jaynes, C. R., and Hayes, J. R. (1982). Treatment of common gynecologic-endocrinologic symptoms by allergy management procedures, *Obstetrics and Gynecology*, 59, 560–564.

Matsumsura, Y., Miquno, K., Miyamoto, T., Suzuki, T. and Oshima, Y. (1972). The effect of ozone, nitrogen dioxide, and sulfur dioxide on experimentally induced allergic respiratory disorder in guinea pigs. *American Review of Respiratory Disease*, **105**, 262–267.

McGrath, J. J. and Smith, W. L. (1984). Respiratory responses to nitrogen dioxide inhalation. *Journal of Environmental Science and Health, Pt A*, **19**, 417–431.

Menzel, D. B. (1976). The role of free radicals in the toxicity of air pollutants (nitrogen oxides and ozone), in *Free Radicals in Biology*, Vol. 2 (Ed. W. A. Pryor), Academic Press, New York, pp. 282–286.

Miller, J. B. (1972). *Food Allergy: Provocative Testing And Injection Therapy*, Thomas, Springfield, Illinois.

Monro, J. (1986). Paper presented at the Fourth Annual International Symposium On Man And His Environment In Health And Disease, Dallas, Texas.

Mustafa, M. G. and Tierney, D. F. (1978). Biochemical and metabolic changes in the lung with oxygen ozone, and nitrogen dioxide toxicity, *American Review of Respiratory Disease*, **118**, 1061–1090.

Nadal, A. and Lee, L. Y. (1977). Airway hyperirritability induced by ozone, in *Biochemical Effects of Environmental Pollutants* (Ed. S. D. Lee), Ann Arbor Science Publishers, Michigan.

Nordin, B. E. C., Smith, D. A., Shimmins, J. and Oxby, C. (1967). The effects of dietary calcium on the absorption and retention of radiostrontium. *Clinical Science*, **32**, 39–48.

National Research Council (1962). *Atmospheric Studies*, National Academy of Sciences, Washington, D.C.

Pelletier, O. (1968). Smoking and vitamin C levels in humans, *American Journal of Clinical Nutrition*, **2**, 1259–1267.

Pfeiffer, C. C. (1975). *Mental And Elemental Nutrients*, Keats Publishing, New Canaan, Connecticut.

Pottigener, P. (1936). *Nutrition And Physical Degeneration*, Thomas, Springfield, Illinois.

Randolph, T. G. (1962). *Human Ecology And Susceptibility To The Chemical Environment*, Thomas, Springfield, Illinois.

Rattner, B. A., Eroschenko, V. P., Fox, G. A., Fry, D. M. and Gorsline, J. (1984). Avian endocrine responses to environmental pollutants. *Journal of Experimental Zoology*, **232**, 683–689.

Rea, W. J. (1977). Environmentally triggered small vessel vasculitis. *Annals of Allergy*, **38**, 245–251.

Rea, W. J. (1978). Environmentally triggered cardiac disease. *Annals of Allergy*, **40**, 243–251.

Rea, W. J. (1980). Cardiovascular disease triggered by foods and chemicals, in *Food Allergy: New Perspectives* (Ed. J. W. Gerrard), Thomas, Springfield, Illinois.

Rea, W. J. and Mitchell, M. J. (1982). Chemical sensitivity and the environment. *Immunology and Allergy Practice*, **157**, 21.

Rea, W. J. and Brown, O. D. (1986). Cardiovascular disease in response to chemicals and foods, in *Food Allergy and Intolerance* (Eds. J. Brostoff and S. J. Challacombe) Baillière, London, pp. 737–750.

Rea, W. J., Smiley, R. E. and Edgar, R. (1981). Recurrent environmentally triggered thrombophlebitis; a five year follow up. *Annals of Allergy*, **47**, 338–341.

Rinkel, H. J., Randolph, T. G. and Zeller, M. (1951). *Food Allergy*, Thomas, Springfield, Illinois.

Samitz, H. H., Scheiner, D. M., and Katz, S. A. (1968). Ascorbic acid in the prevention of chrome dermatitis: mechanism of inactivation of chromium. *Archives of Environmental Health*, **17**, 44–45.

Selye, H. (1946). The general adaptation syndrome and the diseases of adaptation. *Journal of Allergy*, **17**, 23.

Smith, R. L. (1986). Some clinical consequences of inborn errors of drug metabolism. Paper presented at the Fourth Annual International Symposium On Man And His Environment In Health And Disease, Dallas, Texas, 1986.

Speer, F. (1977). *Migraine*, Newlson-Hall, Chicago.

Stokinger, H. E. (1965). Ozone toxicology: A review of research and industrial experience: 1954–1964. *Archives of Environmental Health*, **10**, 719–731.

Stokinger, H. E. and Coffin, D. L. (1968). Biological effects of air pollutants, in *Air Pollution* (Ed. A. C. Stern), American Press, New York.

Symington, I. S., Kerr, J. W. and McLean, D. A. (1981). Type I allergy in mushroom soup processors. *Clinical Allergy*, **11**, 43–47.

Varghese, A. J., Land, P. C., Furrer, R., and Bruce, W. R. (1978). Non-volatile N-nitrose compounds in human faeces, in *Environmental Aspects of N-nitrose compounds*, International Agency for Research on Cancer, TARC Scientific Publications No. 19, pp. 257–264.

Ward, J. M. (1985). Proliferative lesions of the glandular stomach and liver in F 344 rats fed diets containing Arocler 1254. *Environmental Health Perspectives*, **60**, 89–95.

Yunice, A. A. and Linderman, R. D. (1979). Effect of ascorbic acid and zinc sulfate on ethanol toxicity and metabolism, *Proceedings Society for Experimental Biology and Medicine*, **154**, 146–150.

Zaffiri, O., Calà, G., Centi, R. and Salicone, A. (1971). Therapeutic method for acute oxycarbonism (with the method Cala-Zaffiri) with intravenous infusions of high doses of ascorbic acid. *Minerva Anestesiologica*, **37**, 332–339.

Zondek, B. and Bromberg, Y. M. (1947). Clinical reactions of allergy to endogenous hormones and their treatment. *Journal of Obstetrics and Gynaecology of the British Empire*, **54**, 1–19.

Functional Disorders of the Menstrual Cycle
Edited by M. G. Brush and E. M. Goudsmit
© 1988 John Wiley & Sons Ltd

CHAPTER 10

Psychological aspects of premenstrual symptoms

ELLEN M. GOUDSMIT*

*Department of Gynaecology,
London. (Mailing address:
United Medical and Dental Schools, St Thomas's Campus,
London SE1 7EH)*

Introduction

Throughout the ages, women have been considered as inherently unreliable and predisposed to irrational thought and inappropriate action. Since these signs of instability were most noticeable before menstruation, they were thought to be inextricably linked to the female body, in particular, the female reproductive system thus reinforcing the widely held belief that women were mentally and intellectually inferior to men because of their biology (Radcliffe-Richards, 1982; Riven, 1983). The tendency to generalize traits found in some women to women at large has continued, and although there has been a considerable increase in sympathy towards sufferers of premenstrual distress, cycle-related symptoms are still regarded by many doctors as a manifestation of psychological weaknesses (Alexander *et al.*, 1986; Bernsted *et al.*, 1984; Notman 1982). Consequently sufferers who are aware of these attitudes may feel inadequate and ashamed and, fearing disapproval, could be reluctant to seek medical advice.

In this chapter, the most important of the psychogenic and psychosomatic explanations of premenstrual symptoms will be examined, focussing particularly on research aimed at identifying and assessing the type, degree and limits of psychological morbidity amongst sufferers of premenstrual distress.

The Psychoanalytic Approach

Central to this approach is the hypothesis that premenstrual distress is the manifestation of one or more unresolved, unconscious conflict(s). Since the

---

*Formerly attached to the Department of Psychophysiology, University of Amsterdam, The Netherlands

literature is extensive, the following discussion will be limited to some of the more influential and plausible explanations.

One of the earliest hypotheses connecting premenstrual symptoms with the psyche was proposed in 1931 by Karen Horney (1967). She suggested that premenstrual tension was closely related to conflicts evolving from the repressed wish for a child and/or to frustrated libidinal energy. Moreover she claimed that women's menstrual disturbances 'disappear completely during periods of fulfilment of their love life and reappear during periods of external frustration or unsatisfying experiences'. Helene Deutsch (1944), like Horney, believed that the psychological changes which occur during the premenstrual phase were triggered by underlying physiological reproductive events as well as increases in libidinal energy. However, Deutsch placed greater emphasis on the influence of the early experiences of menstruation and the fear of injury, illness and pain which was evoked by the thought and sight of menstrual blood. She maintained that these fears persisted into adolescence and adulthood, recurring every menstrual cycle in certain women as premenstrual or menstrual symptoms.

Similarly, Shainess (1961) suggested that both the menarche and the mother's attitude to it greatly influenced the daughter's later experience of her menstrual cycle and her attitudes towards herself. On the basis of the results from a questionnaire submitted to over 100 women, including her own patients, she concluded that women who suffered from premenstrual tension had not been adequately prepared for menstruation by their mothers and that their experience of the menarche had been an unpleasant one.

Following a slightly different line of thought, Shuttle and Redgrove (1978) proposed that premenstrual symptoms were the manifestation of latent, unconscious disturbances which a woman could not suppress during the premenstruum when she was most 'in accord with herself'. In order to alleviate menstrual distress, the woman had to learn to accept her cyclical bodily changes with its psychological (creative, educative) concomitants. They supported this view, by citing Shuttle's own experiences of dream analysis, which helped her to evaluate and change her own attitudes to menstruation and which led to a significant reduction of her own premenstrual depression.

It is difficult to assess the validity of explanations focussing on unconscious conflicts as the existence of such conflicts cannot be verified either directly or objectively. Hence researchers have been limited to assessing the nature and extent of disturbances which may be attributed to such conflicts. For instance, several studies have investigated women's attitudes towards the conventional female social and sexual roles, menstruation, the menarche and self-image. Paulson (1961) administered questionnaires to a large group of volunteers and found positive correlations between premenstrual symptoms and the following five factors: intrafamilial tension, negative attitudes towards the menarche, difficulty in accepting the female psychosocial and psychosexual roles and a poor self-image. Similarly, Gough (1975) and Paige (1973) postulated a link between premenstrual complaints and traditional femininity whilst Van Assen (1962) noted that many of his patients who reported premenstrual symptoms held negative attitudes towards sexuality and body image.

However, not all the findings are unequivocal. Berry and McGuire (1972) using the Moos Menstrual Distress Questionnaire (MDQ) and a role-acceptance scale found that there were significant negative correlations between role acceptance and some premenstrual symptoms, but not with premenstrual negative affect and behaviour change. Similarly, Slade and Jenner (1980) were unable to show a relationship between premenstrual symptoms and attitude towards femininity although they did find a significant correlation between premenstrual negative affect and the perception of the mother's embarrassment about menstruation.

The relationship between premenstrual distress and early experiences of menstruation which was proposed by Deutsch (1944) and Shainess (1961), has been investigated by several researchers including Paige (1973) and Fugate-Woods et al. (1982). Paige found no relationship between symptoms and a woman's early experiences of menstruation, her parents' attitudes and her mother's own experiences. Similarly, data presented by Fugate-Woods and her co-workers failed to show an association between current premenstrual symptoms and negative recollections of the menarche. Indeed, the women who had positive recollections tended to report more severe premenstrual negative affect. These findings are supported by De Leeuw (1982) who sent questionnaires to over 400 Dutch women but could not find any evidence of a link between the presence and severity of symptoms and attitudes to or knowledge about menstruation.

In one of the few studies using women specifically selected because of their premenstrual symptomatology, Watts et al. (1980) found that women suffering from the premenstrual syndrome (PMS) held more negative attitudes towards their bodies, genitals, sex and masturbation than a control group. However, the patients did not appear to reject or resent feminine role stereotypes or childbearing and rearing and although they held negative attitudes towards the menarche and menses, so did the controls. These findings were partly supported by Spencer-Gardner et al. (1983) whose research showed that women suffering from premenstrual symptoms did not differ in their attitudes towards the traditional role and the menarche from other women investigated. However, contrary to the results of Watts et al., women with premenstrual disturbances did not differ from the comparison group in their attitudes towards their bodies, genitals and sex. These two well designed studies suggest that negative menarcheal experiences, the acceptance of the traditional female role and negative attitudes towards menstruation are not important factors in the aetiology of premenstrual symptoms. However, the women suffering from cycle-related symptoms in these studies did hold a negative view of menstruation as did women recording high scores for premenstrual symptoms reported by Fugate-Woods *et al.* (1982). Whereas the psychoanalysts probably view such negative attitudes as a cause of premenstrual symptomatology, it could also be argued that they are a consequence of the symptoms.

Unfortunately, it is extremely difficult to draw any firm conclusions from the literature as a whole since many of the findings are contradictory and rather confusing. This may be partly due to the markedly different assessment techniques used and samples studied by the various researchers. For instance, some have based their views solely on their own observations and verbal reports from their patients (Deutsch, 1944; Horney, 1967; Van Assen, 1962) whilst others have relied on questionnaires and other self rating instruments.

The many methodological difficulties and inadequacies which have marred much of the research in this area have been comprehensively reviewed by Koeske (1983) and Parlee (1982) and these should be taken into account when interpreting the data.

The Psychosomatic Approach

There has been much discussion in recent years concerning the relationship between a woman's experience of premenstrual symptoms and her ability to cope with internal and external stressors. For instance, Sampson (1983) observed that many of the women who consulted her for premenstrual symptoms reported conflicts, particularly within the marriage, and also felt inadequate as a wife and mother. Similarly Clare (1983) in his study of 691 women found that marital disharmony correlated positively and significantly with premenstrual symptoms while Wood *et al.* (1979) noted that sexual and emotional problems were common amongst women with premenstrual tension.

It has been suggested that stressful life events may adversely affect the physical condition of women predisposing them to greater cycle-related discomfort (Siegel *et al.*, 1979). As yet, there is little empirical support for such a view. Watts *et al.* (1985) found that mean cortisol levels during the luteal phase in women suffering from PMS were higher than those of a control group although all the results were within the normal range. Whether the raised cortisol levels reflected abnormalities in the hypothalamic–pituitary–adrenal axis or increased stress levels is impossible to ascertain from the given data.

Apart from her physical health, a woman's ability to cope with stressful life events may also be affected by her personality and several researchers have tried to identify personality characteristics which may compromise a woman's ability to deal effectively with the demands made upon her during the second half of her menstrual cycle. For example, there is evidence from controlled studies that some women complaining of premenstrual distress have high trait anxiety scores indicating a predisposition to suffer from anxiety (Halbreich and Kas, 1977; Watts *et al.*, 1980; Goudsmit, 1983). Similarly, Coppen and Kessel (1963) and Slade and Jenner (1980) found a positive correlation between certain premenstrual symptoms and neuroticism while Taylor (1979) reported that fifteen subjects with troublesome premenstrual symptoms scored positively on several subscales of the Sixteen Personality Factor Questionnaire indicating that they were suspicious, apprehensive, tense, easily upset and undisciplined.

Premenstrual symptoms have also been correlated with the MMPI scales for schizophrenia, hysteria, hypochondria and psychasthenia suggesting that women who report premenstrual symptoms are more likely than non-sufferers to be seen as emotional, highly strung, prone to worry, serious, sensitive, modest, frank and generally concerned about bodily complaints (Gruba and Rohrbaugh, 1975). More recently, data presented by Spencer-Gardner *et al.* (1983) demonstrated that women suffering from premenstrual symptoms had significantly lower self-esteem and felt less in control over the events in their lives than the comparison group of female students.

Research has also focussed on the relationship between the presence of premenstrual symptoms, neurosis and other forms of psychiatric ill-health. Rees (1953) studied 85 patients attending a psychiatric out-patient department, a psychosomatic and allergy clinic and a group of 61 'normal' women using the Maudsley Medical Questionnaire and the Word Connection Test. Although he found a positive correlation between the intensity of premenstrual symptoms and the severity of neurosis, he observed that premenstrual tension could exist 'in women with little or no evidence of instability in personality adjustment or of neurosis or predisposition to neurosis'. Conversely, many of the women with severe neurosis did not suffer from premenstrual symptoms and he concluded that neurosis or emotional instability in itself was not sufficient to account for premenstrual symptoms.

In another study, Coppen (1965) submitted a general questionnaire and two personality questionnaires to groups of patients suffering from neurosis, affective disorders and schizophrenia. Compared with the controls, women suffering from neurosis complained more frequently of irritability, depression, anxiety and headaches around menstruation and at other times of the menstrual cycle. The schizophrenic group reported far fewer menstrual symptoms than the controls whilst the prevalence of symptoms in women with affective disorders did not differ significantly from those of controls except for menstrual depression.

However, this last finding is only partially supported by those of Diamond *et al.* (1976) who compared the type, severity and frequency of perimenstrual symptoms reported by women with affective disorders to those of a control group. Although there were no differences between the groups for most of the somatic symptoms, the patient group tended to report more affective symptoms. Likewise, Kashiwagi *et al*. (1976) interviewed 81 women attending a neurology clinic and noted that patients with a history of affective disorders were more likely to suffer from psychological premenstrual symptoms than patients with other psychiatric conditions. An association between affective disorders and premenstrual symptoms was also found by Wetzel *et al*. (1975) who charted the medical attendances of a number of college students and discovered that the women recording premenstrual symptoms at the start of the university year were significantly more likely than those who did not report them to seek psychiatric help, particularly for affective disorders during the subsequent four years.

The relationship between premenstrual symptoms and psychiatric ill-health was also investigated by Clare (1983) who studied a large number of women attending their general practitioner and found that of those reporting premenstrual symptoms, approximately half scored positively on the General Health Questionnaire, (indicating the presence of a non-psychotic psychiatric condition). The psychiatrically ill women reported more premenstrual symptoms than the psychiatrically healthy ones, particularly psychological symptoms like depression. However, there was no difference in their respective tendency to complain of physical symptoms such as breast tenderness and weight gain and when symptoms belonging to the negative affect and concentration factors were removed from the analysis, the relationship between psychiatric ill-health and the severity of premenstrual complaints ceased to be significant. Clare suggested that the psychiatrically ill women probably had less severe symptoms than the psychiatrically healthy women but that the former had been sensitized by their condition to the comparatively mild cyclical changes which they consequently identified as symptoms and complained about.

The possibility that some women's perception and reporting of premenstrual symptoms may be coloured by concurrent psychological problems was also considered by Taylor (1979) who speculated that factors such as a fear of pregnancy, the dislike of the inconvenience which accompanies menstruation, and even secondary gain may sensitize certain women to menstrual phenomena so that their subjective appreciation of normal physiological changes are magnified. As a result, they are more likely than other women to report troublesome symptoms.

While the majority of the above studies suggest that some women reporting premenstrual symptoms may have certain psychological difficulties, research has also indicated that there are many women who experience premenstrual distress but who do not suffer from either primary or secondary psychiatric problems, and furthermore do not show any unusual psychological characteristics (Clare, 1983; Haskett *et al*, 1980; Rees, 1953).

For instance, Seagull (1974) found no difference on measures of neuroticism and adequacy of personality functioning between groups reporting severe and mild premenstrual tension. James and Pollitt (1974) administered the Hysteroid-Obsessoid Questionnaire (HOQ) to women with premenstrual symptoms and reported that the correlations between the two factors were weak and non-significant. However, there was a significant correlation between deviation on the HOQ and a tendency to complain and they concluded that there was probably a strong though non-specific relationship between personality extremes and a tendency to complain.

More recently, Laws (1985) claimed that many women focus on PMS instead of facing and dealing with their other problems such as stressful relationships or adverse circumstances. Consequently they find it more difficult to cope with otherwise unobtrusive premenstrual alterations in mood.

Several authors, most notably Clare (1983) and Rees (1953, 1976) have tried to integrate and assimilate the mass of contradictory data into multi-dimensional models. These models focus on the interaction between cycle-related physiological changes and social, cultural, psychological and environmental factors, each differing in the relative importance which they attribute to a particular variable. For instance, Rees (1976) viewed PMS as a somato-psychic disorder in which biological processes, such as a deficiency in the secretion of progesterone, are of primary importance. However, he believed that the severity of the syndrome was a product of the physiological changes plus the reaction of the patient as determined by her personality, stability and emotional state.

The relationship between premenstrual symptomatology, personality variables and 'stress' is obviously a complex one and although studies have tended to concentrate on personality deficiencies and existing psychiatric ill-health, a woman's ability to cope with stressful events and internal biological changes may be compromised by a number of other factors. These include the number and severity of stressors, the absence of social support, dissatisfaction with work and home life, the existence of menstrual taboos and social disapproval of cycle-related conditions. In order to clarify the role of psychosocial factors in the aetiology of premenstrual symptoms a distinction should be made in future research between women whose symptoms recur every month and are limited to the second half of the cycle and those women whose premenstrual symptoms also occur at other times and which may represent an exacerbation of a separate physical or psychological condition (i.e. menstrual distress).

If such a differentiation is not made, the extent to which particular stressors (and personality traits) modify the experience of premenstrual symptoms will remain difficult to ascertain.

The Influence of Attitudes and Beliefs on Symptom Reporting

An issue which has received much attention in recent years is the accuracy of self-reports used to assess premenstrual symptoms. Where studies have used questionnaires to get retrospective and concurrent accounts of cycle-related experiences, there have been some noticeable discrepancies in the scores from the two measures (Moos, 1985; Parlee, 1982). Consequently, doubts were cast on the accuracy of the self-reports used in research and it was suggested that the more pronounced cyclical changes noted in the many retrospective reports may reflect socially-shared beliefs about the discomfort experienced around menstruation (Clare, 1983; Parlee, 1974, 1982; Ruble and Brooks-Gunn, 1982). For instance, Ruble and Brooks-Gunn noted from their research that young girls expected to feel more menstrual pain than is actually experienced and their studies suggest that beliefs about menstrual and pre-menstrual discomfort are acquired early, often before the menarche.

Further evidence that culturally-influenced beliefs may affect responses on menstrual questionnaires was provided by Parlee (1974) who asked a group of female and male students to describe symptoms which 'women sometimes experience' during three different cycle phases. She found that men scored higher than the women on all except one of the eight MDQ subscales, although both groups agreed as to which symptoms tend to change during the cycle and which do not. Discussing the results, she suggested that the women had probably based their responses on their own experiences while the men had probably based theirs on what they had learned about menstruation through a myriad of social sources. However, because of the high correlations between the male and female data, she thought that both groups might have been influenced by stereotypic beliefs about menstruation. This led several researchers to examine the effect of labelling symptoms as menstrual. Cernovetz *et al*. (1979) gave the MDQ to one group of college men and women with the usual instructions and to another group who were told that the symptoms occurred frequently among college students. The scores of the men and the women were generally similar although the women reported *less* distress on six out of the eight MDQ subscales when those symptoms were labelled as menstrual. In contrast, Markum (1976) found that awareness that the symptoms were menstrual ones did not significantly affect the responses.

In another study, Ruble (1977) informed a group of female college students who were all in the premenstrual phase that they were either in the premenstrual phase and about to menstruate or in the intermenstrual phase of the cycle. The 'premenstrual' subjects recorded significantly higher scores than the 'intermenstrual' subjects on items for water retention, pain, change in eating habits and sexual arousal, but there were no differences between the groups on scores for negative affect, concentration, behaviour change, autonomic reactions and arousal. The results from this study are often quoted as evidence that beliefs about the menstrual cycle can influence women's reporting of their experiences (Parlee, 1982; Slade, 1983; Spencer-Gardner *et al*., 1983) even though the actual differences between the two groups were often very small. This was particularly true for psychological symptoms such as tension, irritability and mood swings. Stereotypic beliefs may have played a part, but it is also possible that the responses obtained in this study were influenced by demand characteristics, which as Aubuchon and Calhoun (1985) showed can have a marked effect on the reporting of cycle related symptoms.

The possibility of biased responses on menstrual questionnaires must be considered when interpreting data from women complaining of premenstrual symptoms especially since some studies have found that women classed as sufferers of premenstrual symptoms on the basis of menstrual questionnaires do not show a marked premenstrual increase in symptoms when these are subsequently assessed by other means. For example, one in six of the women classified by Clare (1983) as premenstrual 'complainers' on the basis of their scores on the MDQ had to be reclassed as non-sufferers following a subsequent interview. While it is conceivable that some may exaggerate their experiences, a number of women as Gannon (1981) has pointed out, may underestimate cycle-related changes particularly on retrospective questionnaires, because they are not aware of the temporal relationship between their cycle and the symptoms and consequently do not consider certain symptoms as menstruation related.

Another factor which may give a slightly distorted view of cycle related symptoms is the possibility that some women may place undue emphasis on the negative states, moods and behaviours and will dismiss positive experiences. It is certainly true that many items on menstrual questionnaires refer to unpleasant or uncomfortable changes, probably because many researchers have been concerned with those symptoms seen in medical practice, but as several studies have shown when women are asked about positive aspects of their cycle, they will acknowledge these as well (Abplanalp et al., 1979; Collins, 1985; Parlee, 1982; Sanders et al., 1983).

In conclusion it is very difficult, given the inconsistencies between the various studies, both in methodology and results, to draw any firm conclusions about the extent to which social expectancy, attitudes and beliefs, whether positive or negative, determine actual experience of cyclical events and responses on self-report instruments. More work is needed in this area, particularly research involving women who have been specifically selected on the basis of clear cut premenstrual symptoms.

Discussion

For many years, women complaining of premenstrual symptoms were considered to have a psychological rather than an organic disorder (Vaitukaitis, 1984). The frequent reports of affective symptoms such as anxiety and irritability in studies of premenstrual distress encouraged speculation of a relationship between cycle-related symptoms and psychiatric disorders, and this was further supported by studies revealing a high prevalence of premenstrual complaints in women with affective disorders (De Jong et al., 1985; Halbreich et al., 1983; Warnes and Hill, 1975). Psychological factors have also been implicated as a result of large placebo responses found in some of the controlled clinical trials of drugs used to treat premenstrual symptoms (Abraham, 1984; Magos et al., 1986) and because of the correlational studies linking the incidence of premenstrual symptoms with high scores on personality inventories measuring neuroticism (Coppen and Kessel, 1963; Taylor, 1979). In the literature, sufferers have been portrayed as vulnerable personalities (Dennerstein et al., 1984) who are unable to cope with the demands made upon them (Sampson, 1984). Not surprisingly, Clare (1983) found that women visiting their general practitioner with one or more premenstrual complaint, which was either moderate or severe, were more likely than symptom-free women to have a psychiatric condition diagnosed as their current medical problem by their doctor and they were more likely to have a drug prescribed. More recently Alexander et al. (1986) discovered that half the general practitioners they questioned considered women suffering from premenstrual symptoms to be more hypochondriacal and introverted than women in general.

However, many of the studies which have been quoted in support of a psychogenic or psychosomatic explanation suffer from a number of methodological flaws. For instance, many investigations have employed retrospective questionnaires which are generally considered to be less valid than daily self-reports because they are more susceptible to the effect of memory distortion. Moreover, many of the mood scales used have not been subjected to rigorous testing to assess their validity and reliability and there is a great variation in the definition of PMS adopted by the researchers, from the strict operational definition formulated by Dalton (1984) to the classification into high and low PMS groups on the basis of whether or not subjects were troubled by PMS (Hart and Russell, 1986).

The samples of women which have been recruited have generally been unrepresentative and biased towards nurses and volunteers, very few of whom were selected for their premenstrual symptoms (Lamb et al., 1953; Wilcoxon et al., 1976; Ruble, 1977; Slade, 1983; Aubuchon and Calhoun, 1985). A comparison of the data from Goudsmit (1983) and Golub (1976) indicates that women who attended a hospital department for their premenstrual symptoms reported more severe symptoms than volunteers from the general population. Similarly, Sanders et al. (1983) assessing women who had sought medical help for their premenstrual distress and a group of volunteers found that although both groups showed basically the same pattern of cyclical changes, the out-patients reported more intense changes and their negative experiences began noticeably earlier in the cycle.

Another problem is that of confounding due to similarity of instruments.

The questions asked in order to ascertain the presence of psychiatric illness are often similar to those found in menstrual questionnaires. Because of the possibility of contamination, Gannon (1981) suggested that specific questions assessing particular personality traits were preferable to large scale personality inventories.

Care must also be taken when interpreting the results from correlational studies, for example, the largest correlation coefficient between neuroticism and premenstrual symptoms reported by Coppen and Kessel (1963) was 0.29 which represents approximately 9 per cent of the variance. This does not offer a great deal of support for a proposed relationship between the two factors although this has not deterred many authors from inferring one or from suggesting a causal link between one factor and the other.

The tendency in the literature has been to see personality traits such as emotional oversensitivity and 'stress', as factors which can exacerbate and predispose women to premenstrual distress (Halbreich and Kas, 1977; Sampson, 1983, 1984). However, little mention has been made of the role which premenstrual symptoms may have in exacerbating 'stress' or its effects on personality. For instance, it is possible that high scores on inventories measuring trait anxiety may, at least in part, reflect many years of disabling symptoms which recur every month, last up to two weeks and are difficult to control. The anxiety they provoke could in turn increase the predisposition of women to respond to stressful situations with more anxiety. Likewise, successive episodes of premenstrual distress may lower a woman's self-esteem and undermine her self-confidence (cf. Spencer-Gardner et al., 1983).

Regularly occurring premenstrual symptoms could also cause 'wear and tear' in the woman, producing physical as well as functional damage and this in itself may provoke physiological stress, compromising a woman's ability to cope. One might expect therefore, to see an increase in the duration and severity of symptoms the longer these symptoms last and this would explain the finding by Sanders et al. (1983) that women seeking medical help for their premenstrual disturbances recorded more intense and longer lasting symptoms than a group of slightly younger volunteers.

Since the majority of sufferers reported in the literature are married (Goudsmit, 1988; Haskett et al., 1980; Spencer-Gardner et al., 1983; Dalton, 1984) and many of them are working at home, caring for children (Clare, 1983; Sanders et al., 1983), it has been suggested that such a lifestyle, with its inescapable commitments may make cyclical changes in mood and well being less easy to tolerate, while also aggravating symptoms like irritability and fatigue. Unfortunately, few studies, particularly longitudinal investigations, have focussed on the effects of premenstrual disturbances on a woman's personality and home life and this area deserves further attention.

Perhaps the most important of the methodological issues affecting research on premenstrual symptoms is that of definition. There is still no universally accepted definition of PMS (but see p. 5) although most agree that since some of the symptoms which are reported premenstrually may also occur at other times during the cycle, the term PMS should be restricted for research purposes at least to those symptoms which show a marked increase during the premenstrual phase. It is also important at this stage to differentiate mild and tolerable cyclical phenomena from the moderate and severe symptoms which interfere with a woman's daily life. And since premenstrual symptoms may be affected by concurrent stressful situations, only those women whose symptoms recur monthly and are well-established should be recruited for research purposes.

Adopting the definition and criteria of Dalton (1980, 1984) for the diagnosis of PMS, Goudsmit (1983, 1988) compared women suffering from PMS with women who did not fulfil the set criteria (the menstrual distress group) and a non-symptomatic control group. The type, timing, intensity of and changes in certain symptoms were recorded on days twelve, eighteen, 22 and 26 of the menstrual cycle using a modified version of the MDQ, the State and Trait Anxiety Inventory and the Depression Adjective Check List. The 20 experimental subjects were all patients attending the gynaecology department at St Thomas's Hospital in London and none of them were taking psychotropic drugs, diuretics or hormonal preparations. The control group consisted of ten medical students and members of the hospital staff who were significantly younger than the patient groups.

Although the number of subjects was small, there were clear group differences in the pattern of the scores recorded during the cycle (see Figure 1). The mean scores of the fifteen subjects in the PMS group rose from day eighteen of the cycle and continued to increase as the cycle progressed while the scores of the remaining five women whose symptoms occurred intermittently during the cycle did not show a significant premenstrual increase.

The scores for state anxiety and depression recorded by the PMS group on day twelve were generally low and similar to those reported by women from the general population. In contrast, the scores on day 26 were significantly higher and comparable to those of psychiatric patients. The trait anxiety scores of half the subjects in the PMS group were outside the normal range and showed significant increases from day eighteen onwards. As trait anxiety refers to a personality characteristic, the scores should have remained fairly stable throughout the cycle and the fact that the scores of the PMS group increased, suggests that some of the women may have changed the way in which they perceived themselves as they experienced more discomfort.

The results clearly indicate the differences between women whose symptoms occurred primarily during the second half of the menstrual cycle and those women whose symptoms were present throughout the cycle. Such differences were also found by Haskett et al. (1980) who observed that

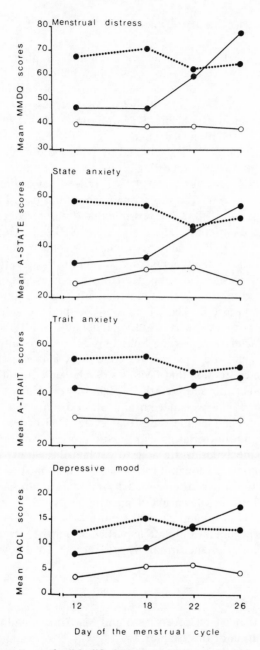

Figure 1. Mean scores on the 'Modified Menstrual Distress Questionnaire' (MMDQ), the 'State and Trait Anxiety Inventory' (STAI) and the 'Depression Adjective Check List' (DACL), recorded on four days during the menstrual cycle by a group of women with PMS (●————●), a group with menstrual distress (●·········●), and a control group (○————○)

women with high MDQ scores during the follicular phase reported more psychological and behavioural symptoms than women recording low follicular MDQ scores. Analysis of the data using a variety of personality tests suggested that the women with the high follicular scores were suffering from non-specific subclinical 'characterologic' or neurotic disturbances which were exacerbated during the premenstruum. Further research is needed to confirm the existence of a 'pure' PMS as defined by Dalton although it is clear from existing studies that women reporting premenstrual symptoms do not form a homogeneous group (Brooks-Gunn, 1986). Indeed, several researchers have claimed that there are subgroups of women who suffer from PMS (Abraham, 1983; Halbreich, *et al*., 1983). It is possible that different symptoms or groups of symptoms have different causes and that as Brooks-Gunn (1986) has suggested, while 'pure' PMS may be primarily a somatic condition, psychosocial factors may be more influential in determining the experience of women with menstrual distress. Again, this needs further investigation.

At present, the literature is littered with confusing and contradictory data, conjecture and supposition. There is a lack of methodologically sound studies which have incorporated a strict operational definition of PMS and this makes it extremely difficult to assess the links between this condition and certain personality characteristics, psychiatric conditions and stressful life events. Evidence for the contention that PMS is a psychogenic condition is generally unconvincing and cannot satisfactorily explain why certain symptoms, particularly physical ones like weight gain and mastodynia, tend to occur solely during the second half of the menstrual cycle. Conversely, there is much support for the multifactorial psychosomatic models, which by allowing for different causal mechanisms are able to explain the variety in number and severity of symptoms, although it can be argued that most of them may have underestimated the role of premenstrual symptoms as stressors.

As yet, very little is known about underlying psychological processes or about the effect of social and cultural factors on the experience of premenstrual symptoms in general and PMS in particular. Further research to increase our understanding of premenstrual distress should prove a worthwhile challenge.

Acknowledgements

I would like to thank Dr Doreen Asso and Ms Anne Dundas for their help with the preparation of this chapter.

References

Abplanalp, J. M., Donnelly, A. F. and Rose, R. M. (1979). Psychoendocrinology of the menstrual cycle: 1. Enjoyment of daily activities and moods. *Psychosomatic Medicine*, **41**, 587–604.

Abraham, G. E. (1983). Nutritional factors in the etiology of the premenstrual tension syndromes. *Journal of Reproductive Medicine*, **28**, 446–464.

Abraham, S. (1984). Premenstrual or postmenstrual syndrome? *Medical Journal of Australia*, **141**, 327–328.

Alexander, D. A., Taylor, R. J. and Fordyce, I. D. (1986). Attitudes of general practitioners towards premenstrual symptoms and those who suffer from them. *Journal of the Royal College of General Practitioners*, **36**, 10–12.

Aubuchon, P. G. and Calhoun, K. S. (1985). Menstrual cycle symptomatology; the role of social expectancy and experimental demand characteristics. *Psychosomatic Medicine*, **47**, 35–45.

Bernsted, L., Luggin, R. and Petersson, B. (1984). Psychosocial considerations of the premenstrual syndrome. *Acta Psychiatrica Scandinavica*, **69**, 455–460.

Berry, C. and McGuire, F. L. (1972). Menstrual distress and acceptance of sexual role. *American Journal of Obstetrics and Gynecology*, **114**, 83–87.

Brooks-Gunn, J. (1986). Differentiating premenstrual symptoms and syndromes. *Psychosomatic Medicine*, **48**, 385–387.

Chernovetz, M. E., Jones, W. H. and Hansson, R. O. (1979). Predictability, attentional focus, sex role orientation, and menstrual-related stress. *Psychosomatic Medicine*, **41**, 383–391.

Clare, A. W. (1983). Psychiatric and Social Aspects of Premenstrual Complaint. *Psychological Medicine. Monograph Supplement 4*, Cambridge University Press, Cambridge.

Collins, A. (1985). *Sex Differences in Psychoneuroendocrine Stress Responses. Biological and Social Influences*. Thesis. Department of Psychology, University of Stockholm.

Coppen, A. and Kessel, N. (1963). Menstruation and personality. *British Journal of Psychiatry*, **109**, 711–721.

Coppen, A. (1965). The prevalence of menstrual disorders in psychiatric patients. *British Journal of Psychiatry*, **111**, 155–167.

Dalton, K. (1980). Progesterone, fluid, and electrolytes in premenstrual syndrome. *British Medical Journal*, **281**, 61.

Dalton, K. (1984). *The Premenstrual Syndrome and Progesterone Therapy*. (2nd edition) Heinemann, London.

De Jong, R., Rubinow, D. R., Roy-Byrne, P., Hoban, C., Grover, G. N. and Post, R. M. (1985). Premenstrual mood disorder and psychiatric illness. *American Journal of Psychiatry*, **142**, 1359–1361.

De Leeuw, E. D. (1982). *Menstruatie: Ervaringen, Kennis en Attituden*. Dissertation. Department of Psychology. University of Amsterdam.

Dennerstein, L., Spencer-Gardner, C. and Burrows, G. D. (1984). Mood and the menstrual cycle. *Journal of Psychiatric Research*, **18**, 1–12.

Deutsch, H. (1944). *The Psychology of Women*. Research Books, London.

Diamond, S. B., Rubinstein, A. A., Dunner, D. L. and Fieve, R. R. (1976). Menstrual problems in women with primary affective illness. *Comprehensive Psychiatry*, **17**, 541–548.

Fugate-Woods, F., Kramer Dery, G. and Most, E. (1982). Recollections of menarche, current menstrual attitudes, and perimenstrual symptoms. *Psychosomatic Medicine*, **44**, 285–293.

Gannon, L. (1981). Evidence for a psychological etiology of menstrual disorders: a critical review. *Psychological Reports*, **48**, 287–294.

Golub, S. (1976). The magnitude of premenstrual anxiety and depression. *Psychosomatic Medicine*, **38**, 4–12.

Goudsmit, E. M. (1983). Psychological aspects of premenstrual symptoms. *Journal of Psychosomatic Obstetrics and Gynaecology*, **2**, 20–26.

Goudsmit, E. M. (1988). Anxiety and depression in the premenstrual syndrome, in *Stress and Anxiety*, Vol. 11, (Eds. C. D. Spielberger, I. G. Sarason and P. B. Defares) Hemisphere, New York, pp. 211–217.

Gough, H. G. (1975). Personality factors related to reported severity of menstrual distress. *Journal of Abnormal Psychology*, **84**, 59–65.

Gruba, G. H. and Rohrbaugh, M. (1975). MMPI correlates of menstrual distress. *Psychosomatic Medicine*, **37**, 265–273.

Halbreich, U., Endicott, J. and Nee, J. (1983). Premenstrual depressive changes. Value of differentiation. *Archives of General Psychiatry*, **40**, 535–542.

Halbreich, U. and Kas, D. (1977). Variations in the Taylor MAS of women with premenstrual syndrome. *Journal of Psychosomatic Research*, **21**, 391–393.

Hart, W. G. and Russell, J. W. (1986). A prospective comparison study of premenstrual symptoms. *Medical Journal of Australia*, **144**, 466–468.

Haskett, R. F., Steiner, M., Osmun, J. N. and Carroll, B. J. (1980). Severe premenstrual tension: delineation of the syndrome. *Biological Psychiatry*, **15**, 121–139.

Horney, K. (1967). Premenstrual tension, in *Feminine Psychology* (Ed. H. Kelman), W. W. Norton, New York, pp. 99–106.

James, H. and Pollitt, J. (1974). Personality and premenstrual tension. *Proceedings of the Royal Society of Medicine*, **67**, 921–923.

Kashiwagi, T., McClure, J. N. and Wetzel, R. D. (1976). Premenstrual affective syndrome and psychiatric disorder. *Diseases of the Nervous System*, **37**, 116–119.

Koeske, R. D. (1983). Lifting the curse of menstruation: toward a feminist perspective on the menstrual cycle. *Women and Health*, **8**, 1–16.

Lamb, W. M., Ulett, G. A., Masters, W. H. and Robinson, D. W. (1953). Premenstrual tension: EEG, hormonal, and psychiatric evaluation. *American Journal of Psychiatry*, **109**, 840–848.

Laws, S. (1985). Who needs PMT? A feminist approach to the politics of premenstrual tension, in *Seeing Red: the politics of premenstrual tension* (Eds. S. Laws, V. Hey and A. Eagan) Hutchinson, London, pp. 16–64.

Magos, A. L., Brincat, M. and Studd, J. W. W. (1986). Treatment of the premenstrual syndrome by subcutaneous oestradiol implants and cyclical oral norethisterone: placebo controlled study. *British Medical Journal*, **292**, 1629–1633.

Markum, R. A. (1976). Assessment of the reliability of and the effect of neutral instructions on the symptom ratings on the Moos Menstrual Distress Questionnaire. *Psychosomatic Medicine*, **38**, 163–172.

Moos, R. H. (1985). *Perimenstrual Symptoms: A Manual and Overview of Research with the Menstrual Distress Questionnaire*. Social Ecology Laboratory, Standford University, Palo Alto, California.

Notman, M. (1982). The psychiatrist's approach, in *Premenstrual Tension. A Multidisciplinary Approach*. (Ed. C. Debrovner) Life Sciences Press, New York, pp. 53–63.

Paige, K. (1973). Women learn to sing the menstrual blues. *Psychology Today*, **7**, 41–46.

Parlee, M. B. (1974). Stereotypic beliefs about menstruation: a methodological note on the Moos Menstrual Distress Questionnaire and some new data. *Psychosomatic Medicine*, **36**, 229–240.

Parlee, M. B. (1982). The psychology of the menstrual cycle. Biological and psychological aspects, in *Behaviour and the Menstrual Cycle*. (Ed. R. C. Friedman) Marcel Dekker, New York, pp. 77–99.

Paulson, M. J. (1961). Psychological concomitants of premenstrual tension. *American Journal of Obstetrics and Gynecology*, **81**, 733–738.

Radcliffe-Richards, J. (1982). PMT—an obstacle in the fight for female equality. *The Listener*, **April 29**, 9–10.

Rees, L. (1953). Psychosomatic aspects of the premenstrual tension syndrome. *Journal of Mental Science*, **99**, 62–73.

Rees, W. L. (1976). Stress, distress and disease. *British Journal of Psychiatry*, **128**, 3–18.

Riven, L. (1983). Premenstrual syndrome: a psychological overview. *Canadian Family Physician*, **29**, 1919–1924.

Ruble, D. N. (1977). Premenstrual symptoms: a reinterpretation. *Science*, **197**, 291–292.

Ruble, D. N. and Brooks-Gunn, J. (1982). A developmental analysis of menstrual distress in adolescence, in *Behaviour and the Menstrual Cycle*, (Ed. R. C. Friedman) Marcel Dekker, New York, pp. 177–197.

Sampson, G. A. (1983). Stress and premenstrual syndrome, in *Premenstrual Syndrome*, (Ed. R. W. Taylor) Medical News Tribune Ltd, London, pp. 43–49.

Sampson, G. A. (1984). The role of the psychiatrist in the treatment of premenstrual syndrome. *Maternal and Child Health*, **March**, 96–101.

Sanders, D., Warner, P., Bäckström, T. and Bancroft, J. (1983). Mood, sexuality, hormones, and the menstrual cycle. 1. Changes in mood and physical state: description of subjects and method. *Psychosomatic Medicine*, **45**, 487–501.

Seagull, E. A. (1974). An investigation of personality differences between women with high and low premenstrual tension. *Dissertation Abstracts International*, **34, 9B**, 4675.

Shainess, N. (1961). A re-evaluation of some aspects of femininity through a study of menstruation: a preliminary report. *Comprehensive Psychiatry*, **2**, 20–26.

Shuttle, P. and Redgrove, P. (1978). *The Wise Wound*, Gollanz, London.

Siegel, J. M., Johnson, J. H. and Sarason, I. G. (1979). Life changes and menstrual discomfort. *Journal of Human Stress*, **5**, 41–46.

Slade, P. and Jenner, F. A. (1980). Attitudes to female roles, aspects of menstruation and complaining of menstrual symptoms. *British Journal of Social and Clinical Psychology*, **19**, 109–113.

Slade, P. (1983). Premenstrual emotional changes in normal women: fact or fiction? *Journal of Psychosomatic Research*, **28**, 1–7.

Spencer-Gardner, C., Dennerstein, L. and Burrows, G. D. (1983). Premenstrual tension and female role. *Journal of Psychosomatic Obstetrics and Gynaecology*, **2**, 27–34.

Taylor, J. W. (1979). Psychological factors in the aetiology of premenstrual symptoms. *Australian and New Zealand Journal of Psychiatry*, **13**, 35–41.

Vaitukaitis, J. L. (1984). Premenstrual syndrome. *New England Journal of Medicine*, **311**, 1371–1373.

Van Assen, F. J. J. (1962). *Premenstruele Spanning*, Thesis. Department of Medicine, University of Leiden.

Warnes, H. and Hill, G. (1975). On the premenstrual syndrome. *Modern Medicine (New Zealand)*, **8**, 45–49.

Watts, S., Dennerstein, L. and Horne, D. J. de L. (1980). The premenstrual syndrome. A psychological evaluation. *Journal of Affective Disorders*, **2**, 257–266.

Watts, J. F. F., Butt, W. R. and Logan Edwards, R. (1985). Hormonal studies in women with premenstrual tension. *British Journal of Obstetrics and Gynaecology*, **92**, 247–255.

Wetzel, R. D., Reich, T., McClure, J. N. and Wald, J. A. (1975). Premenstrual affective syndrome and affective disorder. *British Journal of Psychiatry*, **127**, 219–221.

Wilcoxon, L. A., Schrader, S. L. and Sherif, C. W. (1976). Daily self-reports on activities, life events, moods, and somatic changes during the menstrual cycle. *Psychosomatic Medicine*, **38**, 399–417.

Wood, C., Larsen, L. and Williams, R. (1979). Social and psychological factors in relation to premenstrual tension and menstrual pain. *Australian and New Zealand Journal of Obstetrics and Gynaecology*, **19**, 111–115.

Functional Disorders of the Menstrual Cycle
Edited by M. G. Brush and E. M. Goudsmit
© 1988 John Wiley & Sons Ltd

CHAPTER 11

Cognitive therapy for premenstrual syndrome

CAROL A. MORSE and LORRAINE DENNERSTEIN
Department of Psychiatry,
University of Melbourne,
Austin Hospital,
Heidelberg, Victoria 3084
Australia

Introduction

Premenstrual syndrome (PMS) is the contemporary name for a complex array of symptoms that trouble many women during their reproductive years. Predisposing factors seem to arise from an interaction of biophysical, psychological and social conditions (Dennerstein and Burrows, 1979). Large scale surveys (e.g. Van Keep and Lehert, 1981) have shown that 30–70 per cent of women report emotional distress and 30–60 per cent report physical changes which occur in the late luteal or premenstrual phase of the menstrual cycle. Fewer women than these actually regard these noticeable changes in themselves as a problem, and fewer still seek treatment. Clare (1985) has recently proposed that perhaps only about 10 per cent of women really experience 'true' PMS and that another 20 per cent may seek help for PMS when in fact alternative diagnoses could be made.

The earlier name for the syndrome was premenstrual tension (PMT), which was first described in 1931 by Frank. He had observed female patients complaining of indescribable tension, irritability and depression, with desires 'to find relief by foolish and ill-considered actions', that occurred in cyclical waves prior to menstruation. This description was later modified by Greene and Dalton (1953) and Dalton (1964) and PMS was defined to include recognition of both physical and psychological symptoms that occurred in the premenstrual phase, which were relieved during menstruation, with at least one week that was symptom-free. Those women who report symptoms throughout the cycle with premenstrual exacerbation in severity were regarded as menstrual distress sufferers and not as true PMS-complainants (Dalton, 1980).

Four main categories of premenstrual symptoms have recently been described (Morse and Dennerstein, 1986). These are physical symptoms (pain, swelling, mastalgia); emotional distress (anxiety, depression, irritability, hostility); cognitive failures (concentration loss, memory disturbances); and changed cognitive schemata (loss of self-esteem, inadequate coping, changed self-concept).

Women complaining of PMS are frequently described as experiencing major stress from some social role (e.g. marriage, parenthood or occupation). Experiences of distress from these sources are thought to interact with cyclical hormonal changes resulting in exacerbation of premenstrual negative moods and disruptive behaviours. If these distress sources are resolved then reported symptoms should decrease or disappear. This frequently seems to be the case when, for example, following the resolution of a parent–child conflict, or marital problems, the premenstrual symptoms seem to abate. Unfortunately, however, symptoms often return at a later date when some other stress develops and this suggests that effective coping strategies are fragile due to lack of conviction, inconsistent use, or both.

Women seeking treatment tend to report strain on certain social roles occasioned by their regular premenstrual experiences. This perspective suggests that a negative expectance set occurs at the anticipation of unpleasant premenstrual experiences. This preconception results in raised anxiety levels, feelings of tension and negative moods that appear to respond to cyclical hormonal changes, whether normal or abnormal, resulting in certain symptom patterns. These in turn, may be adversely affected by concurrent social stresses, or alternatively, social relationships may deteriorate from the impact of negative moods and changed behaviours. In all of these equations, each aspect (hormones, symptoms, stress, social roles) can act as both stimulus and response at several levels in chained sequences. This illustrates the contemporary view of psychosomatic conditions (Reiser, 1975) that develop through constant reciprocal interaction with the individual's environment. The important element not yet examined is the individual's belief system or patterns of cognitive style that mediate within the stimulus–response (S–R) equations at every phase.

A Cognitive Approach to Understanding PMS

Women who do seek help commonly report an awareness of premenstrual irritability, feelings of anger, poorly controlled social behaviour, poor physical co-ordination, feelings of tension, restlessness, fatigue, loss of concentration leading to a poor standard of logical thinking and decision-making, weight gain, swelling, sore breasts, feelings of depression, low self-esteem and worthlessness. In addition to these most frequently reported difficulties women may refer to a variety of aches and pains, skin changes, sleep pattern

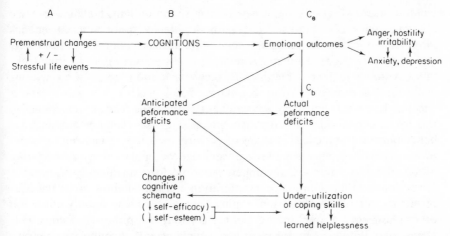

Figure 1. A cognitive model of premenstrual syndrome (A = Activating events; B = Beliefs, cognitions; C_b = Behavioural consequences; C_e = Emotional consequences)

alterations, and appetite problems, usually cravings for certain sweet foods. In essence, they are complaining not only of personal distress that is periodically experienced, but also they are expressing concern about the effects of these changes on important others in their lives (children and partners, in particular). This concern incorporates a partially expressed fear about the permanent damage being done to their important relationships for which they feel responsible but helpless.

A cognitive model has been proposed by Morse and Dennerstein (1986) that provides a framework within which the roles of cognitions in PMS may be conceptualized. The model is presented in Figure 1.

A rational–emotive framework (Ellis, 1962, 1975) is utilized to explain the cause–effect links between symptoms, feelings, thinking, behaviours, and self-concept. In this model, the activating event is the cluster of premenstrual changes that take place and which are experienced as additional strain (stress) with or without concurrent adverse life stresses. Over an uncertain time frame, these changes trigger off specific overlearned stereotypic cognitions at the beliefs level that are characteristic of high-anxious individuals who tend to respond to and interpret their personal and social contexts as overwhelming (i.e. over demanding) and threatening. Statements bordering on the irrational are common such as: 'I can't stand this. Being premenstrual means I'll fall apart! It's terrible! He/she/they (the world) should be more understanding and treat me better.' These 'irrational' beliefs, in turn, create or heighten levels of anxiety, depression, or anger resulting in consequent behaviours that typify these affective states. Behaviours result in secondary or tertiary levels of distress (e.g. feeling guilty about 'out of character' responses to spouse or children, feeling anxious about being anxious and uptight, feeling depressed about behaving as a depressed and apathetic wife and mother etc.). Feedback loops exist between emotions and cognitions so that feeling-states of anxiety and irritability trigger further secondary anxious and irritable thinking (self-talk). Also, anxious, irritable thinking feeds back into (one of) the activating event(s), (e.g. premenstrual phase), the woman labels it as a negative experience, and/or labels her social environment as (more) stressful. In response to this defensive mode of cognitive processing, she anticipates negative behavioural consequences in terms of performance deficits and this anticipation also adversely affects her self-concept (efficacy and esteem). Anticipation of lowered performance and competence to perform adequately often tends to result in actual performance deterioration in a self-fulfilling prophecy. This results in outcomes where usual coping strategies, which are ably utilized at other phases of the menstrual cycle, are severely compromised if not totally abandoned. When she finds herself behaving in ways that contravene her own personal standards, over time it is likely she will feel increasingly trapped in a 'downward spiral' that generates helplessness and hopelessness, leading to secondary levels of depression and lowered self-esteem. With the onset of menstruation, hormonal fluctuations are at a minimum and physical symptoms settle and gradually diminish. At this point the cognitive attributions change.

Simultaneously, menstruation is a visible sign of an underlying 'just' cause for the emotional and behavioural upheavals. Acceptance of the 'justifiable' explanation removes most of the personal responsibility for the recent changes in control. In this way, ascribing to a 'raging hormones' explanation by both men and women results in the dismissal of the woman's own cognitive processes which may be filling an important intermediary role.

Cognitive Processing in Women with Premenstrual Symptoms

The cognitive style of women complaining of premenstrual symptoms presenting to the University of Melbourne PMT Clinic since 1979 is characterized by vigilant perception of both external and internal events and the conceptualization of these as possible threats to interpersonal or emotional well-being. It is impressive that some of these women are very attentive to bodily fluctuations with the result that feelings and sensations are accorded pathological significance. This defensive and threatened cognitive set is characteristic of the anxiety-prone individual who, over time, has learned to respond to her internal environment, mental condition, and interpersonal world as arenas of threat, harm and overwhelming challenge (Beck and Emery, 1985). At the thinking level, demands are interpreted alternatively as threats or harm, either because they are too many in number to be dealt with competently (overload) or because it is believed they require more of the individual's personal capability than she feels able to provide (over extension). In either case, these women recognize that they do not cope premenstrually with their daily life conditions. This provides cause for further emotional distress (being upset because they do not cope, and not coping because they are experiencing premenstrual mood and physical changes). Treatment-seeking women frequently describe their feelings and behaviours as 'like Jekyll and Hyde' when they mean that the benign person becomes transformed into the hideous objectionable creature during the premenstrual phase that is regarded as the 'cause' of all the trouble. In fact, prospective reports of symptoms and behaviours frequently show problematic moods and symptoms at other phases of the cycle also, which then intensify in the late luteal phase (Hart and Russell, 1986; Morse *et al.*, 1987) thus demonstrating an important advantage of this type of assessment. However, only the premenstrual phase is given special attention and negative interpretations by the great majority of investigators.

Cognitive processing of women seeking PMS treatment operates at both general and specific levels. Over all, when these women, as high-anxious individuals, use a general processing style that is defensive and threatened it seems to occur particularly in instances of social importance. In addition, being acutely sensitive to physical changes they pay much attention to the cyclical alterations occasioned by hormonal fluctuations throughout the cycle which are then interpreted negatively at the premenstrual time, coloured by adverse moods. Over time, a purposeful though maladaptive response set becomes established. This means that as the premenstrual phase approaches, these overlearned responses of feelings and behaviours seem to occur automatically i.e. 'without thinking', which sabotage long-term goals whilst seeming to meet immediate and short-term requirements. This really refers to a particular style of coping which in fact, ultimately is self-defeating, both in terms of increased physical symptoms and worsened interpersonal relations. Holroyd and Lazarus (1982) have suggested that negative health outcomes arise from ineffective coping attempts rather than from the presence or absence of social stresses. Different patterns of catecholamine arousal have been identified when threat or challenge is perceived depending on whether the self is viewed as dominant or subordinate at that time (Henry and Stephens, 1977).

The individual who feels unable to manage effectively (coping psychologically) may instead focus on the physical functions of one system or another. In the long term, frequently mobilized physiological activations through psychoneuroendocrine pathways are likely to contribute to system disregulation, as described in the 'exhaustion' stage of the general adaptation syndrome. The PMS sufferer who has developed a defensive cognitive set interacts with the sensations and effects of regular menstrual cycle fluctuations and is more distressed than a woman who is less reactive and sensitized. The combination of physical change and loss of emotional stability often results in the adoption of purposeful though maladaptive behavioural sequences (e.g. resorting to sick-role behaviours or excessive self-demand for exemplary performances). These behavioural changes affect the woman's social environment. This may, in turn, respond with complaints and criticism. Also she commonly experiences secondary guilt about what her 'premenstrual problem' is doing to her important relationships. It seems it is possible to identify PMS-sufferers from nonsufferers, both by the magnitude of experienced premenstrual changes as well as by level of self-esteem, reported stress level, and presence of dysfunctional emotions (Morse *et al.*, 1986). It appears that the PMS treatment-seeker feels uncertain about her personal effectiveness, and she vacillates between nonassertion and aggression. She frequently experiences episodes of low self-esteem and her rejection or disapproval by others is anticipated in a myriad social situations. These perceptions are very influential in determining subsequent behaviours. Because she is vigilant in viewing social interactions negatively, she learns to behave in ways to minimize personal risks, particularly premenstrually, when she regards her capabilities as more fragile than usual. She may avoid overt social activities, resist initiating interactions, break off conversations, behave unassertively and dither in opinion formation and decision making. She may make considerable efforts to hold herself together and complete her paid work with little outward sign of inner turmoil and tension in nerves and muscles. The cost is likely borne through experiences of fatigue, lethargy and increased errors in fine-motor skills. At home with the family, she is likely 'to let it all out' through short-tempered nagging, criticism, and hostility which invites counter-responses from partners and children. Secondary emotional distress then ensues as she feels unloved and unappreciated, guilty about her own loss of control, and helpless in the face of her own biology which is surely the causative factor, and depressed about the reduced possibility of attaining positive outcomes from her daily life. It is highly likely that although she readily reports mood problems premenstrually she is overlooking or dismissing similar experiences at other times when she readily finds an external reason. Only premenstrually can and must the reason be internal, i.e. hormonal.

Cognitive Therapy Procedures

General Considerations

Cognitive therapy consists of the application of empirical procedures to the cognitive, affective, and behavioural processes of women troubled by PMS. A psycho-educational perspective is adopted that is both remedial and preventive. This approach teaches cognitive behavioural techniques to enhance the individual's repertoire of effective coping skills and to reduce the magnitude of distressing emotions. The psychotherapist assumes the role of teacher and the patient becomes a student who is regarded as capable of unlearning old assumptions, beliefs, expectations and behaviours. These are to be replaced by more appropriate self-enhancing thinking and actions that are likely to increase the acquisition of life goals and personal satisfactions. The basic strategy that underpins the therapeutic relationship is one of collaborative empiricism. This is the keynote in established cognitive therapies for other conditions e.g. treatment of depression (Beck *et al.*, 1979). Patient and therapist actively work together to identify problems-in-living that contribute to symptoms and to explore how symptoms adversely affect relationships and competent performance.

Emphasis is placed on a coping model rather than a mastery model with increased self-efficacy as a main goal. The cognitive behavioural programme developed for PMS utilizes a rational–emotive therapy (RET) framework to address the premenstrually magnified emotional and behavioural disturbances. Over time, although women report that their PMS adversely affects their relationships, because the direct A to C connection is clearly identified, what is less obvious to them is that their problems-in-living also adversely affect their premenstrual symptomatology. What is more, their beliefs and selftalk are powerful, though usually unperceived mediating forces that operate centrally throughout (Morse and Dennerstein, 1986).

Women who present to a specialist PMS clinic are often emotionally over-sensitive and have been found to have high anxiety, extraversion, feelings of inadequacy, ineffectual coping and low self-esteem. They express directly or indirectly feelings of powerlessness and an external attribution of good fortune and well-being. Many of these feelings are ubiquitous in women who seek help for a variety of problems and suggest the existence of some predisposition to vulnerability in treatment seeking. This has been noted elsewhere (Cohen, 1979; Morse *et al.*, 1987; Morse 1988). Wolfe 1985 has suggested that the common route lies in biased childhood sex role learning, where female children have been 'steeped . . . in the idea that their worth and happiness should derive from living for and through others'. While the ways in which early learning precedents are well-established are not readily accessible, the fact remains that many adult PMS sufferers exhibit low frustration tolerance, a readiness to over-exaggerate and over-analyze events and their effects and an anxious predisposition through which all aspects are coloured, processed and evaluated.

This results in a readiness to accept blame, to denigrate themselves, to seek external approval, to view their world as full of threats rather than challenges and to utilize fragile coping strategies that easily crumble at the first sign of opposition. On arrival at the clinic, women report multiple instances of cognitive failures (forgetfulness, clumsiness and poor or inappropriate decision making), all of which may be indicative of the over-extended, hypervigilant, cognitively-saturated, anxious individual (Beck and Emery, 1985). They are hyper-sensitive to normal hormonally induced fluctuation in affect and behaviour that occur diurnally (Lyons *et al.*, 1985) as well as cyclically, and they imbue these with pathological significance.

Group Therapy for PMS Sufferers

Small group therapy has been developed over the last four years for up to six women who meet weekly for a twelve week therapy programme. No more than six are taken into any one group, as this number has proven to be the maximum that profitably benefits with one therapist in terms of time and attention with specific problems. Sessions take place weekly for 90 min and meetings are offered during the day and early evening. The small group format is viewed very favourably as a comfortable setting where learning takes place from the therapist, from other members, through modelling, teaching and sharing. Group cohesion is quickly established after the first session which states aims and goals of the programme and addresses ideas and concerns of members about the programme and the group environment. Many groups have continued to remain in contact for on-going self help support long after the therapy programme has terminated. Individual participants have kept in touch by telephone or letter and referred friends and relatives to the clinic for help with similar or related problems.

Major Aspects of the Coping Skills Training for PMS

Coping Skills Training

The group programme is designated as coping skills training because women spontaneously express 'loss of coping' as a major concern when presenting for help, and also because cognitive–behaviour therapy is rather a formal, even foreign sounding terminology. Over time, they come to equate the programme with the ideas expressed in their bibliotherapy (Ellis and Harper, 1975) and they focus on the rational–emotive ideas almost to the exclusion of the behavioural components. From the outset, the circular cause-effect links of PMT as stimulus and response with thinking, feelings and behaviours are explained.

The premenstrual phase is proposed as an internal stressor in certain sensitized women. A basic description is given of ovarian hormone fluctuations and these are linked to common feelings at different phases of the menstrual cycle.

Anxiety-Reduction Techniques

Sessions two, three and four introduce the group to whole body relaxation techniques following Jacobsen's (1942) procedures. Nearly all of session two is devoted to learning relaxation methods. The amount of time in session three given to relaxation is reduced by about half in session four. Concurrently, information and ideas about the nature of anxiety, its sub-categories (ego and discomfort anxieties) and rational–emotive characteristics are increasingly introduced. From session two, each group member is provided with an audio tape of relaxation instructions from the three practice sessions to keep and use at home. Relaxation practice logs are also provided and discussions about effects and problems are invited at the following sessions.

Stress Inoculation and Rational Disputation

Sessions five to seven focus entirely on stress inoculation training in preparing to deal with a stressor, through the stressful experience, and post-event evaluation and self feedback. In addition, rational–emotive restructuring of weekly events takes place through blackboard display and discussion. Initially, on a one-to-one basis, the therapist explains the A–B–C structure (see Figure 1), identifies the rational and irrational beliefs and gradually introduces disputations. Gradually, the therapist shifts the focus by engaging in the role of facilitator, and invites other group members to identify the irrational beliefs and propose disputations to each other's reported events. Group support and help is usually high at these times, but the therapist should be vigilant for any sign of distress that may surface at any time in any individual member. These may be used advantageously to challenge additional underlying irrational beliefs, e.g. 'It's too awful to let these others know the true extent of my problem', or 'I don't know this stuff well enough—the therapist will think I'm stupid, that's too awful'.

Responsible Assertiveness Training

The element of felt powerlessness is challenged through sessions eight to twelve when non-assertion, assertion, and aggression are correctly identified and described. The cognitive elements in appropriate assertiveness are emphasized and behavioural tasks are presented which encourage practice in dealing effectively with demands from self and others, and preplanned expression of feelings, wants, and likes. Efficient non-verbal communication skills are identified and assertive techniques controlling thoughts including broken record, fogging-disarming, thought-stopping, and palliative distraction are taught. The final session includes an overview of progress. Identification of obstacles to progress and continuing goals for success are made. At this last meeting the therapist elicits feedback on the strengths and weaknesses of the programme for future modification.

Homework

Every session includes bibliotherapy which involves reading at least one prescribed chapter from Ellis & Harper (1975). Main points from the readings are required to be written down in a notebook for discussion the following week.

From week two, relaxation exercises and recordings of attempts are required to be carried out on a daily basis. Reports of the past week's events are invited to encourage the identification of the A–B–C components (see Figure 1).

Specific behavioural tasks are provided on a group basis (e.g. replacing a demand on another with a wish or preference), or on an individual basis if a specific problem surfaces and help is requested (e.g. time out and reward contingency programme for a child's unacceptable behaviours). Successes, partial successes and failures are all encouraged to be reported at subsequent sessions for group discussion and generation of alternative strategies. Group members learn from others vicariously and directly.

Follow-up

The therapist contacts each member after three months and after one year to find out about her progress. Each woman knows she can contact the clinic directly at any time for any similar or alternative help.

Case Study

Patricia is a 35-year-old divorced mother of two children. She works full time as a secretary. She has a difficult relationship with her ex-husband, who has remarried, regarding his visiting rights with their children. She feels he does not manage his parental responsibilities satisfactorily and she gets frustrated and angry at being the 'emotional sponge' on whom her children vent their distress arising from their parents' divorce and their insecure paternal relationship. She is involved in a live-in relationship with another man who resists accepting responsibilities within the relationship and who regularly backs out and withdraws if he feels demands are presented to him. She presented to the PMT clinic complaining of severe irritability, uncontrolled anger, confusion, tearfulness, insomnia, fatigue, and low libido for the last one and a half years. These symptoms appeared up to two weeks prior to menses and disappeared up to a week after the end of menstruation. With a 30-day cycle, this meant she experienced only about ten days when she felt better and in control. She was very concerned that her relationship with her children was deteriorating and simultaneously, that the role of single parent was too arduous and she could not sustain it for much longer. Assessment across two consecutive cycles using daily records and both post- and premenstrual measures revealed high stress levels, cognitive failures and depression throughout, with high anxiety and low frustration tolerance particularly peaking in the premenstrual phase i.e. a form of menstrual distress. This resulted in feelings of rising irritation

Table 1. Case study—Patricia's application programme

Problems	RET Perspective	Coping skills
1. Anger and hurt at lover's reluctance to commitment and sharing of responsibilities	Anti-awfulizing about his behaviour, disputing her 'need' for active male support	Worked at increasing her frustration tolerance for his lack of involvement
2. Anger and hurt at ex-husband for his uncertain involvement with their children	Anti-awfulizing about his behaviour. Disputing her 'need' for his active involvement. Disputing her self-pity about her misfortune as a single parent	Considered joining local group of 'Parents Without Partners'. Sought out friends who were coping single parents for role models. Looked for evidence of positive intent in ex-husband and refused to focus on the absences of interest. Discussed parenting expectations assertively with him
3. Anger and hurt at children for their demands on her	Anti-awfulizing about their behaviour. Challenged her low frustration tolerance and discomfort anxiety about their behaviours and demands	Sought specialist help for behaviour problems of elder child. Worked at relationship-building with this child in particular. Worked at accepting childrens' emotional distress rather than rejecting.
4. Self-pity and other-pity (children). Depression and guilt over inadequate mothering	Anti-awfulizing about her own and the children's relationships and life situations. Challenged self-downing and guilts about her parenting efforts. Challenged resignation—low frustration tolerance and giving up tendencies	Explained to children and lover that she was making the best efforts she could. Invited their collaborative efforts. Engaged herself more deliberately in activities with her children

which were expressed in angry, overly critical verbal exchanges, and hostile punishing behaviours to her children and partner. She was depressed and overwhelmed by this situation. Her problems were identified as anxiety about herself as an effective mother; anger about the unfairness of her single parent status both in relation to her ex-husband and present partner; anxiety about the quality and future of her present relationship; negative self evaluations and feelings of depression, self pity and pity for her children's plight for which she felt greatly to blame. Within the structure of the therapy programme she applied herself in the ways listed in Table 1.

In twelve weeks Patricia felt increasingly positive about her relationships in all directions. She believed improvements with her children had certainly appeared. Her ex-husband became more definite in his expressed interest in the children and the older child spent two weeks holiday with him by mutual agreement. She welcomed this but believed she no longer regarded his role in their lives as an imperative. She became more appropriately assertive with her lover and resisted his attempts at emotional manipulation. Consequently, their relationship moved onto a more satisfying plane. She now regards her premenstrual phase as a more normal time, when she may have feelings of sluggishness, fatigue or be 'out of sorts'. She no longer responds inappropriately to these signals, but 'allows' herself to be less on top for a while, confident that she will recover her competence in one or two days.

Summary

This case study supports the notion of PMS as a psychosomatic condition that emerges from an interaction of the person within her environment. Problems in living arising from centrally important relationships became magnified in intensity to overwhelm this woman. The more dissatisfying she found her daily life to be, the more emotional distress was generated. This triggered adverse reactions in the other participants as well as secondary self-defeating experiences in herself. As anxiety, anger and depression appeared, she paid attention to sensations and changes that were labelled with concern as symptoms. When she learned new techniques of emotion control and rational challenging to thoughts and assumptions, she began to experience more control. As she increasingly took charge of her personal and interpersonal environments she felt better about herself, symptoms abated, and she faced the future with increased confidence and a more secure self-concept.

Cobb (1976) has proposed that different kinds of social support are operative in providing buffers against stress and symptom production. These social supports provide feelings of being cared for, experiences of esteem and value and a sense of belonging to a communicative network. These social support characteristics increasingly emerged in the case study example, through the woman's own efforts. This process exemplifies the stated aim of the coping model in a coping skills training. This therapy is easily replicable, inexpensive and cost effective in the small group setting and can be taught to other health professionals. There is increasing patient-demand for non-drug interventions coupled with frequent non-compliance in traditional drug-centred treatment studies (Dennerstein and Morse, 1986; Maddocks et al., 1986). The prospect of control for their own welfare is an appealing concept for an increasing number of women.

References

Beck, A. T. and Emery, G. (1985). *Anxiety Disorders and Phobias: A Cognitive Perspective*, Basic Books, New York.

Beck, A. T., Rush, A. J., Shaw, B. F. and Emery, G. (1979). *Cognitive Therapy of Depression*, Guilford Press, New York.

Clare, A. W. (1985). Hormones, behaviour and the menstrual cycle. *Journal of Psychosomatic Research*, **29**, 225–233.

Cobb, S. (1976). Social support as a moderator of life stress. *Psychosomatic Medicine*, **38**, 300–314.

Cohen, F. (1979). Personality, stress and the development of physical illness, in *Health Psychology: A Handbook* (Eds. J. Stone, F. Cohen and N. Adler) Jossey-Bass, San Francisco.

Dalton, K. (1964). *Premenstrual Syndrome*. Heinemann, London.

Dalton, K. (1980). Progesterone, fluid and electrolytes in premenstrual syndrome. *British Medical Journal*, **281**, 61.

Dennerstein, L. and Burrows, G. D. (1979). Affect and the menstrual cycle. *Journal of Affective Disorders*, **1**, 77–92.

Dennerstein, L. and Morse, C. (1986). Alprazolam in the treatment of premenstrual tension, in *Hormones and Behaviour, Proceedings of the 8th International Congress of Psychosomatic Obstetrics and Gynaecology*. (Eds. L. Dennerstein and I. Fraser), Elsevier/North Holland, Amsterdam, pp. 175–182.

Ellis, A. (1962). *Reason and Emotion in Psychotherapy*. Lyle Stuart, New Jersey.

Ellis, A. and Harper, R. H. (1975). *A New Guide to Rational Living*. Prentice-Hall, Hemel Hempstead.

Frank, R. T. (1931). Hormonal causes of premenstrual tension. *Archives of Neurology and Psychiatry*, **26**, 1053–1057.

Greene, R. and Dalton, K. (1953). The premenstrual syndrome. *British Medical Journal*, **1**, 1007–1014.

Hart, W. G. and Russell, J. W. (1986). A prospective comparison study of premenstrual symptoms. *Medical Journal of Australia*, **14**, 466–468.

Henry, J. P. and Stephens, P. (1977). *Stress, Health and the Social Environment*. Springer-Verlag, Berlin.

Holroyd, K. A. and Lazarus, R. S. (1982). Stress, coping and somatic adaption, in *Handbook of Stress*, (Eds. L. Goldberger and S. Bresnitz) Free Press, New York.

Jacobsen, E. (1942) *You Must Relax*. McGraw-Hill, New York.

Lyons, D., Hartley, L. and Dunn, M. (1985). *Memory and menstrual cycle*. Paper presented to the 1st combined Conference of the Australian and New Zealand Psychological Societies, Christchurch, New Zealand.

Maddocks, S., Hahn, P., Moller, F. and Reid, R. L. (1986). A double-blind placebo-controlled trial of progesterone vaginal suppositories in the treatment of premenstrual syndrome *American Journal of Obstetrics and Gynaecology*, **154**, 573–581.

Morse, C. A. and Dennerstein, L. (1986). Cognitive perspectives in premenstrual syndrome, in *Hormones and Behaviour. Proceedings of the 8th International Congress of Psychosomatic Obstetrics and Gynaecology* (Eds. L. Dennerstein and I. Fraser) Elsevier/North Holland, Amsterdam, pp. 197–203.

Morse, C. A., Dennerstein, L. and Varnavides, K. (1987). Premenstrual syndrome: a comparison of treatment-seekers with volunteers. *Psychological Medicine*, Journal of Affective Disorders (in press).

Morse, C. A. (1988). Menopausal mood disorders. *Contemporary Therapy* (in press).

Reiser, M. F. (1975). *Changing theoretical concepts in psychosomatic medicine* (Ed. M. F. Reiser) American Handbook of Psychiatry, Vol. 4, Basic Books, New York.

Van Keep, P. A. and Lehert, P. (1981). The premenstrual syndrome: an epidemiological and statistical exercise, in *The Premenstrual Syndrome* (Eds. P. A. van Keep and W. H. Utian) MTP Press, Lancaster, pp. 31–42.

Wolfe, J. L. (1985). Women, in *Clinical Applications of Rational-Emotive Therapy*. (Ed. A. Ellis and M. E. Bernard) Plenum, New York, p. 101.

Functional Disorders of the Menstrual Cycle
Edited by M. G. Brush and E. M. Goudsmit
© 1988 John Wiley & Sons Ltd

CHAPTER 12

Investigation and treatment of cyclical benign breast disease

R. E. MANSEL

Department of Surgery,
University of Wales College of Medicine
and University Hospital of Wales,
Heath Park,
Cardiff CF4 4XN

Cyclical breast symptoms are very common in the premenopausal woman with pain (mastalgia) and swelling being the most prominent. Some women also report cyclical 'lumps', although nodularity would be a better term to describe these changes as these are commonly multiple small nodules rather than single dominant lumps. Studies have shown that in the working female population up to 60 per cent of women experience breast pain, usually in the luteal phase of the cycle. A recent report from a breast screening unit where women were questioned about mastalgia showed that 70 per cent of well women reported significant mastalgia every two to three months or more frequently (Leinster *et al.*, 1987). These authors also noted that cyclical breast pain is much commoner than non-cyclical and the incidence of breast pain increases with age until the menopause. Despite this high incidence of mastalgia, only 3.4 per cent of these patients had received any treatment for the symptom. It is thus clear that cyclical mastalgia is a common symptom, as is shown in Table 1 which gives the incidence of this symptom in various groups of women.

The high incidence of cyclical mastalgia in apparently normal working women begs the question, 'what is normality?'. Some authors have even suggested that benign breast disease does not exist (Love *et al.*, 1982), but the major problems are that the terminology of benign breast disease (BBD) is confused and that there is undoubtedly a spectrum which extends from normality to disease. The confusion of terminology is caused by the mixing of

191

pathological and clinical terms, for example fibroadenosis, which is a term derived by pathologists to describe the histological picture of fibrosis and adenosis in the breast, but is used by the clinician to describe painful nodularity in the breast. In fact there is no correlation between the clinical picture of painful lumpy breasts and the pathological description of fibroadenosis, as any of the variety of histological changes seen in BBD such as cystic change, epithelial hyperplasia and sclerosing adenosis can be present in a biopsy taken from a woman with painful nodular breasts. This is graphically shown by the study of Ayers and Gidwani (1983) where they demonstrated that structural changes in the breast (measured by ultrasonography) failed to correlate with clinical symptomatology or with endocrine abnormalities whereas symptoms correlated well with hormonal abnormalities. For the above reasons, the author uses the term cyclical mastalgia to describe the symptom of breast pain and thereby makes no attempt to correlate this with any specific histological change, as no such relationship exists. If the symptom is then discussed on its own merits, then the only clinical decision that is needed, is the severity of the mastalgia and the need for therapy in those cases where the symptom is disturbing the patient's life. In this chapter cyclical nodularity will be taken to be synonymous with cyclical mastalgia as the two so commonly co-exist.

Investigation of Cyclical Mastalgia

The first priority when a patient complains of cyclical pain and nodularity is to exclude cancer by careful clinical examination of the breast looking for a palpable dominant lump or any other visible change which might suggest cancer. In women over 30 years a mammogram should also be performed to exclude a subclinical cancer. The problem of breast cancer is not common below the age of 30 years but rapidly increases thereafter. As the mean age of cyclical mastalgia patients is around 34 years (Preece *et al.*, 1976) there is considerable overlap between the two groups and a history of cyclical pain although suggesting benign disease, does not rule out an underlying asymptomatic cancer.

Table 1. Prevalence of mastalgia[a]

Population	%
Working women	66
General practice	50
Screening clinic	70
Breast clinic	40

[a] Elicited by questionnaire.

A careful history in most cases will identify the pattern of mastalgia whether cyclical or non-cyclical and this is important for therapy as will be shown later. A more convenient and accurate way of delineating the mastalgia pattern is to use a simple pain chart, such as the chart designed for use in the Cardiff Mastalgia Clinic (Figure 1). These charts are readily accepted and are usually completed accurately by the majority of patients. Monitoring of the pattern should be carried out for at least two months as cyclical mastalgia can be episodic with periods of spontaneous resolution. These charts have the additional advantage that an objective record can be kept of the days of mastalgia experienced per cycle and also give an accurate description of cycle length and regularity. After recording for two to three months, a decision can be made after discussion with the patient whether treatment is required for her mastalgia. Factors such as interference with work, sleep or marital relations, are indicators that suggest therapy is required in individual patients. The general irritability caused by mastalgia occurring for three weeks in each cycle is understandable and is often the reason for consultation in the breast clinic. The general concern of these women and their frustration with the lack of any effective therapy until recently, has prompted many clinicians to label these patients as being 'neurotic' a suggestion which Astley Cooper made in the eighteenth century. However, study of the psychoneurotic profiles of

Daily Breast Pain Chart

Name

Record the amount of breast pain you experience each day by shading in each box as illustrated.

Severe pain

Mild pain

No pain

For example:- If you get severe breast pain on the fifth of the month then shade in completely the square under 5. Please note the day your period starts each month with the letter 'P'

Please bring this card with you on each visit.

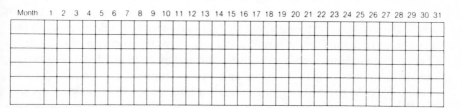

Figure 1. A Cardiff Mastalgia Clinic pain chart used for recording the severity and duration of breast pain

mastalgia patients have failed to confirm this longstanding hypothesis (Preece *et al.*, 1978).

A complete history of the site, onset, and timing of the pain should be taken and note should be made of any symptoms that could indicate cancer. The pattern of mastalgia may be determined by a clear history but if there is doubt, a pain chart (Figure 1) should be given to the patient for two months. Clinical examination of the breasts should be performed to exclude any dominant lump which could require biopsy. The usual findings in cases of cyclical mastalgia are areas of increased density or nodularity, typically in the upper outer quadrant of one or both breasts, which are variably tender depending on the phase of the cycle. In order to assess the extent of the cyclical change, the breasts should be examined both in the follicular and luteal phases of the menstrual cycle.

Hormonal investigations are of no value in the routine case as no clear abnormality has been identified in cyclical mastalgia. Patients with significant galactorrhoea should have their serum prolactin measured to exclude a prolactinoma. Detailed hormonal studies of patients with cyclical mastalgia have failed to show any clear abnormality but several groups have recently demonstrated an enhanced release of prolactin in response to exogenously administered TRH (Kumar *et al.*, 1984; Watt-Boolsen *et al.*, 1985; Dogliotti *et al.*, 1985). This enhanced prolactin release seems to occur selectively in the cyclical pattern of mastalgia as non-cyclical cases failed to show a similar enhanced response (Kumar *et al.*, 1984). It is of interest that when tests of prolactin release were performed prior to treatment of breast pain using endocrine based therapies, a high peak prolactin response correlated with subsequent therapeutic response (Kumar *et al.*, 1985). Thus it appears that these patients have an enhanced responsivity to prolactin releasing agents, but the underlying abnormality has not been identified and may relate to increased biological action of oestrogen although no direct evidence exists to support this idea at the moment.

Treatment of Cyclical Mastalgia

There are several different agents which have been proven in controlled studies to be effective in alleviating pain and nodularity in patients with cyclical mastalgia. Different agents have widely differing side effects and thus the choice of agents depends on the balance between efficacy and side effects. The proven agents that are licensed for use in benign breast disease are danazol, an anti-gonadotrophin, and bromocriptine, a dopamine agonist. Other drugs have been recommended but have major drawbacks at present. The anti-oestrogen tamoxifen was shown to be effective in cyclical mastalgia (Fentiman *et al.*, 1986) but this drug is not licensed for use in benign breast disease and there are theoretical disadvantages such as bone demineralization and elevated serum oestrogen in premenopausal women. Progestogens have been used extensively to treat benign breast disease (not specifically mastalgia), but double blind studies have shown no advantage over placebo treatment. In the evaluation of drugs for cyclical mastalgia, controlled studies are essential as placebo response rates of around 30 per cent are common (Pye *et al.*, 1985). Newer agents such as evening primrose oil and LHRH analogues are currently being investigated in mastalgia in controlled trials. There have been few comparative studies of the different agents but a recent review by Pye *et al.* (1985) showed that danazol was the most effective drug over-all with bromocriptine being next in order.

Danazol is known to be an anti-gonadotropin in the human at high dosage (Greenblatt *et al.*, 1971) but at low dosage, the mode of action is less certain, as menstruation often continues. The drug has many potential actions at both the target tissues and the pituitary ovarian axis. Early studies used doses of 400–600 mg daily but androgenic side effects of acne, hirsutism and voice deepening were troublesome. More recently, much lower doses have been used and our current starting dose is 100 mg twice daily and this is often reduced to a maintenance dose of 50–100 mg daily when a response has been obtained. At these low doses, only about 15 per cent of patients experience side effects.

Bromocriptine which acts by lowering serum prolactin, has been shown to be an active drug for the reduction of breast pain in many controlled studies (Mansel *et al.*, 1978; Durning and Sellwood, 1982). There is no direct correlation between the extent of prolactin suppression produced by the drug and symptom improvement in patients with cyclical mastalgia, who are generally normoprolactinaemic prior to therapy. However, the observation that peak prolactin correlates with response may indicate that the important measure should be the dynamic prolactin response not the basal level. It also appears that bromocriptine is much more effective in cyclical mastalgia compared with non-cyclical mastalgia (Mansel *et al.*, 1978) but this may simply reflect the non-hormonal aetiology of non-cyclical mastalgia—as shown by the normal TRH response in these patients (Kumar *et al.*, 1984). The drug is used continuously throughout the cycle at a dose of 2.5–5 mg daily after starting on a gradual incremental dose scheme to limit side effects. Side effects are common and include dizziness due to postural hypotension and nausea, which can be reduced by taking the drug with food. It is interesting that the side effects of bromocriptine appear to vary widely between different series but this discrepancy should be clarified by a large European multicentre study of bromocriptine in cyclical mastalgia which is currently underway in some fourteen European centres.

The choice of active drug therapy thus lies between these two principal agents and in making this choice, the wishes of the patient should be taken into account. Both agents are potentially teratogenic and thus mechanical methods of contraception should be used while patients are on therapy. Danazol may cause amenorrhoea in a proportion of patients (up to 30 per cent at 300 mg) and patients who dislike the idea of amenorrhoea may not choose to take this drug. Bromocriptine will not interfere with menstruation but does have a slightly higher over-all incidence of side effects. Thus patients with cyclical mastalgia could be started on either drug initially and if side effects occur or the pain fails to respond, they can be switched to the alternative treatment. Once remission of pain has occurred the dose may be reduced and treatment should be continued for four to six months and then stopped to see if the patient remains pain free. Generally some 50 per cent of the patients will experience further mastalgia, although not at the previous level of severity in some, and these patients can be recommenced on a further six months course of treatment if their symptoms are severe enough. This sequence of intermittent courses of therapy may be continued up to the menopause in patients with severe mastalgia.

Newer Agents Under Evaluation

Two new agents are currently being evaluated, evening primrose oil and LHRH agonists either taken as a nasal insufflation or as a depot injection. The rationale behind the use of dietary essential fatty acid (EFA) supplementation by evening primrose oil is the observation that the incidence of breast disease is positively correlated with saturated fat intake in Western populations and essential fatty acid deficiency states appear to correlate with some types of breast disease (Horrobin, 1979). Studies in the Cardiff Mastalgia Clinic have shown low levels of some EFAs in patients with cyclical mastalgia when compared with controls (Table 2). A double blind study of evening primrose oil (Efamol) dietary supplementation in patients with cyclical mastalgia has shown improvement in breast pain when compared with placebo response (Table 3) although the overall magnitude of response was lower than that obtainable with danazol or bromocriptine, and was slower in onset as full responses took up to four months to obtain. The principal advantage of this dietary treatment is the very low (<2 per cent) rate of side effects.

Table 2. Serum fatty acids in cyclical mastalgia patients[b]

Fatty acid	Control $N = 50$ (mean ± S.E.)	Cyclical mastalgia $N = 21$ (mean ± S.E.)
20 : 4n–6	11.36 ± 0.24	8.10 ± 0.48[a]
22 : 4n–6	0.73 ± 0.04	0.23 ± 0.05[a]
22 : 5n–6	1.12 ± 0.09	0.54 ± 0.07[a]

[a] $p < 0.001$ Students's t-test.
[b] Expressed as per cent plasma phospholipids.

Table 3. Results of Efamol treatment in cyclical mastalgia

	Mean linear analogue scores[a]		
Breast symptom	Pre-trial	End two months	End four months
Pain	76	61[b]	52[c]
Heaviness	71	56[b]	49[c]
Tenderness	89	74[b]	53[c]

[a]100 mm scales.
[b]Not significant.
[c]$p < 0.02$ v pretrial score (Wilcoxon's signed ranks test.)

As yet there is no published evidence of treatment of cyclical mastalgia by LHRH agonists, although theoretically these agents will produce a profound and lasting ovarian suppression which is reversible on cessation of treatment. The major disadvantage is the inevitable suppression of menstruation that will occur. It remains to be seen whether this will be acceptable to the patient who requests treatment for her cyclical mastalgia.

References

Ayers, J. W. T. and Gidwani, G. P. (1983). The 'luteal breast', hormonal and sonographic investigation of benign breast disease in patients with cyclical mastalgia. *Fertility and Sterility*, **40**, 779–784.

Dogliotti, L., Faggiuolo, R., Ferusso, A., Orlandi, F., Sandrucci, S., Tibo, A. and Angeli, A. (1985). Prolactin and thyrotrophin response to thyrotropin releasing hormone in premenopausal women with fibrocystic disease of the breast. *Hormone Research*, **21**, 137–144.

Durning, P. and Sellwood, R. A. (1982). Bromocriptine in severe cyclical breast pain. *British Journal of Surgery*, **69**, 248–249.

Fentiman, I. S., Caleffi, M., Brame, K., Chaudary, M. A. and Hayward, J. L. (1986). Double blind controlled trial of tamoxifen therapy for mastalgia. *Lancet*, **i**, 287–288.

Greenblatt, R. B., Dmowski, W. P., Mahesh, V. B. and Scholer, H. F. L. (1971). Clinical studies with an antigonadotropin—danazol. *Fertility and Sterility*, **22**, 102–112.

Horrobin, D. F. (1979). Cellular basis of prolactin action: involvement of cyclical nucleotides, polyamines, prostaglandins, steroids, thyroid hormones, Na/K ATPases and calcium: relevance to breast cancer and the menstrual cycle. *Medical Hypotheses*, **5**, 599–614.

Kumar, S., Mansel, R. E., Hughes, L. E., Edwards, C. A. and Scanlon, M. F. (1985). Prediction of response to endocrine therapy in pronounced cyclical mastalgia using dynamic tests of prolactin release. *Clinical Endocrinology*, **23**, 699–704.

Kumar, S., Mansel, R. E., Hughes, L. E., Woodhead, J. S., Edwards, C. A., Scanlon, M. F. and Newcombe, R. G. (1984). Prolactin response to thyrotropin-releasing hormone stimulation and dopaminergic inhibition in benign breast disease. *Cancer*, **53**, 1311–1315.

Leinster, S. J., Whitehouse, G. H. and Walsh, P. V. (1987). Cyclical mastalgia: clinical and mammographic observations in a screened population. *British Journal of Surgery*, **74**, 220–222.

Love, S. M., Gelman, R. S. and Silen, W. (1982). Fibrocystic 'disease' of the breast—a non-disease? *New England Journal of Medicine*, **307**, 1010–1014.

Mansel, R. E., Preece, P. E. and Hughes, L. E. (1978). A double blind trial of the prolactin inhibitor bromocriptine in painful benign breast disease. *British Journal of Surgery*, **65**, 724–727.

Preece, P. E., Mansel, R. E. and Hughes, L. E. (1978). Mastalgia: psychoneurosis or organic disease. *British Medical Journal*, **1**, 29–30.

Preece, P. E., Hughes, L. E., Mansel, R. E., Baum, M., Bolton, P. M. and Gravelle, I. H. (1976). Clinical syndromes of mastalgia. *Lancet*, **ii**, 670–673.

Pye, J. K., Mansel, R. E. and Hughes, L. E. (1985). Clinical experience of drug treatments for mastalgia. *Lancet*, **ii** 373–377.

Watt-Boolsen, S., Eskildsen, P. C. and Blaehr, H. (1985). Release of prolactin, thyrotrophin and growth hormone in women with cyclical mastalgia and fibrocystic disease of the breast. *Cancer*, **56**, 500–502.

Functional Disorders of the Menstrual Cycle
Edited by M. G. Brush and E. M. Goudsmit
© 1988 John Wiley & Sons Ltd

CHAPTER 13

Hyperprolactinaemia and the menstrual cycle

STEPHEN FRANKS

*Department of Obstetrics and Gynaecology,
St Mary's Hospital Medical School,
London W2 1PG*

Prolactin and the Normal Menstrual Cycle

The physiological role of prolactin in non-lactating women remains obscure. Prolactin has been shown to have a variety of biological effects on the ovary, other endocrine organs and non-endocrine tissue, but the importance of these actions is still unclear. If, however, serum prolactin concentrations are inappropriately elevated, the effects on the reproductive system are profound and this will be discussed below.

The pituitary is clearly the major source of circulating prolactin in women but studies over the last few years have established that the human endometrium is also capable of synthesizing prolactin. High concentrations of prolactin are present in amniotic fluid and the origin of this prolactin is now known to be decidual cells (Golander *et al.*, 1978; Riddick *et al.*, 1978). The non-pregnant uterus can also synthesize prolactin. Prolactin synthesis and secretion can be demonstrated in explants of late secretory endometrium, the source of decidualized endometrial stromal cells (Maslar and Riddick, 1979). Decidual prolactin is similar in structure to that from the pituitary but the sub-cellular localization and mechanism of control are completely different in the two organs, thus dopamine (and its agonists) and TRH will stimulate prolactin secretion from the pituitary but not from the endometrium (Handwerger *et al.*, 1984). Much interest has been aroused in the study of decidual prolactin since it seems possible that the hormone has a role in the maintenance of normal early pregnancy (Riddick and Daly, 1982). As yet, however, there are few data to support this hypothesis. There appears to be a minor cyclical variation in serum prolactin concentrations (Franks and Jacobs, 1983). The most consistent feature is an increase in serum prolactin at midcycle (Franchimont *et al.*, 1976; Bäckström *et al.*, 1982), but this has not been observed in all studies. Discrepancies between the results of different studies could be partly due to the episodic nature of prolactin secretion, but may simply be related to the frequency in blood sampling (Bäckström *et al.*, 1982). The variations during the cycle appear to reflect changes in circulating concentrations of oestradiol, a phenomenon that can also be observed in hyperprolactinaemic women in whom ovulation has been induced with pulsatile LHRH (see below). Differences in endogenous oestrogen concentrations also explain the marked increase in prolactin secretion during pregnancy and the sex-related differences in prolactin responsiveness to exogenous thyrotrophin releasing hormone (TRH) (reviewed by Franks, 1979).

In contrast to the slight cyclical variations in serum prolactin there are marked changes during a 24 h period (Franks, 1979). Prolactin secretion increases dramatically with the onset of sleep to reach levels which are two to three times greater than during the waking hours. The levels fall steadily towards normal on waking, but this does mean that a blood sample taken betwen eight and nine a.m. may not reflect the 'baseline' prolactin concentration. Once this baseline has been reached, however, episodic secretion of prolactin is characterized by fairly low amplitude pulses without fixed periodicity (Sagle *et al.*, 1986). Single blood samples are therefore usually sufficient to assess prolactin secretion.

Hyperprolactinaemic Amenorrhoea

Prevalence and Presentation

Excessive secretion of prolactin is perhaps the most common pituitary disorder. There are a variety of causes of increased secretion of prolactin and the most common of these are summarized in Table 1. Since prolactin secretion is under tonic inhibitory control by hypothalamic dopamine, drugs such as phenothiazines which are dopamine receptor antagonists will stimulate prolactin secretion. It is therefore very important to take account of this in taking a history from a patient with hyperprolactinaemia. The most important single cause of increased prolactin secretion is a prolactin secreting pituitary tumour. Pathological hyperprolactinaemia is one of the most frequent abnormalities in women presenting with amenorrhoea: 13–23 per cent have hyperprolactinaemia (Franks and Jacobs, 1984); 40 per cent of the women with hyperprolactinaemic amenorrhoea have radiological evidence of a pituitary tumour (Jacobs, 1981). More recent studies using high resolution CT scanning to screen patients who have moderate hyperprolactinaemia with normal plain X-rays of the pituitary fossa suggest that these figures may under-estimate the incidence of microadenomas. Nevertheless there is a substantial proportion of patients with hyperprolactinaemic amenorrhoea who have no evidence of a space occupying lesion in the pituitary. The aetiology of hyperprolactinaemia

Table 1. Causes of hyperprolactinaemia

Drug-induced hyperprolactinaemia	
Dopamine receptor antagonists	e.g. Phenothiazines
	Sulpiride
	Metoclopramide
Dopamine depleting agents	e.g. α-methyldopa
	Reserpine
Oestrogens	
Pathological hyperprolactinaemia	
Pituitary tumours	Primary prolactin-secreting
	tumours (prolactinomas)
	Acromegaly
	Nelson's syndrome
	'Functionless' pituitary tumours[a]
Lesions of the hypothalamus or	Granulomatous disease e.g.
pituitary stalk	tuberculosis
	Neoplasms e.g.
	craniopharyngioma
	Irradiation of the pituitary area
	Pituitary stalk section
Primary hypothyroidism	
Chronic renal failure	
'Idiopathic' ('functional')	
hyperprolactinaemia	

[a] Non-hormone-secreting tumours which may cause hyperprolactinaemia by pressure on, or damage to, the pituitary stalk or hypothalamus.

in this group is not yet clear. Galactorrhoea occurs in 30–90 per cent of patients according to the series reported (Edwards and Feek, 1981; Bergh and Nillius, 1982). The wide variation in the prevalence of galactorrhoea is, in part dependent on selective referral of patients with this symptom to certain centres. It is important to realize that the presence or absence of galactorrhoea is not a reliable index of hyperprolactinaemia and diagnosis depends on measurement of serum prolactin concentrations (Franks *et al.*, 1975). Hyperprolactinaemic amenorrhoea may be accompanied by symptoms and signs of oestrogen deficiency (Jacobs *et al.*, 1976) such as superficial dyspareunia and even hot flushes. Visual symptoms due to the presence of a large prolactin secreting pituitary tumour are unusual in women who present with amenorrhoea (less than 10 per cent have suprasellar extention of a pituitary tumour; Jacobs, 1981).

Endocrine Features and Mechanism of Hyperprolactinaemic Amenorrhoea

The typical biochemical profile of patients with hyperprolactinaemic amenorrhoea is of low levels of serum oestradiol and basal gonadotrophin concentra-

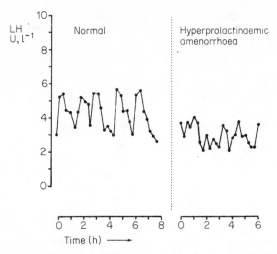

Figure 1. LH concentrations in serial blood samples in a normal subject on day six of an ovulatory menstrual cycle and in a woman with hyperprolactinaemic amenorrhoea. Note the low amplitude, disordered pulse pattern in the patient with hyperprolactinaemia

tions which are either low or normal (Jacobs *et al.*, 1976). The gonadotrophin response to exogenous LHRH is variable but usually falls within the normal range suggesting that pituitary gonadotrophin reserve is normal. There are abnormalities of both negative and oestrogen-mediated positive feedback (Glass *et al.*, 1975; Aono *et al.*, 1976; Jacobs *et al.*, 1976). Characteristic abnormalities of pulsatile pattern of LH secretion in these women (Figure 1) provide further evidence for a hypothalamic disorder (Bohnet *et al.*, 1976).

Despite the impressive evidence for a primary hypothalamic disturbance of gonadotrophin regulation, it has been suggested that there may be a direct effect of raised levels of prolactin on the ovarian response to gonadotrophins (Thorner and Besser, 1977). Preliminary studies of the effects of pulsatile LHRH treatment in women with persistent hyperprolactinaemia showed that it was possible to induce ovulation, thus supporting the concept that the primary disorder is at hypothalamic level (Leyendecker *et al.*, 1980). However Bergh and Nillius (1983) showed that luteal function in most of the cycles treated in their patients was impaired, raising the question of a direct effect of prolactin on the corpus luteum. We therefore undertook a study to confirm that ovulation could be induced by LHRH in the presence of high prolactin concentrations and to make a more detailed study of luteal function in patients with hyperprolactinaemic amenorrhoea (Polson *et al.*, 1986).

A total of twelve cycles of LHRH treatment in five women with hyperprolactinaemia were assessed. The clinical details of the five women are

Table 2. Details of patients with hyperprolactinaemia who were treated with pulsatile LHRH

Patient	Age (years)	Diagnosis	Serum PRL mU l⁻¹ (normal <600)	Number of treatment cycles with LHRH	Ovulation
1	37	Hypothalamic TB	1570	3	3/3
2	36	Prolactinoma	5060	2	1/2
3	28	Idiopathic	1390	5	3/5
4	28	Prolactinoma PCO	7500	1	1/1
5	30	Prolactinoma	10 500	1	1/1

summarized in Table 2. Gonadotrophin releasing hormone (LHRH) was given subcutaneously at 90 min intervals at a dose of 15 μg per pulse. In two women the pulse frequency was reduced to once every 180 min following ovulation. The response to treatment was assessed by pelvic ultrasound and measurements of gonadotrophins, prolactin and oestradiol. Progesterone concentrations were measured during the mid-luteal phase and in one patient serial blood samples were taken at 15 min intervals for 8 h during the mid-luteal phase for measurement of progesterone.

Nine of the twelve cycles were ovulatory and significantly we found that the length of the luteal phase was normal in all ovulatory cycles (mean $\pm$ S.D. 13.6 $\pm$ 1.1; range twelve to sixteen days). Mid-luteal progesterone levels were normal, in the range 25–95 nmol l⁻¹. Figure 2 shows the pituitary and ovarian response to pulsed LHRH therapy in a patient with a large pituitary tumour. The pattern of gonadotrophins and the ovarian response in terms of follicular growth and oestradiol and progesterone secretion were normal despite the fact that serum prolactin concentrations remained high during the treatment. Indeed there was a further increase in serum prolactin in the late follicular phase presumably related to oestrogen stimulation in the pituitary. Analysis of gonadotrophin and progesterone concentrations in another patient showed that not only was progesterone secreted at levels appropriate to the mid-luteal phase but that there was also a marked pulsatility of progesterone in response to preceeding LH pulses, thus our study revealed that luteal function was normal once ovulation had been induced by replacing LHRH in a physiological way.

The mechanism of disordered LHRH secretion is still not entirely understood but abnormalities of hypothalamic dopamine turnover have been implicated (Quigley et al., 1979). Increased activity of endogenous opiate containing neurones may also be important in suppressing gonadotrophin secretion in hyperprolactinaemia. It has been shown that opiate receptor blockade by infusion of naloxone increases LH concentrations in hyperprolactinaemic women (Quigley et al., 1980; Grossman et al., 1982).

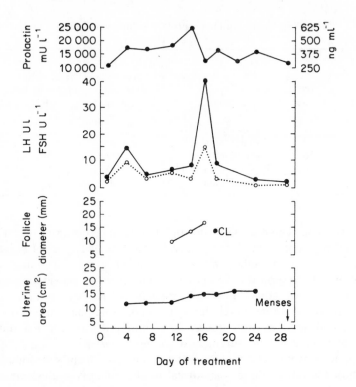

Figure 2. Response to pulsatile LHRH (15 μg per 90 min in follicular phase, 15 μg per 180 min in luteal phase) in patient five. The endocrine results and the ovarian and uterine changes on ultrasound are characteristic of a normal ovulatory menstrual cycle. The mid-luteal progesterone was 34 nmol 1^{-1}. (Polson *et al.*, 1986)

Diagnostic Tests of Prolactin Secretion

Measurement of basal serum prolactin is the most valuable test in establishing the diagnosis. If a raised serum prolactin concentration is found it should be confirmed by a subsequent random sample. The definition of hyperprolactinaemia varies according to the reference laboratory and it is important that the clinician is aware of the reference range of his own laboratory (Jeffcoate *et al.*, 1986). A number of dynamic tests of prolactin secretion have been devised. Both TRH and dopamine receptor antagonists (such as domperidone or metoclopramide) cause significant and reproducible stimulation of prolactin but in practice these tests give little further information about the aetiology of hyperprolactinaemia and the results do not influence management of the patient (Franks, 1983).

Management of Hyperprolactinaemic Amenorrhoea

This has been the subject of a number of recent reviews and it is beyond the scope of this chapter to discuss the details of management (Franks and Jacobs, 1983; Tan and Jacobs, 1986). There are, however, certain important principles which influence the decision to treat and the choice of treatment.

The primary indication for treatment is infertility associated with amenorrhoea, but the patient may also be troubled by galactorrhoea and/or symptoms of oestrogen deficiency. There has been a good deal of discussion about the need for treatment in women who have none of the above symptoms, but who nevertheless are amenorrhoeic. Recent data suggest that patients with untreated hyperprolactinaemia and amenorrhoea have evidence of reduced bone density and may be at risk of developing osteoporosis. The risk appears to be especially high in women with very low serum oestradiol concentrations but is still significant even in those patients whose oestradiol levels fall within the normal range for the early to mid-follicular phase (Klibanski *et al.*, 1980).

The choice of treatment of hyperprolactinaemia includes dopamine receptor agonists (such as bromocriptine), pituitary surgery and radiotherapy. Bromocriptine treatment offers a specific and effective means of controlling serum prolactin concentrations even when hyperprolactinaemia is associated with the presence of a large prolactin secreting pituitary tumour. It is now clear that bromocriptine as well as reducing serum prolactin levels also is able to reduce the volume of the tumour (Nillius, 1980; Bergh and Nillius, 1982, 1984; Tindall *et al.*, 1982; Franks and Jacobs, 1983). This has allowed successful medical treatment of symptomatic large pituitary tumours and our approach to the management of pituitary prolactinomas has therefore altered radically in the last few years.

Treatment with dopamine agonists effectively restores normal fertility in most patients with hyperprolactinaemic amenorrhoea, including those who have large prolactinomas (Franks and Jacobs, 1983).

Because the pituitary expands during pregnancy, patients with large prolactinomas are at risk of developing compression of the optic chiasma during pregnancy. For this reason it was considered necessary, until recently, to perform some form of pituitary ablative therapy—either radiotherapy or surgery—before advising the patient that it was safe to conceive. However recent studies strongly suggest that when bromocriptine is used as primary therapy, the risk of serious complications in pregnancy is very small even in patients with large prolactinomas (in the order of 1 per cent; Tan and Jacobs, 1986). This is presumably because bromocriptine treatment has a protective effect on the lactotroph which is sustained even when the drug is stopped in early pregnancy. The use of bromocriptine as primary treatment for induction of ovulation may be advocated in all cases except perhaps those who have significant suprasellar extension of a tumour prior to treatment. In such cases a 'trial' of bromocriptine might be indicated. In other words bromocriptine is administered for perhaps three months after which the CT scan is repeated. If this then shows significant reduction of tumour volume it may be considered that the patient is 'safe' to conceive.

Pituitary surgery now has a limited place in management of hyperprolactinaemia. The best results from surgery are obtained in those patients with small pituitary tumours, but these women will respond extremely well to bromocriptine and since the rate of 'cure' appears no better following pituitary surgery (Serri et al., 1983) there seems little point in using this as a first line of treatment. In patients with large pituitary tumours surgery is less successful. It is therefore best reserved for the few patients who are intolerant of or fail to respond to dopamine agonist therapy.

Radiotherapy should be restricted to the small minority of patients who have significant residual tumour after surgery for a large prolactinoma. Even in these cases it can be argued that long-term treatment with bromocriptine is preferable. It has been the practice of some groups to perform 'prophylactic' radiotherapy to the pituitary area routinely in patients with pituitary tumours who wish to become pregnant (Thorner et al., 1979). There is no evidence that this is effective and in view of the long term consequences of irradiation (e.g. hypopituitarism and temporal lobe epilepsy) there seems little justification for the continued use of this procedure.

Although the prognosis for normal fertility in women with hyperprolactinaemic amenorrhoea is extremely good, long-term management remains a problem. In patients with moderate hyperprolactinaemia and no radiological evidence of a pituitary tumour there is a significant remission rate, in that 40 per cent of women can be expected to resume normal ovulatory cycles after bromocriptine-induced pregnancy (Jacobs, 1981). This is associated with a significant fall in prolactin concentrations which in many cases reach the normal range. It is not clear whether this 'cure' results from treatment with bromocriptine from pregnancy or from both. It should be noted, however, that remissions have also been recorded in patients with moderate hyperprolactinaemia who have had neither bromocriptine treatment nor been pregnant (March et al., 1981). Indeed the natural history of hyperprolactinaemia is still unclear (Franks and Horrocks, 1984).

In patients with radiological evidence of a pituitary tumour and markedly elevated serum prolactin concentrations it is unusual for serum prolactin to be normalized following prolonged treatment with bromocriptine. The mean prolactin concentrations are usually lower than before treatment but are still significantly elevated (Franks and Horrocks, 1984). The effect of long-term treatment with bromocriptine (i.e. five years or more) on the natural history of prolactinomas remains to be determined, but figures should soon be available to answer this point.

As can be judged from the results presented above it is possible to induce ovulation in infertile patients with persistent hyperprolactinaemia with the use of pulsatile LHRH. This therefore provides an alternative method of treatment of the infertile patient who fails to respond to bromocriptine. Similar results can be obtained by conventional gonadotrophin therapy. Such methods of induction of ovulation are best avoided if the patient has a large pituitary tumour since without the protective effect of bromocriptine the risk of significant expansion of the tumour during the pregnancy must be considered to be high.

Prolactin and Other Menstrual Disturbances

Moderate hyperprolactinaemia is occasionally found in women who have irregular anovulatory menstrual cycles. These are usually patients who have polycystic ovary syndrome in whom the hyperprolactinaemia appears to be secondary to exposure of the pituitary to 'unopposed' oestrogen (Franks *et al.*, 1985). Bromocriptine is also a useful form of therapy in these patients and can be expected to restore ovulatory cycles (Polson *et al.*, 1987). However, clomiphene is a reasonable alternative particularly if bromocriptine is poorly tolerated (Franks *et al.*, 1985).

Raised serum prolactin concentrations have also been identified in association with impaired luteal function. In our experience this is most commonly observed in women who have polycystic ovaries (S. Franks and D. Polson, unpublished).

In some centres measurement of serum prolactin is performed routinely in women with ovulatory infertility. There seems little rational basis for this. Indeed problems may arise when slightly elevated serum prolactin concentrations are identified in this group of women (Jeffcoate *et al.*, 1986). There is no evidence that lowering prolactin levels in women with ovulatory infertility (either with normal or slightly elevated prolactin levels) makes any difference to the chances of conception. It has been suggested that hyperprolactinaemia may influence early pregnancy and increase the risk of miscarriage. This too seems very unlikely since decidual cells in the endometrium produce significant concentrations of prolactin locally and the uterine environment is therefore exposed to a high concentration of prolactin in normal pregnancy.

Summary

Whilst the physiological role of prolactin in the normal menstrual cycle remains unclear, there is no doubt that pathological hypersecretion of prolactin results in disturbed menstrual function. Hyperprolactinaemic amenorrhoea has well defined clinical and biochemical features and can be specifically treated by lowering serum prolactin levels. Dopamine agonists are the first choice of treatment even in patients with pituitary tumours. Moderate hyperprolactinaemia can also be found in patients who have anovulatory menses. These women generally have polycystic ovaries. There is no evidence to suggest that raised serum concentrations of prolactin are important in the aetiology of ovulatory infertility.

References

Aono, T., Myake, A., Schioji, T., Kingusa, T., Onishi, T. and Kurachi, K. (1976). Impaired LH release following exogenous oestrogen administration in patients with amenorrhoea-galactorrhoea syndrome. *Journal of Clinical Endocrinology and Metabolism*, **42**, 696–702.

Bäckström, C. T., McNeilly, A. S., Leask, R. M. and Baird, D. T. (1982). Pulsatile secretion of LH, FSH, prolactin, estradiol and progesterone during the human menstrual cycle. *Clinical Endocrinology*, **17**, 29–42.

Bergh, T. and Nillius, S. J. (1982). Prolactinomas: follow up of medical treatment, in *A Clinical Problem: Microprolactinoma* (Ed. G. M. Molinatti) Excerpta Medica, Oxford, pp. 115–130.

Bergh, T. and Nillius, S. J. (1983). Prolactinomas and pregnancy, in *Proceedings of Symposium on Prolactinomas and Pregnancy. XI World Congress of Fertility and Sterility, Dublin, June 1983*. (Ed. H. S. Jacobs), MTP Press, Lancaster, pp. 51–56.

Bohnet, H. G., Dahlen, H. G., Wuttke, W. and Schneider, H. P. G. (1976). Hyperprolactinaemic anovulatory syndrome. *Journal of Clinical Endocrinology and Metabolism*, **42**, 132–143.

Edwards, C. R. W. and Feek, C. M. (1981). Prolactinoma: a question of rational treatment. (Editorial). *British Medical Journal*, **283**, 1561–1562.

Franchimont, P., Dourcy, C., Legros, J., Reuter, A., Vrindts-Gevaert, Y., Van Cauwenberge, J. R. and Gaspard, U. (1976). Prolactin levels during the menstrual cycle. *Clinical Endocrinology*, **5**, 643–650.

Franks, S., Murray, M. A. F., Jequier, A. M., Steele, S. J., Nabarro, J. D. N. and Jacobs, H. S. (1975). Incidence and significance of hyperprolactinaemia in women with amenorrhoea. *Clinical Endocrinology*, **4**, 597–607.

Franks, S. (1979). Prolactin, in *Hormones in Blood* (Eds. C. H. Gray and V. H. T. James) (3rd edition), Vol. 1, Academic Press, London, pp. 280–332.

Franks, S. (1983). Prolactin secretion, in *A Guide to the Diagnosis of Endocrine Disorders* (Ed. R. A. Donald), Marcel Dekker, New York, pp. 651–655.

Franks, S. and Jacobs, H. S. (1984). Medical treatment of prolactinomas, in *Proceedings of Symposium on Prolactinomas and Pregnancy. XI World Congress of Fertility and Sterility, Dublin, June 1983*. (Ed. H. S. Jacobs), MTP Press, Lancaster, pp. 39–44.

Franks, S. and Horrocks, P. (1983). Treatment of hyperprolactinaemia with bromocriptine and other dopamine agonists: tumour, shrinkages, recurrences and cures, in *Trends in Diagnosis and Treatment of Pituitary Adenomas*. (Eds. S. W. J. Lamberts, F. J. H. Tilders, E. A. van der Veen and J. Assies), Free University Press, Amsterdam, pp. 157–166.

Franks, S., Adams, J., Mason, H. D. and Polson, D. (1985). Ovulatory disorders in women with polycystic ovary syndrome. *Clinics in Obstetrics and Gynaecology*, **12**, 605–632.

Glass, M. R., Shaw, R. W., Butt, W. R., Edwards, R. L. and London, D. R. (1975). An abnormality of oestrogen feedback in amenorrhoea-galactorrhoea. *British Medical Journal*, **3**, 274–275.

Golander, A., Hurley, T., Barrett, J., Hizi, A. and Handwerger, S. (1978). Prolactin synthesis by human chorion-decidual tissue: a possible source of prolactin in the amniotic fluid. *Science*, 202, 311–313.

Grossman, A., Moult, P. J. A., McIntyre, H. Evans, J., Silverstone, T., Rees, L. H. and Besser, G. M. (1982). Opiate mediation of amenorrhoea in hyperprolactinaemia and in weight-loss related amenorrhoea. *Clinical Endocrinology*, 17, 379–388.

Handwerger, S., Markoff, E. and Barry, S. (1984). Regulation of the synthesis and release of decidual prolactin, in *Prolactin Secretion: A Multi-disciplinary Approach*. Proceedings of a Symposium on Frontiers and Perspectives of Prolactin Secretions: A Multi-disciplinary Approach, Mexico City, Mexico, (Eds. F. Mena and C. M. Valverde), Academic Press, New York, p. 57.

Jacobs, H. S., Franks, S., Murray, M. A. F., Hull, M. G. R., Steele, S. J. and Nabarro, J. D. N. (1976). Clinical and endocrine features of hyperprolactinaemic amenorrhoea. *Clinical Endocrinology*, 5, 439–454.

Jacobs, H. S. (1981). Abnormal prolactin secretion in men and women, in *Endocrinology of Human Infertility: New Aspects* (Eds. P. G. Crosignani and B. L. Rubin), Academic Press, London, pp. 129–138.

Jeffcoate, S. L., Bacon, R. R. A., Beastall, G. H., Diver, M. J., Franks, S. and Seth, J. (1986). Assays for prolactin: guidelines for the provision of a clinical biochemistry service. *Annals of Clinical Biochemistry*, 23, 638–651.

Klibanski, A., Neer, R. M., Beitins, M. D., Ridgway, E. C., Zervas, N. T. and McArthur, J. W. (1980). Decreased bone density in hyperprolactinaemic women. *New England Journal of Medicine*, 303, 1511–1514.

Leyendecker, G., Struve, T. and Plotz, E. J. (1980). Induction of ovulation with chronic intermittent (pulsatile) administration of LHRH in women with hypothalamic and hyperprolactinaemic amenorrhoea. *Archives of Gynaecology*, 229, 172–190.

Maslar, I. A. and Riddick, D. H. (1979). Prolactin production by human endometrium during the normal menstrual cycle. *American Journal of Obstetrics and Gynecology*, 135, 751.

March, C. M., Kletzky, O. A., Davajan, V., Teal, J., Weiss, M., Apuzzo, M. L., Marrs, R. P. and Mishell, D. R. (1981). Longitudinal evaluation of patients with untreated prolactin-secreting adenomas. *American Journal of Obstetrics and Gynecology*, 139, 835–844.

Nillius, S. J. (1980). Medical therapy of prolactin secreting pituitary tumours. *Progress in Reproductive Biology*, 6, 194–221.

Polson, D. W., Mason, H. D. and Franks, S. (1987). Bromocriptine treatment of clomiphene resistant patients with polycystic ovary syndrome. *Clinical Endocrinology*, 26, 197–203.

Polson, D. W., Sagle, M., Mason, H. D., Adams, J., Jacobs, H. S. and Franks, S. (1986). Ovulation and normal luteal function during LHRH treatment of women with hyperprolactinaemic amenorrhoea. *Clinical Endocrinology*, 24, 531–537.

Quigley, M. E., Sheehan, K. L., Casper, R. F. and Yen, S. S. C. (1980). Evidence for increased opioid inhibition of luteinizing hormone secretion in hyperprolactinaemic women with pituitary microadenomas. *Journal of Clinical Endocrinology and Metabolism*, 50, 427–430.

Riddick, D. H., Luciano, A. A., Kusmik, W. F. and Maslar, J. A. (1978). De novo synthesis of prolactin by human decidua. *Life Sciences*, 23, 1913.

Riddick, D. H. and Daly, D. C. (1982). Decidual prolactin production in human gestation. *Seminars in Perinatology*, 6, 229.

Sagle, M., Mason, H. D., Polson, D. W., Bridgewater, B., Buchanan, J. and Franks, S.

(1986). 24-Hour pulse patterns of LH and prolactin in normal and anovulatory women. *Journal of Endocrinology*, **108 (supplement)**, Abstract 240.

Serri, O., Rasio, E., Beauregard, H., Hardy, J. and Somma, M. (1983). Recurrence of hyperprolactinaemia after selective transsphenoidal adenomectomy in women with prolactinoma. *New England Journal of Medicine*, **309**, 280–283.

Tan, S. L. and Jacobs, H. S. (1986). Management of prolactinomas—1986. *British Journal of Obstetrics and Gynaecology*, **93**, 1025–1029.

Thorner, M. O. and Besser, G. M. (1977). Hyperprolactinaemia and gonadal function: results of bromocriptine treatment, in *Prolactin and Human Reproduction* (Eds. P. G. Crosignani and C. Robyn), Academic Press, London, pp. 285–302.

Thorner, M. O., Edwards, C. R. W., Charlesworth, M., Dacie, J. E., Moult, P. J. A., Rees, L. H., Jones, A. E. and Besser, G. M. (1979). Pregnancy in patients presenting with hyperprolactinaemia. *British Medical Journal*, **2**, 771–774.

Tindall, G. T., Kovacs, K., Horvath, E. and Thorner, M. O. (1982). Human prolactin producing adenomas and bromocriptine: a histological, immunocytochemical, ultrastructural and morphometric study. *Journal of Clinical Endocrinology and Metabolism*, **55**, 1178–1183.

Functional Disorders of the Menstrual Cycle
Edited by M. G. Brush and E. M. Goudsmit
© 1988 John Wiley & Sons Ltd

CHAPTER 14

Studies on headache related to menstrually linked migraine and allied conditions

RICHARD PETTY

Sections of Vascular Biology and Endocrinology,
MRC Clinical Research Centre,
Northwick Park Hospital,
Watford Road,
Harrow,
Middlesex HA1 3UJ

Fordyce, writing in 1758, was probably the first to report that in some women, headaches recurred regularly with the menstrual period (Greene and Dalton, 1953). It is now estimated that some 30 per cent of women regularly suffer from headaches—usually migrainous—in the few days preceding each menstrual period (Greene, 1967, 1973).

Migraine is much commoner in women than in men—large studies suggest that 75 per cent of sufferers are female (Lance and Anthony, 1966; Olesen, 1978). Furthermore, in an epidemiological study of 2933 women (aged 20–64), 19 per cent had experienced a vascular headache of migraine type during the previous year, the peak incidence of migraine being at 20–45 years of age (Waters and O'Connor, 1971). In women who suffer from migraine, approximately 60 per cent show an association of at least some of their headaches with the perimenstrual phase of the cycle, and less often to the periovulatory phase (Lance and Anthony, 1966; Klee, 1968). Strict menstrual migraine, that is headache that occurs *only* perimenstrually and at no other time, is much less common, occurring in only 14 per cent of female migraine sufferers.

Typically, menstrual migraine starts around the menarche, particularly in the latter group. It tends to cease after the menopause, although there is no predictable change in the pattern of the headache attacks at this time (Epstein *et al.*, 1975). The premenstrual syndrome is a common accompaniment

(Magos *et al.*, 1983). The comprehensive study of 1955 headache sufferers, by Nattero (1982), supports the contention that female hormones may influence migraine. In this study, 68 per cent of the sufferers were female; a chronological connection with menstruation was found in 55 per cent, while there was an absence of premenstrual tension in 54 per cent. There was a positive correlation between menstrual headache and the absence of headache during pregnancy. Indeed, this, and other studies, have shown that over 70 per cent of women with menstrually linked headaches cease to have attacks in pregnancy (Friedman and Merritt, 1959; Somerville, 1972a,b; Nattero, 1982).

In those in whom headaches only occur perimenstrually, fluid retention as part of a periodic syndrome is particularly likely. Although these observations suggest a role for the menstrual cycle in the aetiology of migraine, migraine can be cyclical in either sex (Medina and Diamond, 1982). However, a hormonal influence on migraine would seem certain—apart from the female preponderance of the disorder and its frequent association with the menstrual cycle, migrainous headaches also show an increased frequency in the first trimester of pregnancy and in the early postpartum period (Stein *et al.*, 1984). Furthermore, oral contraceptives and oestrogen replacement therapy may increase the incidence of migraine (Pluvinage, 1975). The typical 'female-ness' of migraine, and the probable association of migraine with hormonal factors is emphasized by the slight male predominance in the prepubertal incidence of migraine (Prensky, 1976). The higher prevalence of migraine in adulthood is mainly due to the prevalence in adult females.

There are no specific clinical features which distinguish hormone-related migrainous headaches from other forms of migraine. An accurate diagnostic classification of headaches is based primarily on the clinical history, only occasionally with help from diagnostic tests. Although difficult, a precise definition of headache type is crucial to the investigation of the symptom (see Lance, 1978, for discussion). The most commonly used classification of headache is that proposed by the Ad Hoc Committee on the Classification of Headache (Friedman *et al.*, 1962; Table 1).

The migrainous headache syndromes, and tension headache are those most likely to be encountered in the context of menstrually linked headaches (Table 2). Any investigation into menstrual headaches should aim to use precise diagnostic criteria, and to define both the frequency and severity of the headaches, and whether or not they only occur in relation to menstru-ation, or also at other times. Although such a classification seeks to clearly differentiate betwen headache types, there is increasing evidence to suggest that migraine and tension headache represent two ends of a spectrum of headache disorders (Featherstone, 1985).

A parental history of migrainous headaches is obtained in 50–60 per cent of patients with migraine, and in 10–20 per cent of headache-free individuals

Table 1. Classification of headache (modified from Friedman *et al.*, 1962)

1. Vascular headaches
   Migraine
   (a) Classical
   (b) Common
   (c) Hemiplegic and ophthalmoplegic
   Cluster
   Non-migrainous vascular headaches:
     Toxic vascular
     Hypertensive
2. Muscle-contraction headache
3. Combined headache: vascular and muscle contraction
4. Headache of delusional, conversion or hypochondriacal states
5. Traction headaches, e.g. from mass lesions
6. Headache due to cranial inflammation, including arteritis
7. Headache due to ocular, nasal and sinusal, dental or other cranial or neck structures
8. Cranial neuritides
9. Cranial neuralgias

Table 2. Headache—clinical features

MIGRAINE
Recurrent attacks of headache, widely varied in intensity, frequency and duration. Commonly unilateral in onset.

CLASSICAL MIGRAINE
Headache with sharply defined, transient, visual, or other sensory or motor prodromes or both.

COMMON MIGRAINE
Headache without striking prodromes, and less often unilateral than classical migraine.

HEMIPLEGIC OR OPHTHALMOPLEGIC MIGRAINE
Headache in which sensory and motor phenomena persist during and after the headache.

CLUSTER HEADACHE
Headache which is unilateral, on the same side, usually associated with flushing, sweating, rhinorrhoea, and increased lacrimation. The headache lasts for no more than 2 hours, but usually occurs in closely packed groups, separated by long remissions. Very rare in women.

MUSCLE CONTRACTION HEADACHE (includes tension headache)
Ache or sensation of tightness, pressure or constriction, widely varied in intensity, frequency and duration. May be very long-lasting. Usually bilateral and suboccipital.

(Selby and Lance, 1960; Lance and Anthony, 1966; Ziegler, 1978). These figures may be under-estimates: in one study in which extensive histories were obtained by personal interview of the families of 100 women with migraine, 90 per cent had a family history of migraine (Dalsgaard-Nielsen, 1965). The incidence of parental migraine in this study was 73 per cent, 57 per cent maternal and 16 per cent paternal. This probably reflects the approximately four-fold higher incidence of migraine in women than in men. There is no evidence that menstrual migraine is hereditary, although there have not been any studies which have addressed this problem directly. In migraine in general the mode of inheritance is not clear, largely because of the few twin studies which have been performed. The current view is that migraine is an autosomal dominant condition with incomplete penetrance. The exception to this is the special case of familial hemiplegic migraine, in which affected family members sustain virtually identical stereotyped attacks. Analysis of several families indicate an autosomal dominant inheritance (Bradshaw and Parsons, 1965).

Headache Precipitants

I shall discuss in detail the precipitation of headache by hormonal changes, but it is important to appreciate that there are many other factors which may do so (see Raskin and Appenzeller, 1980, for discussion).

   Certain foods are said to induce migraine. The most widely accepted dietary triggers are the tyramine-containing cheese and red wine. Phenylethylamine in chocolate is alleged to be another agent which may provoke migrainous headaches. Doubt has been cast upon these as the agents responsible for provoking migraine (Glover *et al.*, 1983). Dietary provocation of migraine appears to occur only in a small proportion of migraine sufferers, and some studies have appeared to show that most patients who claim to be sensitive to some foods are not so on formal blind testing (Moffat *et al.*, 1974). There are, however, persistent reports of sensitivity to a wide variety of foods in migraine (Monro, 1982; Hanington, 1983). The finding of a deficiency of platelet phenolsulphotransferase in patients demonstrably sensitive to cheese, chocolate, citrus fruit and wine, (Littlewood *et al.*, 1982), supports a physical cause for this form of dietary triggering of migraine, but it has been suggested that some cases of dietary triggering of migraine may be the result of the development of a conditioned taste aversion (Jessup, 1978).

   Some have suggested that the reproducible provocation of headache by stereotyped stimuli is one of the most useful ways of approaching the clinical diagnosis of migraine (Raskin and Appenzeller, 1980). Headache occurring monthly, the day before or on the first day of the menstrual flow, and usually at other times also (Epstein *et al.*, 1975), is so highly characteristic of migraine as to be virtually pathognomonic.

   It is important to point out that any of the precipitants of migraine, including the menstrual cycle, are only rarely 100 per cent reproducible. This facet of the disorder has frustrated all attempts to achieve an objective diagnostic test for migraine. It may be that anybody can get a migraine attack if they are subjected to sufficient triggers. The current view is that a genetic predisposition to migraine results in a lowering of a threshold of response to triggers.

The Pathophysiology of Menstrual Migraine

There have been few studies which have addressed the mechanism of menstrual migraine. In a statistical analysis of data obtained in a series of 720 women with migraine, (Nattero, 1982), χ-square analysis revealed two populations, with either menstrual or non-menstrual migraine. Statistically significant differences were found between the two groups with regard to pattern, familial background, history of headache, premenstrual stress, relationship with menstruation and pregnancy, duration of crises, frequency, topography, site and accompanying symptoms.

Some authors have stated that true menstrual migraine is always of the 'common' variety (Sachs, 1970), although others have found that classical or complicated migraine may occur in these patients. In a large study of menstrual migraine in patients attending the Princess Margaret Migraine Clinic, the present author found classical migraine in 11 per cent of women who only experienced migraine in relation to the menstrual cycle.

It will be helpful to preface discussion of the pathophysiology of menstrual migraine by a brief summary of the current views on the pathophysiological mechanisms of migrainous headaches in general.

The conventional view of migraine is that it is a primary vascular disturbance. The aura is said to be the result of vasoconstriction in the cerebral vasculature, primarily of the posterior cerebral vessels, followed by reactive vasodilation of the intra- and extracranial vessels. This dilatation of extracranial vessels which have previously been rendered sensitive to distension, by local accumulation of pain-producing substances, is said to cause the pain of migraine (Dalessio, 1980). This vascular origin of migraine was originally suspected from the observation that arteries and veins on the forehead and temples were prominent during the attack, and pressure on the scalp vessels, or the common carotid artery eased the pain to some extent. However, based upon a re-analysis of early work, the extracranial vascular concept has been criticized by Blau (1978). Other studies have not shown any relationship between temporal pulse amplitude and intensity of migraine headache (Brazil and Friedman, 1956; Heyck, 1969). A study of the extracranial circulation of 66 migrainous patients, assessed during unilateral headache by recording the pulse amplitude of the superficial temporal artery and its main frontal branch, by facial thermography, and by changes in the intensity of headache when temporal or carotid arteries were compressed, concluded that dilatation of the superficial temporal artery and its branches contribute substantially to migraine headache in only a minority of patients (Drummond and Lance, 1983).

The concept of vascular constriction being responsible for the migranous aura, followed by reactive dilatation which causes the pain of migraine, implies that neurological symptoms should be contralateral to the headache. This is very rarely the case. The neurological symptoms and headache are almost invariably ipsilateral (Peatfield *et al.*, 1981).

Experimentally, many workers have shown decreased cerebral blood flow (rCBF) when the aura is present and hyperaemia during the headache (Skinhoj, 1973). There is evidence of elevation of extracranial blood flow during migraine headache (Sakai and Meyer, 1978). However, subsequent studies using the intracarotid injection of 133-xenon, showed a different pattern (Olesen *et al.*, 1980), namely that the symptoms of the migrainous aura are preceded by decreases of cerebral blood flow, often by many hours. Furthermore, in classical migraine, variations in cerebral blood flow moved across the cortex at approximately 2 mm min^{-1} (Lauritzen *et al.*, 1983). This same group failed to find abnormalities of cerebral blood flow in common migraine (Olesen *et al.*, 1981).

The vascular hypothesis of migraine has been elegantly reviewed and criticized by Bruyn (1982). He points out that the typical visual displays of migraine do not occur with occlusions of the posterior cerebral vessels, and many of the patterns of neurological involvement do not correspond to single arterial territories of the cerebral cortex. He hypothesizes that the visual displays of migraine could be explained by involvement of the lateral geniculate bodies. Similarly the complex sensory and motor phenomena which accompany some attacks could be explained by involvement of the thalamic nuclei. The vegetative, autonomic symptom-complex of mood changes, nausea, anorexia, vomiting, diarrhoea, fluid retention and polyuria, followed by sleep, suggest a disturbance of the hypothalamus (reviewed by Johnson, 1978).

The involvement of blood vessels in the production of migraine headaches seems certain. However, as we have discussed, headache is only one of many events in the spectrum of the disorder, and regional changes in cerebral blood flow, oedema of arterial walls, and 'ischaemic symptoms' are not synonymous with a primary vascular cause. As noted above, a decrease in cerebral blood flow precedes, often by many hours, any symptom of the 'ischaemic aura', and there is no evidence that this oligaemia is caused by a vasoconstrictive mechanism. Indeed, if a major arterial trunk were constricted for several hours, cerebral infarction would be the rule, and not the exception. A further difficulty for the vascular hypothesis arises from the observation that regional cerebral blood flow is sometimes increased over both sides of the brain during the headache phase, although the headache itself is most often unilateral.

It is therefore clear that vascular instability of the large cerebral arteries is no longer tenable as a hypothesis for the initiating event in migraine (see Fisher, 1971 for review).

The Biochemical Hypotheses of Migraine

There have been several hypotheses implicating various biochemical agents in the pathophysiology of migraine. These can be roughly divided into the amine and the platelet hypotheses.

Many vasoactive amines have been isolated from the extracellular fluid surrounding the superficial temporal arteries during the migraine attack. These include acetylcholine, noradrenaline, bradykinin, histamine, and substance P. All have been implicated as the pain-producing peripheral agents in relation to dilated large scalp arteries (Fanchamps, 1974).

Platelets drawn during migraine attacks retain their ability to take up 5-hydroxytryptamine (5-HT, serotonin) and contain normal levels of adenine nucleotides; however, plasma specimens drawn during attacks have the capacity to release 5-HT from normal platelets (Anthony and Lance, 1975; Dvilansky et al., 1976). This circulating factor which released 5-HT from platelets remains unidentified. The responses of cerebral vessels to 5-HT have been studied extensively, and it has been hypothesized that 5-HT release is responsible for the putative vasoconstrictor phase of the migraine attack. In the subsequent painful (dilated) phase, the levels of 5-HT were found to be low, and were thought to account for the vasodilatation.

Increased platelet aggregability (Couch and Hassanein, 1977), increased release of platelet Factor 4, and β-thromboglobulin (Gawel et al., 1979) associated with a decrease in the platelet levels of 5-HT and monoamine oxidase, have been confirmed in migraine attacks. These observations have formed the basis of the hypothesis that migraine is a haematological disorder that is due to abnormal platelet function (Hanington et al., 1981, 1982a). The observation that oral contraceptive medications induced changes in platelet behaviour appeared to support this hypothesis (Hanington et al., 1982b).

Unfortunately, this attractive hypothesis is weakened by the considerable variability in platelet function that occurs in normal non-migrainous subjects with age, exercise, emotional stress, and many drugs. A recent study of platelet function in common and classical migraine sufferers during treatment with the agents propranolol, metoprolol, and the β-2-selective antagonist Li-32468, found no correlation between headache and platelet function as measured by aggregation to adensoine diphophate (ADP) and adrenalin, and platelet secretion of adenosine triphosphate (ATP), casting further doubt on the platelet theory of migraine (Steiner et al., 1985).

The Neural Hypothesis

If the aura is not a result of spreading cerebral ischaemia, what may be causing it? Dynamic studies support Roy and Sherrington's hypothesis (1890), that altered cerebral metabolism causes variation in the calibre of cerebral vessels, and not vice versa. Using [^{14}C]deoxyglucose, Sokoloff (1978) showed that focal metabolic alterations occurred first, and were followed by vascular reactions within seconds. A possible candidate is 'spreading cortical depression' of Leao (1944) (see also Gardner Medwin, 1981; Pearce, 1985). This is a wave of excitation, followed by depression, which moves over the surface of the cerebral cortex at approximately 2 mm of cortical surface per minute. This is associated with local arterial dilatation, rather than constriction. The rate of movement of this wave, and of its associated vascular disturbance, corresponds closely to the speed of movement of vascular flow observed by Olesen et al. (1981) while measuring cerebral blood flow during induced migraine attacks. Marshall (1959) reviewed the phenomenon, and pointed out that the spreading depression reaction only occurs in the presence of pathology, such as exposure of the cerebral cortex. However, Leao himself reported that, in rabbits, spreading depression could be precipitated by retinal stimulation with flashing lights.

Several abnormalities of neurotransmitters have been proposed to be the central aetiological factor in migraine. Sicuteri et al. (1978), have suggested that headache derives from a failure of cerebral mechanisms to cope with noxious stimuli, both cerebral and psychic. These workers have referred to a 'central biochemical dysnociception'. According to this view, headache of all types is a result of breakdown of intrinsic neurotransmitter defence mechanisms. This 'central' hypothesis has been extended to include disturbances of endogenous opioids, induced by hormonal alterations (Sicuteri 1980, 1982; Sicuteri et al., 1976). Recently, several workers have produced evidence of hypothalamic dysfunction in menstrual migraine. Petraglia et al. (1983) examined eighteen migraine sufferers in either the middle or late phase of the menstrual cycle, and found that naloxone did not induce the expected rise in luteinizing hormone (LH). Interpretation of this study is difficult, and further work is needed in this important area. Facchinetti et al. (1983) measured LH, FSH, prolactin, oestradiol and progesterone at different phases in the cycle in fifteen control women and in nine women suffering from perimenstrual migraine. The migraine sufferers showed markedly reduced progesterone levels throughout the luteal phase of the cycle, in association with persistently elevated oestrogen levels. Interestingly, these patients responded well to prophylactic treatment with dihydroergotamine retard, without any alteration in this hormonal abnormality.

Recently, Lance and colleagues (1983), have postulated that migraine represents activation of the locus coeruleus in the brain stem, and have produced experimental evidence in monkeys showing that electrical stimulation of this area leads to dilatation of the external carotid vessels and constricts intracerebral vessels by means of a non-cholinergic transmitter. This concept supports the notion of migraine as a disorder that arises via a neural mechanism in the brainstem.

Burnstock (1981), has reviewed experimental work, and suggests that the regulation of the microcirculation is mediated by purinergic nerves which release adenosine triphosphate (ATP) and its breakdown products adenosine monophosphate (AMP), and adenosine. All three are potent vascular dilators and also stimulate pain receptors both in cerebral vessels and more peripherally. This hypothesis again fails to explain the association of ipsilateral neurological symptoms and headache.

The most persuasive of the neurotransmitter hypotheses, is that altered reactivity of brainstem 5-HT containing neurones and the synaptic turnover of serotonin may be important to the mechanism of recurring headache (Raskin and Appenzeller, 1980). There are many lines of evidence in support of this hypothesis:

1. Reserpine, which releases 5-HT from neurones, is a potent precipitator of attacks within 4–6 h in most migraine sufferers, but only occasionally, and to a lesser degree in normal subjects (Anthony et al., 1967).
2. Drugs that block central 5-HT receptors, or alter the activity of 5-HT-containing neurones are amongst the most effective agents for treating migraine (Fozard, 1982).
3. Migraine is relieved by 5-HT and its metabolic precursors (Kangasniemi et al., 1978).

Additional evidence in support of some role for 5-HT came from the observation that urinary levels of 5-hydroxyindoleacetic acid (5-HIAA), a serotonin metabolite, were increased in some patients during headache attacks (Sicuteri et al., 1961), and the previously mentioned finding of a fall in platelet 5-HT, with a concomitant rise in urinary 5-HIAA, in 85 per cent of patients during headache attacks (Anthony and Lance, 1975). Although these findings cannot be reflecting brainstem levels of 5-HT, and indeed CSF levels of 5-HT are undetectable during migraine attacks (Curzon et al., 1969), they may indicate a generalized disorder of 5-HT metabolism.

There have not been studies of monaminergic status in menstrual migraine, but serum levels of dopamine β-hydroxylase activity has been measured in menstrual migraine (Magos et al., 1985). Serum β-hydroxylase has been shown to be an index of peripheral sympathetic activity (Geffen, 1974; North and Murlow, 1976). The enzyme was found to be elevated during the headache free interval in migraine, but not in muscle contracton headache (Gotoh et al., 1976), and also to rise during migraine headaches (Anthony, 1981). In the study of menstrual migraine sufferers, mean values of serum dopamine β-hydroxylase were higher than in control subjects but this difference failed to reach statistical significance (Magos *et al.*, 1985). The levels of the enzyme were significantly lower in the premenstrual phase, compared with the ovulatory phase of the cycle, as in normal subjects (Lamprecht *et al.*, 1974) implying that there is no obvious dysfunction of sympathetic activity in menstrual migraine. It remains possible that excessive fluctuations in the levels of the enzyme may be related to menstrual migraine.

In a study of eleven migraine sufferers, whose attacks appeared, or were exacerbated, at the time of menstruation, Lehtonen *et al.* (1979), measured visual evoked potentials (VEP), as well as oestrogen, progesterone, FSH and LH. The VEPs of the migraine patients were consistently abnormal, compared with a group of healthy controls, and were not dependent on the hormonal cycle, with the exception of 10 flash s^{-1} responses which increased in the post-ovulatory period in controls but not in the migraine sufferers. There were no significant differences in the hormonal levels of the controls and those with migraine. Similarly, in patients who sustain migrainous attacks accompanied or preceded by focal visual symptoms, VEP latencies, as obtained with pattern reversal stimuli, are prolonged compared to controls during headache-free periods (Kennard *et al.*, 1978). The particular significance of this study is that VEPs may be altered by the monoaminergic status of the brain (Schafer and McKean, 1975).

Migraine Pathophysiology—Summary

The results from the studies summarized above lead to the concept that while there is undoubtedly a vascular element in migraine, it rarely, if ever, has a causal role. Vascular dilatation appears to be an accompaniment of many migraine attacks, but this dilatation is only perceived as painful since there has been a lowering of the level at which painful stimuli are perceived. This lowering of sensory threshold may be a consequence of altered reactivity of brainstem 5-HT containing neurones, and altered regulation of the synaptic turnover of 5-HT. Certainly any hypotheses of the causation of migraine require that there are alterations of both central sensory processing and vascular reactivity.

Hormonal Measurements

Various measurements of hormonal status have been made in patients with menstrually-linked migraine. The premenstrual phase is characterized by falling levels of oestradiol and progesterone. Since these two hormones tend to fall together, withdrawal of one or both could precipitate migraine (Edelson, 1985). During the early 1970s, Somerville (1971, 1972a,b) reported a series of careful studies of women who suffered from menstrual migraine during a normal ovulatory cycle. He then manipulated the cycles by injecting either oestradiol or progesterone during the premenstrual phase in order to examine the effect of the withdrawal of each hormone separately. Progesterone and oestradiol levels were measured in all subjects and related to the clinical features of the disorder. The injection of oestradiol valerate during the premenstrual phase resulted in menstruation at the normal time, but a delay in the development of headache for between three and nine days. These migraine attacks were closely related to the phase of oestradiol withdrawal. However, the injection of progesterone during the premenstrual phase delayed menstruation but resulted in migraine attacks at the normal time. This work revealed that the falling oestrogen level seemed to be the significant precipitant. It was demonstrated that several days of oestrogen exposure were needed before withdrawal provoked migraine.

Oral Contraceptives and Headache

The oral contraceptive may be associated with vascular headache (Mears and Grant, 1962). The figures in the literature relating to the incidence of headache in women on oral contraceptives vary from 0.2 to 60 per cent (Whitty et al., 1966; Pluvinage, 1975; Dalton, 1976). In only one study (Markush et al., 1975), was this association not found.

A review of the literature on the oral contraceptive and headache, suggests that the severity and frequency of attacks increase in 18–40 per cent of cases of established migraine sufferers with the use of the oral contraceptive. Furthermore, established migraine sufferers show an increased incidence of attacks during the drug-free interval of the cycle, but in those who develop vascular headaches for the first time while taking the oral contraceptive, there is no such tendency for an exacerbation during the drug-free interval. There appear to be a small number of migraine sufferers who improve if they take the oral contraceptive. These patients have not yet been studied in detail. A family history of migraine is found less commonly in those who develop migraine for the first time on taking oral contraceptives. These observations suggest that oestrogens may lead to the development of the migraine syndrome. It is also recognized that when migraine is precipitated for the first time by the oral contraceptive, it may occur in the early cycles but it may occur for the first time after prolonged use. It is common knowledge in headache clinics that stopping oral contraceptive use does not result in immediate relief in all cases. In some individuals the headaches may continue for up to one to two years (Welch et al., 1984). The author has encountered several patients who first developed vascular headaches while taking oral contraceptives, and who continued to have headaches indefinitely after stopping the oral contraceptive. It is not yet clear whether the use of low dosage oestrogen formulations is associated with a reduced frequency of this side effect, although there are indications that they are associated with fewer migrainous headaches.

These observations, and others outlined below, led Welch *et al*. (1984), to propose the novel theory that oestrogen exerts its effect by modulating sympathetic control of the cerebral vasculature. Kudrow (1975) has studied the effect of oestrogens, administered for gynaecological reasons, on the migraine syndrome. He studied 300 patients, 87 of whom were taking oestrogen in various doses and in a cyclical pattern of administration; 47 per cent were found to have more than four attacks of migraine per month. 58 per cent of these patients were said to be improved following reduction of dosage and decycling of the oestrogen therapy. The greater the initial frequency of headache, the better the response to the therapy adjustment.

Epstein *et al*. (1975), reported a significant difference in mean plasma oestrogen and progesterone levels in migraine patients compared with controls. Although the levels of oestrogen and progesterone were higher in migraine sufferers than in controls, there was no significant difference betwen levels in menstrually related compared with non-menstrually related migraine sufferers. In this study there was no clear temporal relationship between the fall in oestrogen or progesterone levels with precipitation of migraine attacks. This study therefore failed to confirm Somerville's earlier study, but this may be explained since in the study by Epstein *et al*., (1975) the migraine sufferers suffered multiple attacks each month, but with a menstrual exacerbation, rather than the group in Somerville's studies who only had premenstrual headache.

In a small study of four women suffering common migraine progesterone and oestrogen levels, as well as aldosterone, were assayed, and compared with the levels found in six normal women (Horth *et al*., 1975). Only progesterone levels were significantly elevated compared with controls one to three days before menstruation. These data suggested that women with menstrual migraine menstruated earlier than normal women for their oestrogen–progesterone status, in that the levels reflected patterns normally observed two to four days earlier. There was in addition an abnormally high level of aldosterone in two migrainous women premenstrually, which may be a factor involved in premenstrual fluid retention.

Oestrogens may cause arteriolar hypertrophy in women who are susceptible to headache. This has been found in a study of endometrial biopsies of patients who were taking oral contraceptives (Grant, 1968). In this study, the incidence of headache closely correlated with the incidence of highly developed arterioles in the endometrial biopsies. The appearance of these arterioles appeared to depend on a critical ratio of progesterone and oestrogen. As mentioned previously, there is evidence that migrainous women who use oral contraceptives are at increased risk of cerebral infarction (Irey *et al*., 1978). Similar intimal hyperplasia to that seen in the endometrium has been found in the cerebral vasculature of women who had been using oral contraception and who died as a consequence of cerebral infarction (Irey *et al.*, 1978). This arterial intimal hyperplasia has also been observed in the pulmonary, portal and coronary circulations in women taking oral contraceptives (Irey and Norris, 1973). This effect of oestrogen on endometrial arterioles may relate to the study by Hockaday *et al.* (1967), in which hand blood flow was significantly increased in women taking oral contraceptives. There was, however, no alteration in reflex responsiveness of the vessels in either controls or migraine sufferers.

Welch *et al.* (1984), propose the unifying hypothesis that migraine is a result of fluctuating levels of oestrogen acting via the sympathetic nervous system. They cite the evidence suggesting an α-denervation sensitivity in migraine, namely iris adrenergic impairment (Fanciullacci, 1979). However, the finding of reduced dopamine β-hydroxylase in the premenstrual phase (Magos *et al.*, 1985) is against a major involvement of the sympathetic nervous system. Oestrogen itself is capable of potent direct and indirect vascular actions (Altura and Altura, 1977). Oestrogens augment the vasoconstrictor activity of adrenaline and noradrenaline in normal mice in systemic vascular beds. This effect may be caused by a stimulation of the production of noradrenaline receptors in vascular smooth muscle, which has been shown to follow exposure to oestrogen (Gorski and Gannon, 1976), by increasing DNA transcription. This attempt at producing a unifying hypothesis involving oestrogens and the sympathetic nervous system clearly fails to explain all the observations on migraine in general, and menstrual migraine in particular, but it does have the merit of being testable. Further experiments are required in this important area.

Prolactin has been suggested to be implicated in the genesis of migraine (Parantainen, 1975; Horrobin, 1973). The levels of prolactin have been investigated in several studies of migraine sufferers. Basal prolactin levels in menstrual migraine are consistently higher in menstrual migraine sufferers, but the levels do not reach statistical significance (Nattero *et al.*, 1979). In a more dynamic test of prolactin secretion, five women with common migraine were studied (Nattero *et al.*, 1986). The response of prolactin to the administration of 0.5 g L-dopa was followed for 120 min. The migrainous group showed a significant reduction in inhibition of prolactin secretion, compared with five age and sex matched controls. This suggests a reduced responsiveness of pituitary prolactin producing cells to the action of dopaminergic agents. The mechanism of this, and its relevance to the aetiology of menstrual migraine remains obscure.

There have been several recent studies suggesting a role for prostaglandins in the aetiology of menstrual migraine. Infusion of prostaglandin E_1, in very high concentrations, (>0.1 μg kg^{-1} min^{-1}) can produce a migraine-like headache, with nausea, and sometimes preceded by characteristically migrainous visual symptoms in non-migraine sufferers (Carlson *et al.*, 1968). In low concentrations (<0.1 μg kg^{-1} min^{-1}) prostaglandin E$_1$ is a potent vaso-constrictor, while in high concentrations it has a predominantly vasodilator action (Horrobin, 1977). Some of the agents known to be of value in the treatment of migraine inhibit prostaglandin synthase or antagonize the actions of some prostaglandins. Oestrogens stimulate the secretion of some prostaglandins both directly and indirectly (Horrobin, 1977). Furthermore, 5-HT releases prostaglandins from the lung, an effect blocked by the drugs methysergide and ergotamine tartrate (Sandler, 1975), both of which are effective in the treatment of migraine (see below).

Treatment of Menstrual Headache

The treatment of menstrual migraine is difficult. Most who have dealt with the problem agree that this form of headache is particularly refractory to conventional treatment regimes. Few studies have dealt specifically with the problems of treating menstrual migraine, but many of the conventional approaches used in the management of headaches in general have been used with menstrual migraine sufferers. Since the therapeutic approach to migraine in general is applicable to menstrual migraine, some comments concerning headache treatment are appropriate.

General Measures

After establishing the diagnosis of headache type, reassurance that there is no evidence of progressive or life-threatening disease is important, and frequently leads to a dramatic improvement in headaches. Migraine is frequently associated with precipitating factors, although these are far less common with other headache types. In some, prolonged fasting may be a precipitating factor and a regularization of meal times may be helpful. In others, 'weekend headaches', or headaches resulting from sleeping too long in the mornings, may be helped by getting up at the same time on each day of the week.

A proportion of patients describe attacks being caused by dietary constituents. The most common of these appear to be cheese, chocolate, citrus fruit, coffee, and alcohol, sometimes only of a specific type. Exclusion of these from the diet is worth a trial in most migraine sufferers. Considerable improvement has followed avoidance of these foods in some patients (Lance, 1978; Monro, 1982; Egger *et al.*, 1983). It appears that many women develop food sensitivities only in the pre-menstruum, and although this has not been confirmed in formal studies, the author has had success with initiating limited dietary exclusions only at this time.

The association of migraine and oral contraceptives has already been discussed. If other acceptable contraceptive measures are possible, the oral contraceptive is best stopped in patients with severe, recurrent migraine.

Treatment of the Acute Attack of Headache

Simple analgesics such as aspirin or paracetamol are often effective, particularly if taken in an effervescent preparation and with metoclopramide. Gastric stasis, with a consequent reduction in drug absorption is common at even the earliest stages of a migraine attack (Volans, 1978), and metoclopramide not only suppresses nausea, but also enhances absorption in migraine (Tfelt-Hansen et al., 1980). The use of effervescent preparations or metoclopramide is of less value in tension headache, where gastric stasis is not a feature. It is important to initiate treatment as early as possible, at the first sign of an acute attack. Several studies have emphasized the value of derivatives of fenamic acid—mefenamic acid (Peatfield et al., 1983), flufenamic acid (Vardi et al., 1976), and finally, tolfenamic acid, which has been shown in a double blind trial to be as effective as ergotamine, but without its side effects (Hakkareinen et al., 1979). Fenamic acid derivatives appear to inhibit the actions as well as the synthesis of prostaglandins (Vardi et al., 1976). Other non-steroidal anti-inflammatories especially naproxen, have been shown to have a useful action in the treatment of acute attacks (Johnson et al., 1985) and the prophylaxis of migraine (Behan and Conelly, 1986).

Ergotamine preparations have a place in the treatment of patients with severe but infrequent attacks. They should, however, be used no more than once or twice each month. Not only may the ergot compounds exacerbate the nausea and vomiting, but more frequent doses tend to be cumulative, and can induce a chronic background headache.

Prophylactic Medication

Prophylaxis is usually recommended for those having more than two attacks of migraine each month, in whom migraine is interfering with the quality of life. In the patient with severe menstrual migraine, this rule is often relaxed. Prophylactic medication taken for the second half of the menstrual cycle may be effective, and is often recommended since the acute attack of menstrual migraine may not respond to the conventional measures outlined above.

Clonidine was the first drug marketed specifically for migraine prophylaxis. Despite promising reports in the early 1970s, it is probably no better than placebo in the majority of patients (Boisen et al., 1978). It has been suggested that it may be of use in patients whose attacks are clearly linked to constituents of the diet.

The drugs of first choice in migraine prophylaxis are pizotifen and propranolol. Pizotifen is considered to block 5-HT receptors, though it may also have a partial agonist action. It produces a significant improvement in some 70 per cent of patients (Peet, 1977; Mikropoulos, 1978). In some patients there may be a relapse after some months on the drug, but in others, interference with an established pattern of headache may lead to long-term benefit. The principal side effects are weight gain and drowsiness, but both can be largely avoided by administering the drug as a single dose in the evening.

Propranolol appears to be the most effective of the β-blockers in treating migraine. Timolol has some beneficial action, as does metoprolol (Vilming et al., 1985). Alprenolol, pindolol, and acebutolol, have little action in migraine. These observations suggest that the action of propanolol is independent of its β-blocking activity. Indeed a trial of D-propranolol, which retains the membrane stabilizing properties of L-propranolol, but has no action at β-receptors, showed this compound to be almost as effective as the racemic form—DL-propranolol—which is in common use (Stensrud and Sjaastad, 1976). There also appears to be no association between the degree of lipid solubility of a β-blocker and its efficacy in migraine.

Methysergide is probably the most potent of specific prophylactic agents, but is usually maintained as the drug of last choice, because of the possible association of its long-term use with retroperitoneal fibrosis. It is recommended that it should be used in interrupted courses of five months duration, separated by a drug free month. Since this practice has been adopted, there have been no further reports of retroperitoneal fibrosis associated with its use.

The calcium antagonists verapamil, nimodipine and flunarizine have been attracting considerable interest as prophylactic agents since they were first shown to have some useful action in the early 1980s (Meyer and Hardenberg, 1983; Amery et al., 1985). Their mode of action in migraine is by no means certain. They may be having effects on the cerebral vasculature—indeed, on the strength of their apparent efficacy it has been postulated that cerebral ischaemia is a crucial element in the genesis of the migraine attack (Amery, 1982). It is also possible that they have an action within the central nervous system. The calcium antagonists are lipid soluble, and penetrate the blood–brain barrier to a variable extent.

The calcium antagonist flunarizine has been compared with the dopamine receptor antagonist domperidone and the prostaglandin synthase inhibitor suprofene, in 100 women with menstrual migraine (Conigliaro et al., 1985). There are few details given in the published abstract, but it appears that in 30 of these patients migraine was only associated with menstruation, while in the remainder headache also occurred on other days of the month. Significant results were only obtained with flunarizine. Those who only had headache in association with the menstrual period showed little improvement, while those in whom headache also occurred at other times showed a significant improvement. This study does not give details of the exact numbers of responders, or the levels of significance applied, and the results must be treated with caution. It would be of interest if the results confirm the previously mentioned concept that women with exclusively menstrual migraine represent a specific and distinct sub-group of migraine.

Benzodiazepines are still sometimes used for the prophylaxis of migraine, but only potassium clorazepate appears to be of use, and then only in cases in which stress is a precipitating factor. Benzodiazepines may, however, have a more important role in the treatment of tension headache, particularly if part of a comprehensive treatment programme.

Various other agents have been used for a migraine prophylaxis, and the following are occasionally used:

1. Indoramin, an α-blocking agent, has received favourable reports (Wainscott et al., 1975; Pearce et al., 1978).
2. Aspirin has been reported to have prophylactic effect when given in high dose (600 mg twice daily). This dose inhibits both platelet and vessel wall prostaglandin synthesis, and its mode of action is unclear (O'Niell and Mann, 1978).
3. Amitriptyline may sometimes be successful in patients resistant to conventional therapy, either alone or in combination with other agents. Its action appears to be independent of its antidepressant actions (Couch et al., 1976). Amitriptylline has been shown to be the most effective prophylactic agent for the treatment of chronic tension headache (Lance and Curran, 1964).
4. Slow release dihydroergotamine was assessed in 20 women with migraine which occurred only, or predominantly in association with menstruation. Of the sixteen women who completed the study, there was a significant reduction in the headache index as determined by severity and duration of headache (D'Alessandro et al., 1983).
5. Fenoprofen calcium, a prostaglandin synthetase inhibitor, has been shown, in an uncontrolled study of 84 women, to have a 25 per cent efficacy when used in the premenstrual and menstrual phases (Diamond, 1984).
6. Lisuride, an isoengonyl derivative with dopaminergic and serotoninergic properties, has been examined in a double-blind study of 30 women with menstrual or premenstrual migraine. Lisuride achieved a significant reduction in the intensity and duration and intensity of migraine attacks, but patients were not divided into those with attacks occurring only in association with the menstrual cycle and those who had attacks at other times (Zuddas et al., 1983).
7. Bromocriptine was studied in seven women with menstrual migraine. The frequency and severity of attacks was reduced in all of them (Hockaday et al., 1975).

Hormonal Interventions

The putative association of migraine in general, and menstrual migraine in particular, with high levels of oestrogen, or oestrogen withdrawal, has led to several attempts to adjust hormonal status for therapeutic purposes.

The first of these was the use of methylnortestosterone or allyloestrenol (Lundberg, 1962). Of 84 patients, 55 (who included six men) became free of migraine attacks, but continuous therapy caused amenorrhoea in most cases. In those who received cyclical therapy, menstrual disturbances occurred in 36 out of 76 women, and in addition nine reported acne, hirsutism or hoarseness. Another progestogenic agent, flumedroxone, was subjected to a controlled trial, in which its effect was compared with that of methysergide over a period of nine months in 35 patients (Hudgson *et al.*, 1967). There was no significant difference between the number of attacks per month experienced before the trial period and the number of monthly attacks while taking flumedroxone. This was in sharp contrast to the improvement which occurred in all but three patients taking methysergide.

Gonadotrophic hormone has been regularly used in the treatment of migraine for many years. However, when studied in a formal setting, improvement was noted in only ten of 26 patients (Lance, 1978).

On the basis of the persuasive evidence implicating oestrogen withdrawal in the pathogenesis of menstrual migraine, and the promising results obtained by Somerville (1975a,b) in oestrogen-withdrawal headache, oestradiol implants have been used (Magos *et al.*, 1983). In all 24 patients were studied, of whom five had classical migraine and nineteen common migraine. All patients complained of regular attacks immediately before or during menstruation, although it was not specified if any belonged to the sub-group which only has attacks in association with the menstrual period. The dose of oestradiol was started at 100 mg, which was usually reduced to a maintenance dose. Implants were repeated at an average interval of 6.2 months. Patients were also given cyclical progestogens to induce regular withdrawal periods and prevent endometrial hyperplasia. All but one patient noted an improvement in their menstrual migraine following treatment. Eleven (46 per cent) became completely headache-free, and nine (37 per cent) gained almost complete symptomatic improvement. All but one reported some degree of improvement. These results are impressive, but some caution is required in the interpretation of short term studies using implants, which have a very high placebo response rate (Magos *et al.*, 1986). A high placebo response rate (up to 65 per cent) has been noted in all studies of prophylactic hormone therapy (Lundberg, 1969).

Non-pharmacological Treatments

Relaxation and biofeedback. There is a growing body of literature on the positive effect of behavioural treatment, specifically relaxation and biofeedback, with or without additional coping techniques, on headache pain (Blanchard *et al.*, 1980). These techniques appear to be particularly effective for tension headache. Two studies have evaluated these treatments in menstrual headache. In the first (Solbach *et al.*, 1984) there were four groups. Patients were allocated to:

1. No treatment group.
2. Autogenic phrases.
3. Electromyographic feedback.
4. Thermal biofeedback.

Multivariate analysis failed to reveal a significant difference between the four groups. This implies that non-drug treatments have a lesser influence on menstrual migraine than they do on migraines not associated with menstruation. In previous studies, males and females have shown a comparable response rate, which excludes the possibility that women as a whole are refractory to these treatment modalities.

The second investigation (Szekely *et al.*, 1986) subdivided patients into those with migraine, muscle contraction, mixed and cluster headache, and used either relaxation with electromyographic and thermal biofeedback, or person-centred insight therapy. Again there was no significant difference between the two groups, or between the number and severity of headaches before or after treatment.

Acupuncture. One investigation, which used the local injection of anaesthetic or of saline into the muscles of the head and neck during attacks of common migraine, reported a significant improvement in headache severity (Tfelt-Hansen *et al.*, 1981). Several studies have examined the effects of both traditional Chinese acupuncture, and simple needling of tender points about the head and neck, both to treat acute attacks of headache, and to provide prophylaxis against further attacks (Cheng, 1975; Bischko, 1978; Jensen and Jensen, 1982; Loh *et al.*, 1984). The results suggest that acupuncture may be valuable in some cases, but each study has had some design flaws. In particular, there has been little attention to the problem of administering a suitable placebo treatment, and there was a variable mixture of different headache types. No study has yet addressed the problem of whether acupuncture is of value in menstrual headache.

Hypnosis. Hypnosis has been claimed to be of value in the treatment of headache. Only one formal study has been undertaken, but this study, although claiming a positive effect of hypnosis, was flawed both by patient selection criteria, and the use of a control group which would not normally be accepted (Anderson *et al.*, 1976). Further studies are required to establish whether hypnosis is of value in the treatment of menstrual headache.

Pyridoxine. The value of pyridoxine (vitamin B_6), as a treatment for the premenstrual syndrome, is discussed elsewhere in this volume. There have been no formal studies of its value in menstrual headache, although in a small open study of 47 women with common or classical migraine, who showed a regular menstrual exacerbation of attacks, the author found a significant improvement in headache index. Further studies are required to establish the value of pyridoxine in the prophylaxis of menstrual headache.

Acknowledgements

I gratefully acknowledge the helpful comments of Drs Jeremy Pearson and Deirdre Gillespie who read and criticized earlier versions of this chapter.

References

Altura, B. M. and Altura, B. T. (1977). Vascular smooth muscle and neurohypophyseal hormones. *Federation Proceedings*, **36**, 1853–1860.
Amery, W. K., Caers, L. I. and Aerts, T. J. L. (1985). Flunarizine, a calcium entry blocker in migraine prophylaxis. *Headache*, **25**, 249–254.
Amery, W. K. (1982). Brain hypoxia: the turning point in the genesis of the migraine attack?, *Cephalalgia*, **2**, 83–109.
Anderson, J. A. D., Basker, M. A. and Dalton, R. (1975). Migraine and hypnotherapy. *International Journal of Clinical and Experimental Hypnosis*, **23**, 48–58.
Anthony, M., Hinterberger, H. and Lance, J. W. (1967). Plasma serotonin in migraine and stress. *Archives of Neurology*, **16**, 544–552.
Anthony, M. and Lance, J. W. (1975). The role of serotonin in migraine, in *Modern Topics in Migraine*, (Ed. J. Pearce) Heinemann, London, pp. 107–123.
Anthony, M. (1981). Biochemical indices of sympathetic activity in migraine. *Cephalalgia*, **1**, 83–89.
Behan, P. O. and Connelly, K. (1986). Prophylaxis of migraine: a comparison between naproxen sodium and pizotifen. *Headache*, **26**, 237–239.
Bischko, J. (1978). Acupuncture in headache. *Research and Clinical Studies on Headache*, **5**, 72–85.
Blanchard, E. B., Andrasik, F., Ahles, T. A., Teders, J. J. and O'Keefe, D. (1980). Migraine and tension headache: A meta-analytic review. *Behaviour Therapy*, **11**, 613–631.
Blau, J. N. (1978). Migraine and vasomotor instability of the meningeal circulation. *Lancet*, **ii**, 1136–1139.
Boisen, E., Deth, S., Hubbe, P., Jansen, J., Klee, A. and Leunbach, G. (1978). Clonidine in the prophylaxis of migraine. *Acta Neurologica Scandinavica*, **58**, 288–295.
Bradshaw, P. and Parsons, M. (1965). Hemiplegic migraine: a clinical study. *Quarterly Journal of Medicine*, **34**, 65–85.

Brazil, P. and Friedman, A. P. (1956). Craniovascular studies in headache. A report and analysis of pulse volume tracings. *Neurology*, **6**, 96–102.

Bruyn, G. W. (1982). Cerebral cortex and migraine. *Advances in Neurology*, **33**, 151–169.

Burnstock, G. (1981). Pathophysiology of migraine: a new hypothesis. *Lancet*, **i**, 1397–1399.

Carlson, L. A., Ekelund, L.-G. and Oro, L. (1968). Clinical and metabolic effects of different doses of prostaglandin E_1 in man. *Acta Medica Scandinavica*, **183**, 423–431.

Cheng, A. C. K. (1975). The treatment of headaches employing acupuncture. *American Journal of Chinese Medicine*, **3**, 181–185.

Conigliaro, S., Rosa, R., Filppi, M. C., Meratti, L. and Taddei, M. T. (1985). The flunarizine on treatment of the menses migraine. Comparison with dopamine and prostaglandin inhibitor (Domperidone and suprofene). *Cephalalgia*, **Supplement 5**, 544.

Couch, J. R. and Hassanein, R. S. (1977). Platelet aggregability in migraine. *Neurology*, **27**, 843–848.

Couch, J. D., Ziegler, D. K. and Hassanein, R. S. (1976). Amitryptiline in the prophylaxis of migraine. *Neurology*, **26**, 121–127.

Curzon, G., Barrie, M. and Wilkinson, M. I. P. (1969). Relationships between headache and amine changes after administration of reserpine to migrainous patients. *Journal of Neurology, Neurosurgery and Psychiatry*, **32**, 555–561.

D'Alessandro, R., Gamberini, G., Lozito, A. and Sacquegna, T. (1983). Menstrual migraine: intermittent prophylaxis with a timed-release pharmacological formulation of dihydroergotamine. *Cephalalgia*, **Supplement 1**; 156–158.

Dalessio, D. J. (Ed.) (1980). *Wolff's Headache and Other Head Pain*, (4th edition) Oxford University Press, Oxford.

Dalsgaard-Nielsen, T. (1965). Migraine and heredity. *Acta Neurologica Scandinavica*, **41**, 287–300.

Dalton, K. (1976). Migraine and oral contraceptives. *Headache*, **16**, 247–251.

Diamond, S. (1984). Menstrual migraine and non-steroidal anti-inflammatory agents. *Headache*, **24**, 52.

Drummond, P. D. and Lance, J. W. (1983). Extracranial vascular changes and the source of pain in migraine headache. *Annals of Neurology*, **13**, 32–37.

Dvilansky, A., Rishpon, S., Nathan, I., Zolotow, Z. and Korczyn, A. (1976). Release of platelet 5-hydroxytryptamine by plasma taken from patients during and between migraine attacks. *Pain*, **2**, 315–318.

Edelson, R. N. (1985). Menstrual migraine and other hormonal aspects of migraine. *Headache*, **25**, 376–379.

Egger, J., Wilson, J., Carter, C. M., Turner, M. W. and Soothill, J. F. (1983). Is migraine food allergy? *Lancet*, **ii**, 1424.

Epstein, M. T., Hockaday, J. M. and Hockaday, T. D. R. (1975). Migraine and reproductive hormones throughout the menstrual cycle. *Lancet*, **ii**, 543–547.

Facchinetti, F., Sances, G., Volpe, A., Sola, D., D'Ambrogio, G., Sinforiani, E. and Genazzini, A. R. (1983). Hypothalamus pituitary-ovarian axis in menstrual migraine: effect of dihydroergotamine retard prophylactic treatment. *Cephalalgia*, **Supplement 1**, 159–162.

Fanchamps, A. (1974). The role of humoral mediators in migraine headache. *Canadian Journal of Neurological Science*, **1**, 189–195.

Fanciullacci, M. (1979). Iris adrenergic impairment in idiopathic headache. *Headache*, **19**, 8–13.

Featherstone, H. J. (1985). Migraine and muscle contraction headaches: a continuum. *Headache*, **25**, 194–198.

Fisher, C. M. (1971). Cerebral ischaemia—less familiar types. *Clinical Neurosurgery*, **18**, 267–335.

Fozard, J. R. (1982). Basic mechanisms of antimigraine drugs. *Advances in Neurology*, **33**, 295–308.

Friedman, A. P., Finley, K. M., Graham, J. R., Kunkle, E. C., Ostfeld, A. M. and Wolff, H. G. (1962). Classification of headache. The Ad Hoc Committee on the Classification of Headache. *Archives of Neurology*, **6**, 173–174.

Friedman, A. P. and Merritt, H. H. (1959). *Headache: Diagnosis and Treatment*, Davis, Philadelphia.

Gardner Medwin, A. R. (1981). Possible roles of vertebral neuroglia in potassium dynamics, spreading depression and migraine. *Journal of Experimental Biology*, **95**, 111–127.

Gawel, M., Burkitt, M. and Clifford Rose, F. (1979). The platelet release reaction during migraine attacks. *Headache*, **19**, 323–327.

Geffen, L. B. (1974). Serum dopamine beta hydroxylase as an index of sympathetic function. *Life Sciences*, **14**, 1593–1604.

Glover, V., Littlewood, J., Petty, R. G., Sandler, M., Peatfield, R. and Clifford Rose, F. (1983). Biochemical predisposition to dietary migraine. The role of phenolsulphotransferase. *Headache*, **23**, 53–58.

Gorski, J. and Gannon, F. (1976). Current models of steroid hormone action: a critique. *Annual Reviews of Physiology*, **38**, 425–450.

Gotoh, F., Tadashi, K., Sakai, F., Yamamoto, M. and Takeoka, T. (1976). Serum dopamine beta hydroxylase activity in migraine. *Archives of Neurology*, **33**, 565–567.

Grant, E. C. G. (1968). Relation between headaches from oral contraceptives and development of endometrial arterioles. *British Medical Journal*, **3**, 402–405.

Greene, R. (1967). Menstrual headache. *Research and Clinical Studies on Headache*, **1**, 62–73.

Greene, R. (1973). The endocrinology of headache: the Sandoz lecture, in *Background to Migraine*, (Ed. J. N. Cumings) Heinemann, London, pp. 82–92.

Greene, R. and Dalton, K. (1953). The premenstrual syndrome. *British Medical Journal*, **1**, 1007–1014.

Hakkareinen, H., Vapaatalo, H., Gothoni, G. and Parantainen, J. (1979). Tolfenamic acid is as effective as ergotamine during acute migraine attacks. *Lancet*, **ii**, 326–328.

Hanington, E., Jones, R. J., Amess, J. A. L. and Wachowicz, B. (1981). Migraine: a platelet disorder. *Lancet*, **ii**, 720–723.

Hanington, E., Jones, R. J. and Amess, J. A. L. (1982a). Migraine and platelets. *Lancet*, **i**, 1248.

Hanington, E., Jones, R. J. and Amess, J. A. L. (1982b). Platelet aggregation in response to 5-HT in migraine patients taking oral contraceptives. *Lancet*, **i**, 967–968.

Hanington, E. (1983). Migraine, in *Clinical Reactions to Food* (Ed. M. H. Lessof) John Wiley, Chichester, pp. 155–180.

Heyck, H. (1969). Pathogenesis of migraine. *Research and Clinical Studies on Headache*, **2**, 1–28.

Hockaday, J. M., MacMillan, A. L. and Whitty, C. W. M. (1967). Vasomotor-reflex response in idiopathic and hormone-dependent migraine. *Lancet*, **i**, 1023–1026.

Hockaday, J. M., Peet, K. M. S. and Hockaday, T. D. R. (1975). Bromocriptine in migraine. *Headache*, **16**, 109–114.

Horrobin, D. F. (1973). Prevention of migraine by reducing prolactin levels? *Lancet*, i, 777.

Horrobin, D. F. (1977). Hypothesis: prostaglandins and migraine *Headache*, **17**, 113–117.

Horth, C. E., Wainscott, G., Neylan, C. and Wilkinson, M. I. P. (1975). Progesterone, oestradiol and aldosterone levels in plasma during the menstrual cycle of women suffering from migraine. *Journal of Endocrinology*, **65**, 24P–25P.

Hudgson, P., Foster, J. B. and Newell, D. J. (1967). Controlled trial of demigran in the prophylaxis of migraine. *British Medical Journal*, **2**, 91–93.

Irey, N. S. and Norris, H. J. (1973). Intimal vascular lesions associated with female reproductive steroids. *Archives of Pathology*, **96**, 227–234.

Irey, N. S., McAllister, H. A. and Henry, J. M. (1978). Oral contraceptives and stroke in young women: a clinicopathologic correlation. *Neurology*, **28**, 1216–1219.

Jensen, L. B. and Jensen, S. B. (1982). Effect of acupuncture on tension headache and urinary catecholamine excretion. *Scandinavican Journal of Dental Research*, **90**, 397–403.

Jessup, B. (1978). The role of diet in migraine: conditioned taste aversion. *Headache*, **18**, 229.

Johnson, E. S. (1978). A basis for migraine therapy—the autonomic theory reappraised. *Postgraduate Medical Journal*, **54**, 231–242.

Johnson, E. S., Ratcliffe, D. M. and Wilkinson, M. (1985). Naproxen sodium in the treatment of migraine. *Cephalalgia*, **5**, 5–10.

Kangasniemi, P., Falck, B., Langvik, V.-A. and Hyyppa, M. T. (1978). Levotryptophan treatment in migraine. *Headache*, **18**, 161–166.

Kennard, C., Gawel, M., Rudolph, N. de M. and Rose, F. C. (1978). Visual evoked potentials in migraine subjects. *Research and Clinical Studies on Headache*, **6**, 73–80.

Klee, A. (1968). *A Clinical Study of Migraine with Particular Reference to the Most Severe Cases*, Munksjaard, Copenhagen.

Kudrow, L. (1975). The relationship of headache frequency to hormone use in migraine. *Headache*, **15**, 36–40.

Lamprecht, F., Raymond, J., Little, B. and Zahn, T. P. (1974). Plasma dopamine beta hydroxylase (DBH) activity during the menstrual cycle. *Psychosomatic Medicine*, **36**, 304–310.

Lance, J. W. (1978). *Mechanism and Management of Headache*, Butterworths, London.

Lance, J. W. and Anthony, M. (1966). Some clinical aspects of migraine. A prospective survey of 500 patients. *Archives of Neurology*, **15**, 356–361.

Lance, J. W. and Curran, D. A. (1964). Treatment of chronic tension headache. *Lancet*, i, 1236–1238.

Lance, J. W., Lambert, G. A., Goadsby, P. J. and Duckworth, J. W. (1983). Brainstem influences on the cephalic circulation: experimental data from cat and monkey of relevance to the mechanism of migraine. *Headache*, **23**, 258–265.

Lauritzen, M., Olsen, T. S., Lassen, N. A. and Paulson, O. B. (1983). Changes in regional cerebral blood flow during the course of classic migraine attacks. *Annals of Neurology*, **13**, 633–641.

Leao, A. A. P. (1944). Spreading depression of activity in cerebral cortex. *Journal of Neurophysiology*, **7**, 359–390.

Lehtonen, J., Hyyppa, M. T., Kaihola, H.-L., Kangasniemi, P. and Lang, A. H. (1979). Visual evoked potentials in menstrual migraine. *Headache*, **19**, 63–70.

Littlewood, J., Glover, V., Sandler, M., Petty, R., Peatfield, R. and Clifford Rose, F.

(1982). Platelet phenolsulphotransferase deficiency in dietary migraine. *Lancet*, **i**, 983–986.

Loh, L., Nathan, P. W., Schott, G. D. and Zilkha, K. J. (1984). Acupuncture versus medical treatment for migraine and muscle tension headaches. *Journal of Neurology, Neurosurgery and Psychiatry*, **47**, 333–337.

Lundberg, P. O. (1962). Migraine prophylaxis with progestogens. *Acta Endocrinologica*, **40 (Supplement 68)**, 1–22.

Lundberg, P. O. (1969). Prophylactic treatment of migraine with flumedroxone. *Acta Neurologica Scandinavica*, **45**, 309–326.

Magos, A. L., Brincat, M., Zilkha, K. J. and Studd, J. W. W. (1985). Serum dopamine beta-hydroxylase activity in menstrual migraine. *Journal of Neurology, Neurosurgery and Psychiatry*, **48**, 328–331.

Magos, A. L., Zilkha, K. J. and Studd, J. W. W. (1983). Treatment of menstrual migraine by oestradiol implants. *Journal of Neurology, Neurosurgery and Psychiatry*, **46**, 1044–1046.

Magos, A. L., Brincat, M. and Studd, J. W. W. (1986). Treatment of the premenstrual syndrome by subcutaneous oestradiol implants and cyclical norethisterone: placebo controlled study. *British Medical Journal*, **292**, 1629–1633.

Markush, R. E., Karp, H. R., Heyman, A. and O'Fallon, W. M. (1975). Epidemiologic study of migraine symptoms in young women, *Neurology*, **25**, 430–435.

Marshall, W. H. (1959). Spreading cortical depression of Leao. *Physiological Reviews*, **39**, 239–279.

Mears, E. and Grant, E. C. G. (1962). 'Anovlar' as an oral contraceptive. *British Medical Journal*, **2**, 75–79.

Medina, J. L. and Diamond, S. (1982). The concept of cyclical migraine, in *Migraine Research*, Vol. 1 (Ed. F. Clifford Rose) Pitman, London, pp. 9–12.

Meyer, J. S. and Hardenberg, J. (1983). Clinical effectiveness of calcium entry blockers in prophylactic treatment of migraine and cluster headaches. *Headache*, **23**, 266–277.

Mikropoulos, H. E. (1978). Toleration and effectiveness of pizotifen in migraine. *Research and Clinical Studies on Headache*, **6**, 167–172.

Moffat, A. M., Swash, M. and Scott, D. F. (1974). Effect of chocolate in migraine: a double-blind study. *Journal of Neurology, Neurosurgery and Psychiatry*, **37**, 445–448.

Monro, J. (1982). Food allergy and migraine. *Clinics in Immunology and Allergy*, **2**, 137–164.

Nattero, G. (1982). Menstrual headache. *Advances in Neurology*, **33**, 215–226.

Nattero, G., Bisbocci, D. and Ceresa, F. (1979). Sex hormones, prolactin levels, osmolarity and electrolyte patterns in menstrual migraine—relationship with fluid retention. *Headache*, **19**, 25–30.

Nattero, G., Corno, M., Savi, L., Isaia, G. C., Priolo, C. and Mussetta, M. (1986). Prolactin and migraine: Effect of L-dopa on plasma prolactin levels in migraineurs and normals. *Headache*, **26**, 9–12.

North, R. H. and Murlow, P. J. (1976). Serum dopamine beta hydroxylase as an index of sympathetic nervous system activity in man. *Circulation Research*, **18**, 2–5.

O'Niell, B. P. and Mann, J. D. (1978). Aspirin prophylaxis in migraine. *Lancet*, **ii**, 1179–1181.

Olesen, J. (1978). Some clinical features of the acute migraine attack. An analysis of 750 patients. *Headache*, **18**, 268–271.

Olesen, J., Tfelt-Hansen, P., Henriksen, L. and Lassen, B. (1981). The common migraine attack may not be initiated by cerebral ischaemia. *Lancet*, **ii**, 438–440.

Olesen, J., Larsen, B. and Lauritzen, M. (1980). Focal hyperaemia followed by spreading oligaemia and impaired activation of rCBF in classic migraine attacks. *Annals of Neurology*, **9**, 344–352.

Parantainen, J. (1975). Prolactin, levodopa, and migraine. *Lancet*, **i**, 467.

Pearce, J., Pearce, I. and Faux, G. A. (1978). Alpha-adrenergic activity and blockade in migraine, in *Current Concepts in Migraine Research*, (Ed. R. Greene) Raven, New York, pp. 49–52.

Pearce, J. M. S. (1985). Is migraine explained by Leao's spreading depression? *Lancet*, **ii**, 763–766.

Peatfield, R. C., Petty, R. G. and Clifford Rose, F. (1983). Double blind comparison of mefenamic acid and acetaminophen (paracetamol) in migraine. *Cephalalgia*, **3**, 129–134.

Peatfield, R. C., Gawel, M. J. and Clifford Rose, F. (1981). Asymmetry of the aura and pain in migraine. *Journal of Neurology, Neurosurgery and Psychiatry*, **44**, 846–848.

Peet, K. M. S. (1977). The use of pizotifen in severe migraine—a long term study. *Current Medical Research Opinion*, **5**, 192–198.

Petraglia, F., Martignoni, E., Sola, D., Cicoli, C., Facchinetti, F., Nappi, G. and Genazzini, A. (1983). Evaluation of central opioid tonus in menstrual migraine. *Cephalalgia*, **Supplement 1**, 98–100.

Pluvinage, R. (1975). Headache, including migraine, and oral contraception, in *Background to Migraine* (Ed. J. N. Cumings), Heinemann, London, pp. 150–153.

Prensky, A. L. (1976). Migraine and migrainous variants in pediatric patients. *Pediatric Clinics of North America*, **23**, 461–471.

Raskin, N. and Appenzeller, O. (1980). *Major Problems in Internal Medicine XIX. Headache*, W. B. Saunders, Philadelphia.

Roy, C. S. and Sherrington, C. S. (1890). On the regulation of the blood supply of the brain. *Journal of Physiology*, **11**, 85–108.

Sachs, O. (1970). *Migraine*, Faber and Faber, London.

Sakai, F. and Meyer, J. S. (1978). Regional cerebral hemodynamics during migraine and cluster headache measured by the ^{133}Xe inhalation method. *Headache*, **18**, 122–132.

Sandler, M. (1975). Monoamines and migraine: a path through the wood?, in *Vasoactive Substances Relevant to Migraine*. (Eds. S. Diamond, D. J. Dalessio, T. R. Graham and J. L. Medina), Thomas, Springfield, Illinois, pp. 3–18.

Schafer, E. W., and McKean, C. M. (1975). Evidence that monoamines influence human evoked potentials. *Brain Research*, **99**, 49–58.

Selby, G. and Lance, J. W. (1960). Observations on 500 cases of migraine and allied vascular headache. *J. Neurology, Neurosurgery and Psychiatry*, **23**, 23–32.

Sicuteri, F. (1980). Opioids, pregnancy and the disappearance of headache. *Headache*, **20**, 220–221.

Sicuteri, F. (1982). Natural opioids in migraine. *Advances in Neurology*, **33**, 65–74.

Sicuteri, F., Del Bene, E. and Fonda, C. (1976). Sex, migraine and serotonin interrelationships. *Monographs on Neurological Sciences*, **3**, 94–101.

Sicuteri, F., Fanciullacci, M. and Michelacci, S. (1978). Decentralization supersensitivity in headache and central panalgesia. *Research and Clinical Studies on Headache*, **6**, 19–33.

Sicuteri, F., Testi, A. and Anselmi, B. (1961). Biochemical investigations in headache: increase in hydroxyindole acetic acid excretion during migraine attacks. *International Archives of Allergy and Applied Immunology*, **19**, 55–58.

Skinhoj, E. (1973). Haemodynamic studies with the brain during migraine. *Archives of Neurology*, **29**, 95–98.

Sokoloff, L. (1978). Local cerebral energy metabolism: its relationship to functional activity and blood flow, in *Cerebral Vascular Smooth Muscle and its Control. Ciba Foundation Symposium 56*. (Eds. K. Elliot and M. O'Connor), Elsevier, Amsterdam, pp. 171–191.

Solbach, P., Sargent, J. and Coyne, L. (1984). Menstrual migraine headache: results of a controlled, experimental, outcome study of non-drug treatments. *Headache*, **24**, 75–78.

Somerville, B. W. (1971). The role of progesterone in menstrual migraine. *Neurology*, **21**, 853–859.

Somerville, B. W. (1972a). The role of estradiol withdrawal in the etiology of menstrual migraine. *Neurology*, **22**, 355–365.

Somerville, B. W. (1972b). A study of migraine in pregnancy. *Neurology*, **22**, 824–828.

Somerville, B. W. (1975a). Estrogen-withdrawal migraine. I. Duration of exposure required and attempted prophylaxis by premenstrual estrogen administration. *Neurology*, **25**, 239–244.

Somerville, B. W. (1975b). Estrogen-withdrawal migraine. II. Attempted prophylaxis by continuous estradiol administration. *Neurology*, **25**, 245–250.

Stein, G., Morton, J., Marsh, A., Collins, W., Branch, C., Desaga, U. and Ebeling, J. (1984). Headaches after childbirth. *Acta Neurologica Scandinavica*, **69**, 74–79.

Steiner, T. J., Joseph, R. and Clifford Rose, F. (1985). Migraine is not a platelet disorder. *Headache*, **25**, 434–440.

Stensrud, P. and Sjaastad, O. (1976). Short-term clinical trial of propranolol in racemic form (Inderal), D-propranolol and placebo in migraine. *Acta Neurologica Scandinavica*, **53**, 229–232.

Szekely, B., Botwin, D., Eidelman, B. H., Becker, M., Elman, N. and Schemm, R. (1986). Non-pharmacological treatment of menstrual headache: relaxation-biofeedback behaviour therapy and person-centred insight therapy. *Headache*, **26**, 86–92.

Tfelt-Hansen, P., Lous, I. and Olesen, J. (1981). Prevalence and significance of muscle tenderness during common migraine attacks. *Headache*, **21**, 49–54.

Tfelt-Hansen, P., Olesen, J., Aebelhoft-Krabbe, A., Melgaard, B. and Vellis, B. (1980). A double-blind study of metoclopramide in the treatment of migraine attacks. *Journal of Neurology, Neurosurgery and Psychiatry*, **43**, 369–371.

Vardi, Y., Rabey, I. M., Steifler, M., Scwartz, A., Lindner, H. R. and Zor, U. (1976). Migraine attacks—alleviation by an inhibitor of prostaglandin synthesis and action. *Neurology*, **26**, 447–450.

Vilming, S., Standnes, B. and Hedman, C. (1985). Metoprolol and pizotifen in the prophylactic treatment of classical and common migraine. A double-blind investigation. *Cephalalgia*, **5**, 17–23.

Volans, G. N. (1978). Migraine and drug absorption. *Clinical Pharmokinetics*, **3**, 313–318.

Wainscott, G., Volans, G. N., Wilkinson, M. and Faux, G. A. (1975). Indoramin in prevention of migraine. *Lancet*, **ii**, 32.

Waters, W. E. and O'Connor, P. J. (1971). Epidemiology of migraine and headache in women. *Journal of Neurology, Neurosurgery and Psychiatry*, **34**, 148–153.

Welch, K. M. A., Darnley, D. and Simkins, R. T. (1984). The role of estrogen in migraine: a review and hypothesis. *Cephalalgia*, **4**, 227–236.

Whitty, C. W. M., Hockaday, J. M. and Whitty, M. M. (1966). The effect of oral contraceptives on migraine. *Lancet*, **i**, 856–859.

Ziegler, D. K. (1978). The epidemiology and genetics of migraine. *Research and Clinical Studies on Headache*, **5**, 21–33.

Zuddas, A., Mulas, S., Del Zompo, M. and Corsini, G. U. (1985). Usefulness of Lisuride on menstrual migraine in a double blind trial. *Cephalalgia*, **Supplement 3**, 514–515.

Functional Disorders of the Menstrual Cycle
Edited by M. G. Brush and E. M. Goudsmit
© 1988 John Wiley & Sons Ltd

CHAPTER 15

Recent progress in the aetiology of dysmenorrhoea and menorrhagia

MARGARET C. P. REES

Nuffield Department of Obstetrics and Gynaecology,
John Radcliffe Hospital,
Oxford OX3 9DU

Introduction

Menstruation, a periodic discharge of sanguinous fluid and a sloughing of the uterine lining in a female, is an event characteristic of the reproductive cycle in humans and most subhuman primates (Scommegna and Dmowski, 1977). Dysmenorrhoea, menstrual pain, and menorrhagia, excessive blood loss, are two common menstrual disorders. The names of these conditions are derived from the Greek (men = month, dys = difficult and rhegynai = to burst forth). Dysmenorrhoea can be classified as either primary or secondary. Primary dysmenorrhoea is defined as painful menstruation occurring in the absence of pelvic pathology, while secondary dysmenorrhoea is usually associated with pelvic pathology, such as endometriosis, pelvic inflammatory disease or submucous leiomyomas. With regard to menorrhagia, while it may be associated with pelvic pathology, no significant abnormality is found in approximately 50 per cent of women having a hysterectomy for the condition. Furthermore, the majority of women with unexplained menorrhagia have apparently normal ovulatory cycles. Primary dysmenorrhoea and menorrhagia in the absence of pelvic pathology can be considered to be two functional disorders of menstruation and recent progress in the study of the factors involved in their aetiology will be discussed in two separate sections.

Primary Dysmenorrhoea

Primary dysmenorrhoea is one of the commonest gynaecological disorders and it is thought to affect about 50 per cent of women. Estimates in the United States suggest that 140 million working hours are lost annually in that country due to dysmenorrhoea. In general, primary dysmenorrhoea occurs in nulliparous women in the presence of ovulatory cycles. It usually appears six to twelve months after the menarche when ovulatory cycles become established. The pain usually consists of lower abdominal cramps and backache and there may be associated gastrointestinal disturbances (vomiting, diarrhoea), headache and faintness. These symptoms are usually present during the first two days of menstruation.

Primary dysmenorrhoea is associated with spastic uterine hypercontractility characterized by excessive amplitude and frequency of contractions and a high 'resting' tone between contractions. Also, uterine work appears to be greater in women with dysmenorrhoea. During contractions endometrial blood flow decreases, and there seems to be a good correlation between minimal blood flow and maximal colicky pain, favouring the concept that ischaemia due to hypercontractility causes primary dysmenorrhoea (Lundstrom, 1981; Lumsden, 1985).

It is now generally agreed that the myometrial hypercontractility pattern associated with primary dysmenorrhoea is associated with excessive prostaglandin production. In addition abnormal vasopressin levels have been implicated. These two possible aetiological factors have recently received considerable attention and will be discussed here. Others have been reviewed elsewhere (Dawood, 1981; Lumsden, 1985).

Prostaglandins

Prostaglandins were first discovered in accessory genital glands and human semen independently by Goldblatt (1933) and Von Euler (1935) and the term prostaglandin was first coined by Von Euler in 1935. Their association with menstruation was first reported by Pickles *et al.* (1965), who found high concentrations of prostaglandin $F_{2\alpha}$ ($PGF_{2\alpha}$) and prostaglandin E_2 (PGE_2) in endometrium and menstrual fluid. Later Wiqvist *et al.* (1971) demonstrated that administration of $PGF_{2\alpha}$ to women during the luteal phase resulted in menstrual bleeding.

Chemistry. Prostaglandins are 20-carbon polyunsaturated fatty acids containing a five-membered carbon ring with two seven- and eight-membered carbon side chains. Depending on the ring structure, prostaglandins are named A to I. The designations PGF_{α} and PGF_{β} differentiate the alternate stereochemistries of the hydroxyl group (OH) at C9. Prostaglandins belong to the '1', '2' or '3' series depending on whether they contain one, two or three double bonds in their side chains (Figure 1). The principal series in mammalian tissues is the '2' series. Thromboxane A_2 (TXA_2) is an unstable vasoconstrictor substance formed from prostaglandin endoperoxides by platelets and does not have the basic prostaglandin structure.

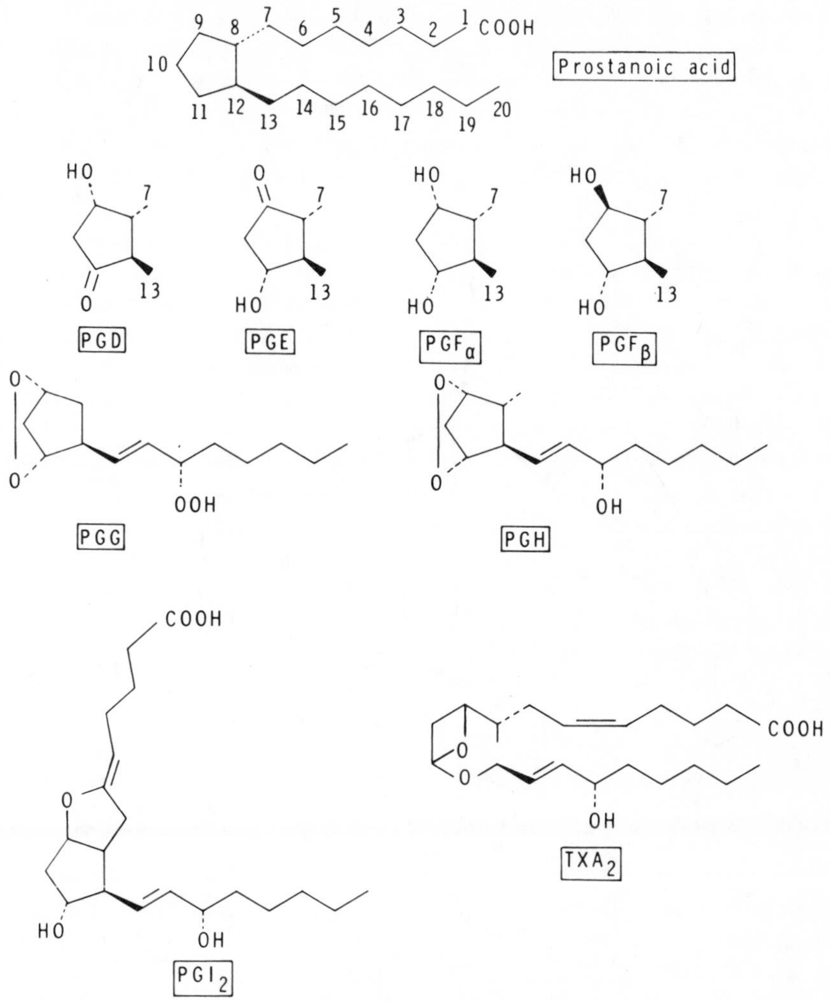

Figure 1. Prostaglandin structures

Biosynthesis. Prostaglandin synthetic pathways have been extensively described and this short account is based on a recent review (Green, 1986; Figure 2). Prostaglandins are not stored in cells but are rapidly synthesized once the substrate fatty acid precursor arachidonic acid becomes available to the appropriate synthetic enzymes. Arachidonic acid is not present as a free carboxylic acid in cells but is abundant in ester linkage at the 2-position of phospholipids. Consequently before commencement of prostaglandin biosynthesis arachidonic acid must be liberated from cellular phospholipids by the

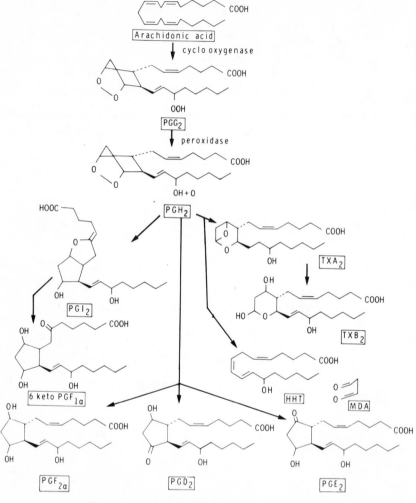

Figure 2. Prostaglandin biosynthetic pathways

action of phospholipases released by lyososomes. Once released from phos-pholipids free arachidonic acid is metabolized either by a cyclo-oxygenase mediated pathway to prostaglandins or by a lipoxygenase pathway to leukot-rienes. Both enzymes systems are present in human uterine tissues (Figure 3) and leukotriene release has recently been demonstrated (Demers *et al*., 1984; Rees *et al*., 1986). In prostaglandin synthesis arachidonic acid is first con-verted to the endoperoxide intermediates PGG_2 and PGH_2 through the action of the cyclo-oxygenase and peroxidase enzymes. Immunohistochemical

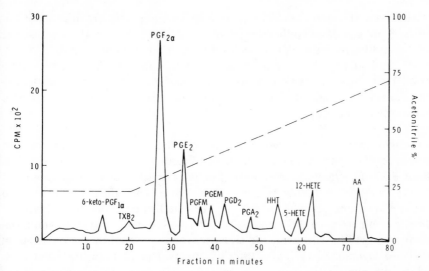

Figure 3. High pressure liquid chromatography profile of endometrial arachidonic acid products. Prostaglandins (PGs) are produced as well as the lipoxygenase products 5-HETE and 12-HETE. Reproduced by permission of Longman Group Ltd from Demers *et al.*, 1984, *Prostaglandins, Leukotrienes and Medicine*, **14**, 175–180

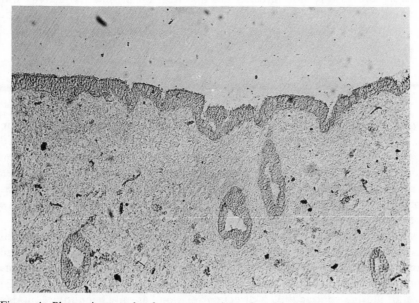

Figure 4. Photomicrograph of a cross section of endometrium in the luteal phase treated with anticyclo-oxygenase antiserum. Specific staining is seen in the surface and glandular epithelium (×6.5). Reproduced by permission from Rees *et al.*, 1982, *Prostaglandins*, **23**, 207–214

studies have shown the cyclo-oxygenase enzyme to be present in endometrial surface and glandular epithelium (Rees *et al.*, 1982) (Figure 4). The unstable PGG_2 and PGH_2 are rapidly converted to the primary prostaglandins $PGF_{2\alpha}$, PGE_2 and PGD_2. PGH_2 is also converted to either TXA_2 or prostacyclin (PGI_2) through the action of thromboxane and prostacyclin synthetase respectively. Human uterine tissue has the capacity to produce all these substances (Figure 3).

Prostaglandins and menstruation.   Prostaglandins play a part in menstruation and in regulating the amount of menstrual bleeding. Individual prostaglandins have differing effects on myometrial activity and haemostasis (Lundstrom, 1981; 1986; Smith, 1980; Wiqvist *et al.*, 1983). The effects on myometrial activity of various prostaglandins have been studied both *in vitro* and *in vivo*. *In vitro*, in general, PGE_2 inhibits and $PGF_{2\alpha}$ stimulates human myometrial strip contractility. However, the situation is complicated by the observation that prostaglandins may have differing effects depending on the layer from which the myometrial strips were obtained. *In vivo* $PGF_{2\alpha}$ administration stimulates uterine contractility during all phases of the menstrual cycle while PGE_2 may produce either inhibition during menstruation or stimulation during the follicular and luteal phases. PGI_2, *in vitro* has an inhibitory effect while *in vivo* intravenous infusion has no effect on myometrial activity but injection directly into the uterus causes a gradual but prolonged stimulation of contractility. Finally TXA_2 is a potent stimulator of myometrial activiy *in vitro*.

With regard to haemostasis PGE_2, PGD_2 and PGI_2 cause vasodilatation while $PGF_{2\alpha}$ and TXA_2 cause vasoconstriction. Platelet aggregation is promoted by TXA_2 and inhibited by PGD_2 and PGI_2.

Prostaglandins and dysmenorrhoea.   Prostaglandins have been implicated in the aetiology of dysmenorrhoea since Pickles *et al.* (1965) showed increased levels of $PGF_{2\alpha}$ and PGE_2 with an increased $PGF_{2\alpha}/PGE_2$ ratio in menstrual fluid in women with dysmenorrhoea compared with women with pain-free periods. Since then many workers have confirmed Pickles' original observation (Rees *et al.*, 1984a). Furthermore, high levels of prostaglandins have been found in endometrium, and endometrial jet washings collected from dysmenorrhoeic women (Lundstrom, 1981). In addition *in vitro* synthesis of $PGF_{2\alpha}$ from arachidonic acid is significantly greater in endometrium obtained from dysmenorrhoeic women than from pain-free controls. However, studies where $PGF_{2\alpha}$ levels in menstrual fluid have been examined in relation to the level of uterine contractility, a direct correlation has only been found on day two of menstruation (Lumsden *et al.*, 1983).

The involvement of prostaglandins in dysmenorrhoea has led to the use of prostaglandin synthetase inhibitors for its treatment. These drugs can be classified chemically into four main groups (a) salicylates, (b) indoleacetic acid analogues (indomethacin), (c) aryl propionic acid derivatives (ibuprofen, naproxen), and (d) fenamates (mefenamic acid, flufenamic acid, meclofenamic acid). Prostaglandin synthetase inhibitors act at the level of the prostaglandin synthetic enzyme cyclo-oxygenase and therefore affect the synthesis of all rather than individual prostaglandins. Studies with mefenamic acid have shown inhibition of prostaglandin synthesis by human endometrium both *in vitro* and *in vivo* (Fraser, 1983). In addition there is evidence that fenamates may also have the ability to antagonize the effects of already formed prostaglandins.

Prostaglandin synthetase inhibitors are usually administered only during menstruation and many studies have shown them to produce subjective relief of pain. Furthermore, objective studies in which intra-uterine pressure was measured have shown a reduction of both frequency and amplitude of contractions during administration of the prostaglandin synthetase inhibitor mefenamic acid (Smith and Powell, 1982). Commencing treatment before the onset of menstruation seems to have no demonstrable advantage over starting treatment when bleeding begins. This observation is compatible with the short plasma half-life of prostaglandin synthetase inhibitors. The advantage of starting treatment at the onset of menstruation is that it prevents the patient treating herself when she is unknowingly pregnant, which would only become apparent when a period is missed. Thus potential teratogenic effects at this stage can be avoided.

Vasopressin

Increased plasma levels of vasopressin have been found in dysmenorrhoeic women compared with pain-free controls (Strömberg *et al.*, 1981). Vasopressin stimulates myometrial activity both *in vitro* and *in vivo*. It is thought that the action of vasopressin may be partly mediated by prostaglandins. The increased levels of vasopressin in dysmenorrhoea has lead to the development of vasopressin antagonists, but these are not available for routine use (Strömberg *et al.*, 1983).

Menorrhagia

Menstrual blood loss is usually considered to be excessive if more than 80 ml is lost per menstruation. Population studies have demonstrated that the upper limit of normal is 80 ml per cycle which is the ninetieth percentile of measured blood loss. Furthermore, with continuing losses above this level there is an increased incidence of iron deficiency anaemia. A measured blood loss of more than 80 ml can therefore be considered as menorrhagia (Hallberg *et al.*, 1966). In the clinical situation a diagnosis of menorrhagia mainly depends on the patient's subjective assessment of her bleeding. However, recent studies measuring menstrual blood loss have shown that this assessment is fallible and as few as 38 per cent of women with a complaint of menorrhagia in fact have the problem in objective terms (Fraser *et al.*, 1984). It is therefore essential to measure menstrual blood loss when exploring possible aetiological factors in menorrhagia.

Abnormal prostaglandin levels and haemostatic mechanisms have recently been implicated in menorrhagia and will be discussed here. Other possible factors have been discussed elsewhere (Shaw and Roche, 1980; Smith, 1985).

Prostaglandins

Abnormal prostaglandin levels have been implicated in menorrhagia since it was reported that elevated concentrations of both $PGF_{2\alpha}$ and PGE_2 were present in endometrium collected from women complaining of heavy periods (Willman *et al.*, 1976). However, there was no objective measurement of menstrual blood loss in this report. Since then other studies of endometrial and menstrual fluid prostaglandins, in which menstrual blood loss was measured suggest increased $PGF_{2\alpha}$ and PGE_2 production during menstruation (Rees *et al.*, 1984a,b) A shift from $PGF_{2\alpha}$ towards PGE_2 has been suggested (Smith, 1985) but has not been confirmed by others (Rees *et al.*, 1984b). In addition the role of prostacyclin in menstrual bleeding has received attention. It has been observed that endometrium from women with menorrhagia was more effective than endometrium from women with normal menstrual blood loss at enhancing production of 6-keto-$PGF_{1\alpha}$ (a metabolite of PGI_2) by a control preparation of myometrium (Smith, 1985).

The implication of excessive prostaglandin levels in menorrhagia has led to the use of prostaglandin synthetase inhibitors in its treatment. The effectiveness of these agents was first demonstrated by Anderson *et al.* in 1976. It was observed that mefenamic acid given during menstruation reduced blood loss from a pre-treatment mean of 119 ml to 60 ml. These findings have been confirmed in other studies. Furthermore, it has been demonstrated that mefenamic acid reduces endometrial concentrations of both $PGF_{2\alpha}$ and PGE_2 (Fraser, 1983).

With regard to scheduling, most studies have started treatment at the onset of menstruation. Again, this avoids possible teratogenic effects. Thus prostaglandin synthetase inhibitors provide suitable therapy for women who have excessive menstrual bleeding but wish to conceive since therapy can be limited to menstruation.

Haemostasis

Uterine haemostasis in relation to menstruation and menstrual bleeding has been recently received considerable attention. It has been known for many years that menstrual blood is fluid, does not clot normally and can be kept in a test tube for several weeks without any visible clot formation. It has been suggested that the mechanisms by which uterine haemostasis is achieved may differ from those found in other tissue systems. Recent morphological studies of uterine haemostasis during menstruation show that haemostatic plugs are only present for a limited period in early menstruation and are smaller than in other tissues (Christiaens et al., 1982). It is therefore believed that the contribution of platelets, coagulation factors and fibrinolysis to uterine haemostasis differs from that usually found in peripheral haemostasis. Furthermore, an abnormality of these mechanisms may be implicated in menorrhagia.

With regard to platelet function, menstrual fluid platelets appear to be 'spent' (Rees et al., 1984c). They are unable to aggregate and metabolize arachidonic acid via the cyclo-oxygenase pathway. Furthermore, ultrastructural studies of menstrual fluid platelets have shown them to be degranulated. Since degranulated platelets have also been found in endometrial haemostatic plugs it appears that menstrual fluid platelets have already been involved in uterine haemostasis before being shed (Christiaens et al., 1982). A relationship between measured menstrual blood loss and platelet function has been explored. No differences were noted between venous and menstrual platelet samples obtained from women with either a light or a heavy loss (Rees et al., 1984c). Platelet abnormalities are therefore an unlikely primary factor in the aetiology of menorrhagia.

Coagulation and fibrinolysis has received considerable attention with respect to uterine bleeding. Plasminogen activator has been demonstrated in endometrium, myometrium and menstrual fluid. In women with menorrhagia and a normal sized uterus, the concentration of plasminogen activator in endometrium is significantly increased as compared with that found in women with normal menstrual blood loss (Rybo, 1966). However, more recent methodology examining coagulation and fibrinolytic activities in menstrual fluid have failed to reveal any clear cut differences between normal and menorrhagic women (Rees et al., 1985). Further studies are required to explore endometrial activity. Heparin-like activity has been found in uterine fluid (Foley et al., 1978). However, patients with menorrhagia do not appear to have significantly higher levels than women with normal menstrual blood loss.

The suggestion that fibrinolytic activity may be abnormal in menorrhagia has led to the use of antifibrinolytic agents such as tranexamic acid and ε-aminocaproic acid. Taken during menstruation they have been found to be effective in reducing menstrual blood loss (Nilsson and Rybo, 1967). The average reduction of menstrual blood loss is 50 per cent. However, there have been some recent reservations regarding their use since systemic fibrinolytic activity is slightly reduced and intracranial thromboses have been reported (Agnelli et al., 1982).

Conclusion

Although menorrhagia and dysmenorrhoea have received considerable attention in recent years, further research is needed. Factors such as the lipoxygenase pathway and prostaglandin receptors require investigation. It is likely that a multifactorial approach will be crucial to further understanding. At present the statement of Hartmann (1932) remains valid: 'Indeed the problem of menstruation itself was then and still is a challenge to biology, for the process common to man and the other higher primates is in its essential physiology still an enigma.'

References

Agnelli, G., Gresele, P., De Cunto, M., Gallai, V. and Nenci, G. G. (1982). Tranexamic acid, uterine contraceptives and fatal cerebral arterial thrombosis. Case report. *British Journal of Obstetrics and Gynaecology*, **89**, 681–682.

Anderson, A. B. M., Haynes, P. J., Guillebaud, J. and Turnbull, A. C. (1976). Reduction of menstrual blood loss by prostaglandin synthesis inhibition. *Lancet*, **1**, 774–776.

Christiaens, G. C. M. L., Sixma, J. J. and Haspels, A. A. (1982). Hemostasis in menstrual endometrium; a review. *Obstetrical and Gynaecological Survey*, **37**, 281–303.

Dawood, M. Y. (1981). Hormones, prostaglandins and dysmenorrhoea, in *Dysmenorrhoea*, (Ed. M. Y. Dawood), Williams and Wilkins, Baltimore, pp. 21–52.

Demers, L. M., Rees, M. C. P. and Turnbull, A. C. (1984). Arachidonic acid metabolism by the non-pregnant human uterus. *Prostaglandins, Leukotrienes and Medicine*, **14**, 175–180.

Foley, M. E., Griffin, M. D., Zuzel, M., Aparicio, S. R., Bradbury, K., Bird, C. C., Clayton, J. K., Julius, D. M., Scott, J. S., Rajah, S. M. and McNichol, G. P. (1978). Heparin like activity in uterine fluid. *British Medical Journal*, **2**, 322–324.

Fraser, I. S. (1983). The treatment of menorrhagia with mefenamic acid. *Research and Clinical Forums*, **5**, 93–99.

Fraser, I. S., McCarron, G. and Markham, R. (1984). A preliminary study of factors influencing perception of menstrual blood loss volume. *American Journal of Obstetrics and Gynecology*, **149**, 788–793.

Goldblatt, M. W. (1933). A depressor substance in seminal fluid. *Journal of the Society of Chemical Industry*, **52**, 1056–1066.

Green, K. (1986). Structure, biosynthesis and metabolism, in *Prostaglandins and their inhibitors in Clinical Obstetrics and Gynaecology*, (Eds. M. Bygdeman, G. S. Berger and L. G. Keith), MTP Press, Lancaster, pp. 13–28.

Hallberg, L., Hogdahl, A. S. M., Nilsson, L. and Rybo, G. (1966). Menstrual blood loss—a population study. *Acta Obstetrica et Gynecologica Scandinavica*, **45**, 320–351.

Hartmann, C. G. (1932). Studies in the reproduction of the Monkey Macacus (Pithecus) rhesus, with special reference to menstruation and pregnancy. *Contributions to Embryology of the Carnegie Institute, Washington, D.C.*, **23**, 1–161.

Lumsden, M. A., Kelly, R. W. and Baird, D. T. (1983). Is prostaglandin $F_{2\alpha}$ involved in the increased myometrial contractility of primary dysmenorrhoea. *Prostaglandins*, **25**, 683–692.

Lumsden, M. A. (1985). Dysmenorrhoea, in *Progress in Obstetrics and Gynaecology*, Vol. 5. (Ed. J. Studd), Churchill Livingstone, Edinburgh, pp. 276–292.

Lundstrom, V. (1981). Uterine activity during the normal cycle and dysmenorrhoea, in *Dysmenorrhoea*, (Ed. M. Y. Dawood), Williams and Wilkins, Baltimore, pp. 53–74.

Lundstrom, V. (1986). The uterus, in *Prostaglandins and their Inhibitors in Clinical Obstetrics and Gynaecology*, (Eds. M. Bygdeman, G. S. Berger and L. G. Keith), MTP Press, Lancaster, pp. 59–82.

Nilsson, L. and Rybo, G. (1967). Treatment of menorrhagia with an antifibrinolytic agent: tranexamic acid (AMCA). A double blind investigation. *Acta Obstetrica et Gynecologica Scandinavica*, **46**, 572–577.

Pickles, V. R., Hall, W. J., Best, F. A. and Smith, G. N. (1965). Prostaglandins in endometrium and menstrual fluid from normal and dysmenorrhoeic subjects. *British Journal of Obstetrics and Gynaecology*, **72**, 185.

Rees, M. C. P., Parry, D. M., Anderson, A. B. M. and Turnbull, A. C. (1982). Immunohistochemical localization of cyclooxygenase in the human uterus. *Prostaglandins*, **23**, 207–214.

Rees, M. C. P., Anderson, A. B. M., Demers, L. M. and Turnbull, A. C. (1984a). Prostaglandins in menstrual fluid in menorrhagia and dysmenorrhoea. *British Journal of Obstetrics and Gynaecology*, **91**, 673–680.

Rees, M. C. P., Anderson, A. B. M., Demers, L. M. and Turnbull, A. C. (1984b). Endometrial and myometrial prostaglandin release during the menstrual cycle in relation to menstrual blood loss. *Journal of Clinical Endocrinology and Metabolism*, **58**, 813–818.

Rees, M. C. P., Demers, L. M., Anderson, A. B. M. and Turnbull, A. C. (1984c). A functional study of platelets in menstrual fluid. *British Journal of Obstetrics and Gynaecology*, **91**, 667–672.

Rees, M. C. P., Cederholm-Williams, S. A. and Turnbull, A. C. (1985). Coagulation factors and fibrinolytic proteins in menstrual fluid. *British Journal of Obstetrics and Gynaecology*, **92**, 1164–1169.

Rees, M. C. P., Di Marzo, V., Tippins, J. R., Morris, H. R. and Turnbull, A. C. (1986). Human endometrium and myometrium release leukotrienes. *British Journal of Clinical Pharmacology*, **21**, 585.

Rybo, G. (1966). Plasminogen activators in the endometrium. *Acta Obstetrica et Gynecologica Scandinavica*, **45**, 429–459.

Scommegna, A. and Dmowski, W. P. (1977). Menstruation, in *Scientific Foundations of Obstetrics and Gynaecology*, (Eds. E. E. Philipp, J. Barnes and M. Newton), Heinemann, London, pp. 127–136.

Shaw, S. T. and Roche, P. C. (1980). Menstruation, in *Oxford Reviews of Reproductive Biology*, Vol. 2 (Ed. C. A. Finn), Clarendon Press, Oxford, pp. 41–96.

Smith, B. J. (1980). The prostanoids in hemostasis and thrombosis. *American Journal of Pathology*, **99**, 743–803.

Smith, R. P. and Powell, J. R. (1982). Intrauterine pressure during dysmenorrhoea therapy. *American Journal of Obstetrics and Gynecology*, **143**, 286–292.

Smith, S. K. (1985). Menorrhagia, in *Progress in Obstetrics and Gynaecology*, Vol. 5, (Ed. J. Studd), Churchill Livingstone, Edinburgh, pp. 293–308.

Strömberg, P., Forsling, M. L. and Akerlund, M. (1981). Effect of prostaglandin inhibition on vasopressin levels in women with primary dysmenorrhoea. *Obstetrics and Gynecology*, **58**, 206–208.

Strömberg, P., Akerlund, M., Forsling, M. L. and Kindahl, H. (1983). Involvement of prostaglandins in vasopressin stimulation of the human uterus. *British Journal of Obstetrics and Gynaecology*, **90**, 332–337.

Von Euler, V. S. (1935). Uber die Spezifische Blutdrucksenkende Substanz des Menslichen Prostata-und Samenblasen secretes. *Klinishe Wochenschrift*, **14**, 1182–1187.

Willman, E. A., Collins, W. P. and Clayton, S. G. (1976). Studies in the involvement of prostaglandins in uterine symptomatology and pathology. *British Journal of Obstetrics and Gynaecology*, **83**, 337–341.

Wiqvist, N., Bygdeman, M. and Kirton, K. (1971). Non-steroidal infertility agents in the female in *Nobel Symposium 15. Control of Human Fertility*, (Eds. E. Diczfalusy and V. Barell), Almquist and Wiskell, Stockholm, pp. 137–167.

Wiqvist, N., Lindblom, B., Wikland, M. and Wilhelmsson, L. (1983). Prostaglandins and uterine contractility. *Acta Obstetrica et Gynecologica Scandinavica*, **Supplement 113**, 23–29.

Functional Disorders of the Menstrual Cycle
Edited by M. G. Brush and E. M. Goudsmit
© 1988 John Wiley & Sons Ltd

CHAPTER 16

Endocrinological aspects of the aetiology and management of endometriosis

W. H. MATTA and R. W. SHAW*

*Academic Department of Obstetrics and Gynaecology,
Royal Free Hospital School of Medicine,
Rowland Hill Street,
London NW3 2QG*

Introduction

The first report of what we now know as endometriosis appeared in 1860 by Von Rokitansky who called it 'adenomyoma', a misnomer that persisted, in the sporadic reports that followed, for nearly 60 years. It was Sampson in 1921 who is credited with being the first to define the disease accurately. The following year Blair Bell coined the terms 'endometriosis' and 'endometrioma' (Whitfield, 1986). The enigmatic nature of this ubiquitous condition has intrigued clinicians during the past six decades, because of the many controversial aspects relating to its aetiology, pathogenesis, natural history, relationship to infertility, prognosis and management.

Endometriosis is characterized by the presence of functioning endometrial glands and stroma outside the uterine cavity. The terms 'endometriosis interna' (usually denoting adenomyosis) and 'endometriosis externa' are best avoided as they are essentially two unrelated conditions.

Endometriosis is the second commonest gynaecological surgical diagnosis, after uterine fibroids; it is encountered in between 10 and 25 per cent of women undergoing laparotomy for gynaecological symptoms in Britain and the United States (Jeffcoate, 1975; Tyson, 1974). The incidence of endometriosis in the general female population is probably between 1 and 2 per cent (Simpson *et al.*, 1980; Strathy *et al.*, 1982). The exact incidence of the condition is difficult to determine because the disease may exist asymptomati-

---

*Correspondence to Professor R. W. Shaw

cally in many women, and because of the different criteria accepted for diagnosis in various reports. Some will use the clinical history and examination alone, now generally accepted as unreliable, others will corroborate clinical suspicion by visualization of the lesions, whilst others will use the more definitive criterion of histopathological confirmation at biopsy.

An apparent increase in the diagnosis of this condition in the past two decades may be explained to some extent by the increased use of diagnostic endoscopy in gynaecological practice.

Pathogenesis and Aetiological Factors

Although there have been numerous theories attempting to explain the pathogenesis of endometriosis, none of them so far can explain all the diverse facets of this complex and apparently multifactorial disease. There have been at least a dozen theories, hence the term 'a disease of theories' has been attributed to endometriosis.

Viable endometrial tissue may be transplanted by reflux menstruation through the fallopian tubes into the peritoneal cavity (Sampson, 1927a), by lymphatic or vascular embolization into distant sites (Sampson, 1927b) or by iatrogenic means (Szlachter *et al.*, 1980), where it may be implanted on susceptible recipient tissues. Another hypothesis is that coelonic epithelium may be transformed into endometrium-like tissue under the influence of certain stimuli (Meyer, 1919) such as prolonged oestrogen stimulation.

In addition to the above mechanical mechanisms, more recent work has suggested that genetic predisposition and immunological factors may influence the susceptibility of some women to develop endometriosis. Familial preponderance for endometriosis has been indicated by reports showing that 7–10 per cent of first or second degree relatives of patients with endometriosis have developed the disease (Simpson *et al.*, 1980; Ranney 1971a). In addition, patients with endometriosis have been found to have specific cellular immunological deficiencies, indicating that endometriosis may be the result of an autoimmune reaction to an as yet unspecified endometrial antigen (Weed and Arquembourg, 1980).

Endocrinological Aspects of Endometriosis

Hormone Responsiveness of Endometriotic Tissue

There is ample clinical and experimental evidence that endometriotic tissue responds to exogenous and endogenous oestrogen and progestogens, in a similar fashion to that of the normally situated endometrium, although this response may invariably be less profound and less predictable. This slight variation in response may be partly due to the differences in the hormone receptor contents of both tissues and in the vascular supply, which may be influenced by the presence of adhesions and fibrous scarring in the case of the endometriotic deposits.

The clinical evidence of the hormone dependency of endometriotic tissue appears to be based on the observations that the condition occurs almost exclusively during the reproductive years. It does not occur before puberty and it is very uncommon after the menopause or surgical oophorectomy; pregnancy and conditions with prolonged amenorrhoea appear to have a beneficial effect on the disease and the symptoms of the disease are often cyclical in nature.

There have been three reports of men who developed endometriosis in the urinary bladder following prolonged oestrogen intake for several years after surgical treatment for prostatic carcinoma (Oliker and Harris, 1971; Pinkert et al., 1979; Shrodt et al., 1980). Further evidence of the influence of oestrogenic stimulation was the report of the development of endometriosis in a woman with a rudimentary uterus and endometrial aplasia (El-Mahgoub and Yasseen, 1980).

In studies on experimental endometriosis in monkeys, Scott and Wharton (1957) have shown that the presence of oestradiol is required for the maintenance of endometrial tissue. Dizerega et al. (1980) found in studies on castrated cynomolgus monkeys, that endometrial tissue transplanted into the peritoneum required no steroid hormones for its initiation, but either oestrogen or progesterone or both were necessary for its growth and maintenance.

Contrary to the above, there have been reports suggesting that endometriosis may develop in the absence of ovarian activity. Djursing et al. (1981) described a case of extensive active endometriosis in a post-menopausal woman with evidence of marked hypo-oestrogenism. Doty et al. (1980) reported endometriosis in a patient with 46 XY gonadal dysgenesis. There have been reports of post-menopausal women developing endometriosis some years after the menopause, and without taking oestrogen replacement therapy (Ranney, 1971b; Punnonen et al., 1980). The latter group also suggested that extra-glandular oestrogen production related to obesity in 70 per cent of their patients may explain the occurrence of endometriosis in these patients.

Endometriotic tissue has classically been described as being morphologically (Roddick et al., 1960), and histologically (Prakash et al., 1965), similar to the endometrium. In more recent studies, however, its appropriate cyclical response to ovarian steroids, in both the follicular and secretory phases, has been contradicted. Electron microscopic studies (Schweppe and Wynn, 1981), nuclear oestrogen binding studies (Gould et al., 1983), and cytosolic oestrogen and progesterone receptor studies (Vierikko et al., 1985) have all indicated that ectopic endometrium responds differently from the normal endometrium to endogenous ovarian hormones. The oestrogen and proges-

Table 1. Effects of various hormonal states upon normal and ectopic endometrium

Hormonal state	Effects on endometrium	Effects on endometriotic tissue
Androgenic state: e.g. danazol and its metabolites, gestrinone	Atrophy	Atrophy and regression
Progestational state: e.g. pregnancy, exogenous progestogens, pseudo-pregnancy treatment (gestrinone)	Secretory activity Decidualization	Secretory activity Decidualization Necrobiosis and resorption
Oestrogenic state: e.g. exogenous oestrogens	Proliferative activity Hyperplasia	Proliferative activity Hyperplasia
Hypo-oestrogenic state: e.g. post-menopause, post-oophorectomy, pseudo-menopause regimes, LHRH agonists	Atrophic changes	Atrophy, regression and resorption

terone receptors in the endometriotic tissue fail to show the significant differences shown by the normal endometrium in the different phases of the cycle (Vierikko *et al.*, 1985).

Janne *et al.* (1981), studying receptors in 41 patients with endometriosis, found that 20 per cent did not show detectable levels of receptors, 30 per cent showed oestrogen and progestin cytosol receptors, and 50 per cent progestin receptors only.

The effects of various hormonal states on both the normal endometrium and the endometriotic tissue are shown in Table 1.

Hyperoestrogenism and the administration of exogenous oestrogen induces proliferation and hyperplasia in both the endometrium and endometriotic tissue.

On the other hand, hypo-oestrogenic states, as occur clinically following surgical gonadectomy or following the menopause, induce atrophy of the endometrium, and atrophy and regression of the endometriotic tissue (Dizerga *et al.*, 1980). Androgens have the same effects as hypo-oestrogenism on both endometrial and endometriotic tissue. This probably partly explains how danazol causes regression of endometriotic tissue.

Progesterone and exogenous progestogens oppose the effects of oestrogen on the endometrial tissue by inhibiting the replenishment of cytosol oestrogen receptors and by induction of 17β-hydroxysteroid-dehydrogenase, which favours conversion of oestradiol to oestrone. Progestogens also induce secretory activity of the endometrial glands and decidual reaction in endometrial stroma in both the normally and ectopically situated endometrium.

Natural pregnancy or pseudo-pregnancy (as induced by the continuous use of high doses of progestogens or the oestrogen–progestogen contraceptive pill) are associated with high levels of cirulating progestogen, resulting in growth arrest, secretory changes and decidualization of the endometrium, and eventually in necrobiosis of endometriotic tissue (Kistner, 1958, 1959).

Endocrine Disorders and Endometriosis

Normal ovarian function appears to occur in most women suffering from endometriosis. There have, however, been many reports in the literature linking endometriosis with a variety of endocrinological abnormalities such as anovulation, altered gonadotrophin secretion, luteal phase deficiency, luteinized unruptured follicle (LUF) syndrome, hyperprolactinaemia and galactorrhoea.

Anovulation. The co-existence of anovulation and endometriosis is well documented, occurring in 10–27 per cent of patients with endometriosis (Soules *et al.*, 1976; Acosta *et al.*, 1973; Dmowski *et al.*, 1976). Menstrual irregularities often accompany both conditions. Pre-menstrual spotting often occurs in patients with endometriosis (Wentz, 1980).

Abnormal gonadotrophin secretion. Hypothalamic–pituitary dysfunction, as a possible contributory factor to infertility associated with endometriosis has been suggested by Cheesman *et al.* (1982) who showed that 26 of 29 patients with endometriosis had two LH peaks two or three days apart. Bayer and Seibel (1986) showed no difference in the frequency of multiple LH peaks or in the mean peak LH values between patients with and without endometriosis. These authors have shown, furthermore, that the onset of the LH peak in patients with endometriosis tended to occur in the early morning, as compared with patients without endometriosis when the onst of LH peaks tended to be more heterogenous.

We have studied the pulsatile LH and FSH secretion patterns in six patients with endometriosis, when blood was sampled every 10 min for 6 h, in the early follicular phase. There was no difference in the pulse frequency and amplitude when compared with control patients.

Disordered prolactin secretion. That patients with endometriosis may have altered prolactin secretion, was suggested by Muse *et al.* (1982) who showed that although baseline serum prolactin levels were normal, there was an increased response to the standard thyroid releasing hormone (TRH) test, when compared with controls. Galactorrhoea in association with endometriosis has also been reported (Hirschowitz *et al*., 1978; Hargrove and Barham, 1980).

Luteal phase dysfunction.   Luteal phase deficiency was found only in 8.8 per cent of 68 infertile patients with endometriosis, compared with 5.3 per cent of 75 infertile patients without endometriosis (Pittaway *et al*., 1983). Brosens *et al*. (1978) have found a 25 per cent incidence of short luteal phase associated with poor serum progesterone levels.

Luteinized unruptured follicle (LUF) syndrome.   Brosens *et al*. (1978) and Marik and Hulka (1978) have reported a high incidence of cycles with luteinized unruptured follicles (LUF) both in women with endometriosis and in women with unexplained infertility. Furthermore, there is a correlation between the presence of the LUF syndrome and lower oestradiol and progesterone concentrations in the peritoneal fluid during the luteal phase as compared with women with normal ovulation (Brosens *et al*., 1978). The hypothesis was put forward, therefore, that the low concentration of progesterone in the peritoneal fluid in women with LUF syndrome favours the implantation and growth of endometrial cells. Koninckx *et al*. (1980) therefore believe that endometriosis is the result of the LUF syndrome, which itself would be the main cause of infertility associated with endometriosis.

The association between LUF and low peritoneal progesterone concentrations has been confirmed by several investigators, but the frequency of LUF in patients with endometriosis has been controversial. Vanrell *et al*. (1982) and Dmowski *et al*. (1980) have found no correlation between the LUF syndrome and endometriosis and/or unexplained infertility. It also remains unclear whether high concentrations of progesterone in the peritoneal fluid following normal ovulation, does indeed prevent the implantation or growth of endometrial cells in the peritoneal cavity.

Possible oocyte maturation defect.   Patients with endometriosis undergoing *in vitro* fertilization seem to respond less favourably than other groups. Wardle *et al*. (1985) found that the fertilization rate of oocytes from patients with endometriosis was approximately half that of patients with tubal factors or unexplained infertility. If fertilization occurred, however, the pregnancy rates were similar in all groups. This may suggest that a possible functional defect in the oocytes from patients with endometriosis may contribute to the infertility in those patients. Chillik and Rosenwaks (1985) have also reported a 48.7 per cent pregnancy rate in patients with minimal and mild endometriosis, and a 15.9 per cent in patients with moderate to severe disease.

Peritoneal Fluid Environment and Endometriosis

It has been suggested that the peritoneal fluid volume and its contents may be adversely affected by the presence of endometriotic tissue in the pelvis, with possible consequent interference with tubo-ovarian function, and/or fertilization and early conceptus.

The role of peritoneal fluid oestrogen and progesterone contents in the luteal phase has been discussed in relation with the LUF syndrome.

Prostaglandins and Prostanoids

The role of prostaglandins and its metabolites present in the peritoneal fluid, in the pathogenesis and symptomatology of endometriosis is controversial. Meldrum et al. (1977) have noted increased levels of prostaglandin $F_{2\alpha}$ ($PGF_{2\alpha}$) in the peritoneal fluid of patients with endometriosis. Other investigators (Drake et al., 1981; Ylikorkala and Vünikka, 1983) have also found that patients with endometriosis had increased peritoneal fluid volume as well as increased concentrations of the prostaglandin metabolites thromboxane B_2 and 6-keto-PG $F_{1\alpha}$ although the timing in the menstrual cycle was not taken into consideration in these studies. Other investigators, on the other hand, (Rock et al., 1982; Sgarlata et al., 1983) have found no increase in either the volume of peritoneal fluid or its concentrations of PGE_2, $PGF_{2\alpha}$ or 15-keto 13,14-dihydroprostaglandin $F_{2\alpha}$ and thromboxane B_2. Schmidt (1985) has suggested that the reasons for the controversy in these conflicting reports reside in both the timing of peritoneal fluid sampling and the quality control of the assay systems, as the short life of prostaglandins demands immediate preservation of the samples and emphasis upon the more stable metabolites. The mechanisms by which the changes in peritoneal fluid prostaglandin content would influence endometriosis and/or associated infertility remain unclear. Furthermore, the increased secretion of $PGF_{2\alpha}$ from endometriotic implants is thought likely to be the main cause of dysmenorrhoea commonly associated with the disease. This is probably why the use of prostaglandin-synthetase inhibitors may often be useful in alleviating this symptom.

Peritoneal Macrophages

The role played by peritoneal fluid macrophages in women with endometriosis, has aroused much interest in recent years. Women with endometriosis-associated infertility were found to have significantly higher concentrations of macrophages in the peritoneal fluid than do either fertile women or infertile women without endometriosis (Haney et al., 1981; Halme et al., 1983). An increase in the number of peritoneal fluid macrophages was also found in women with non-mechanical causes of infertility (Olive et al.,

1985). The number of tubal macrophages was also significantly higher in patients with endometriosis than in normal fertile patients (Haney *et al.*, 1983). The macrophages from patients with endometriosis appear to be highly phagocytic against spermatozoa *in vitro* compared with those from fertile women or infertile women without endometriosis (Muscato *et al.*, 1982). They are also able to survive better *in vitro* than those from fertile controls (Halme *et al.*, 1986). Peritoneal fluid from patients with endometriosis was shown to have a cytotoxic effect on *in vitro* cleavage of mouse embryos (Morcos *et al.*, 1985).

Thus, these findings on the quantitative and qualitative properties of macrophages in the peritoneal fluid from patients with endometriosis may explain the mechanism of infertility and possibly the increased incidence of spontaneous early abortions.

Endometriosis and Infertility

There has been much controversy about the association between endometriosis and infertility. Infertility occurs in between 30 and 40 per cent of patients suffering from endometriosis (Kistner, 1975). In infertile women, on the other hand, endometriosis was found at laparoscopy in between 15 and 25 per cent of all cases (Cohen, 1976; Jones and Rock, 1977); and in 70–80 per cent of women with otherwise unexplained infertility (Kistner, 1977). It has also been estimated that endometriosis may be the only factor causing infertility in 6–15 per cent of infertile women (Spangler and Jones, 1971).

The pathogenesis of infertility in patients with endometriosis remains poorly understood and is probably multifactorial. It is, perhaps, easier to explain the occurrence of infertility in women with the more severe degrees of endometriosis by obvious anatomical distortions, such as periadnexal adhesions and ovarian tissue destruction by endometriomas. These mechanical factors may interfere with the release or pick-up of oocytes. Furthermore, it is not uncommon to find some associated pathology affecting fertility such as chronic salpingitis, which was found in approximately one-third of patients with endometriosis by Czernobilsky and Silverstein (1978), uterine fibroids, cornual endometrial polyps, adenomyosis or proximal tubal obstruction.

The role of minimal endometriosis in causing infertility has been controversial. Reports of spontaneous cure as evidenced by the reported pregnancy rates of up to 75 per cent (Schenken and Malinak, 1982; Portuondo *et al.*, 1983; Garcia and David, 1977; Seibel *et al.*, 1982) have encouraged some clinicians to pursue a policy of expectant management, questioning whether there indeed is any association between the two conditions in those patients.

Several possible mechanisms have been postulated to explain why infertility occurs in women with mild endometriosis. These have been discussed in other parts of this chapter, and are summarized in Table 2. It is difficult, however, to

Table 2. Possible mechanisms causing infertility associated with minimal/mild endometriosis

Coital function	Dyspareunia causing reduction in coital frequency and penetration
Spermatozoal function	Superficial ejaculation due to deep dyspareunia
	Phagocytosis by macrophages (intra-uterine and intra-tubal)
	Inactivation by intra-uterine antibodies (immune response
Ovarian function	Endocrinopathies: anovulation
	LUF syndrome
	altered LH peaks
	altered prolactin secretion
	Luteolysis caused by prostaglandin F
	?Oocyte maturation defects (evidence from IVF studies)
Tubal function	Prostaglandin-induced alteration in tubal and cilial motility may alter ovum pick-up, sperm progression and transport of fertilized egg
Implantation	Interference by endometrial antibodies
	Luteal phase deficiency
Early pregnancy loss	Increased early spontaneous abortion due to prostaglandin-induced uterine contractility, immune response, or macrophage phagocytic activity

understand whether these different mechanisms are a cause or result of endometriosis itself.

There have been reports suggesting that endocrinopathies resulting in anovulation, luteal phase deficiency, the LUF syndrome or altered gonadotrophin and prolactin secretion, have been associated with endometriosis with varying frequency. Other reports suggest that endometriosis is an autoimmune phenomenon resulting in a possible anti-endometrial antibody reaction, which may interfere with spermatozoal progression in the uterine cavity, with poor implantation, or even the possible rejection of an early conceptus causing spontaneous abortion. Because the fallopian tubes and ovaries are immersed in peritoneal fluid, it is possible to postulate that a hostile peritoneal fluid environment may adversely affect fertility. The increase in the number and activity of macrophages in the peritoneal fluid reported in patients with endometriosis, may lead to increased phagocytosis of spermatozoa. The increased secretion of prostaglandins and prostanoids by endometriotic tissue suggest that they may alter tubal motility, cilial activity, ovum pick-up and transport or even lead to spontaneous abortion by increasing uterine contractility. In addition, prostaglandin $F_{2\alpha}$ may induce luteolysis.

We can presume that deep dyspareunia may lead to reduction in coital frequency or to inadequate penetration which may be a contributory factor to infertility.

Increased incidence of spontaneous abortions in patients with endometriosis has been reported to range between 10 and 51 per cent (Naples et al., 1981; Rock et al., 1981; Olive et al., 1982; Wheeler et al., 1983; Groll, 1984). It has also been suggested that medical or surgical treatment of endometriosis may decrease abortion rates (Metzger et al., 1986).

Diagnosis

The common perceptions that endometriosis occurs typically in nulliparous caucasian women in their fourth decade and of higher socio-economic status have now been discredited in several reports. Endometriosis should be suspected in any patient presenting with infertility or with worsening dysmenorrhoea, dyspareunia or pelvic pain, regardless of her age, ethnic origin, parity or socio-economic status.

It is now well established that direct visualization of endometriotic lesions by either laparoscopy or laparotomy, preferably with biopsy histopathological confirmation, is the only acceptable means of diagnosing the disease with certainty. It is no longer acceptable to rely on the clinical history and examination alone, as this may be misleading. The widespread use of diagnostic laparoscopy in the past decade or so has remarkably increased the accuracy with which endometriosis is diagnosed. Conservative surgical procedures may also be performed via the laparoscope. A post-treatment laparoscopy should be highly recommended to confirm resolution of the lesions and/or to decide on further course of action should it be necessary.

Various classifications (Riva et al., 1961; Acosta et al., 1973; Kistner et al., 1977) have been proposed over the past three decades, which attempt to standardize the criteria upon which the severity of endometriosis should be based. This would help in the critical assessment of the performance of various forms of treatment and provide meaningful prognostic indicators. None of these classifications received wide acceptance, and they all suffered from various pitfalls, which made it difficult to compare treatment results. The most recent attempt to provide a standard classification for uniform use has been the Revised American Fertility Society Classification of Endometriosis (1985).

Treatment

Management should be individualized according to the patient's circumstances in terms of fertility wishes, severity of the symptoms, extent of the disease and age.

Treatment may be surgical, medical or a combination of both. When medical treatment is used in combination with surgery, it may be used before, after or both before and after surgery.

The indices used to assess the efficacy of a particular treatment modality include:

1. The degree of resolution of endometriotic lesions as assessed by pre- and post-treatment laparoscopy using a standardized classification scoring system and histological confirmation.
2. Pregnancy rate for those patients who wish and are able to conceive.
3. The rate of symptomatic relief during and after treatment.
4. The rate of recurrence of endometriosis over a specified period of time.

Prophylactic Measures

These may be considered in selected patients especially those with a past history or first degree family history of endometriosis. They may be encouraged to conceive and breast feed if this is desirable to them or to use a combined oestrogen–progestogen oral preparation as these may delay the onset of occurrence or recurrence of endometriosis. Measures to prevent the iatrogenic obstruction to menstrual flow and the transplantation of endometrial tissue into the peritoneal cavity or external genitalia may also be taken in the susceptible patients (Ranny, 1975).

Expectant Management

The role of expectant management in patients with minimal endometriosis, especially when they desire to conceive, has been controversial. Seibel *et al*. (1982) in a prospective study, found no significant difference between danazol treatment and no treatment after initial diagnostic laparoscopy in terms of pregnancy rate. This compared with a retrospective study by Schenken and Malinak (1982) who reported that twelve of sixteen patients with mild endometriosis had conceived within one year without treatment which was comparable with a similar conception rate in another group treated with conservative surgery. On the other hand, Buttram and Betts (1979) reported 73 per cent pregnancy rate within fifteen months from conservative surgery in 56 patients with a mean duration of infertility of 37 months. Of those who conceived, 36 per cent did so within three months and 56 per cent within six months. It has also been shown in a prospective randomized double-blind placebo controlled study that 47 per cent of seventeen patients with minimal disease deteriorated within six months when no treatment was given, whilst 24 per cent had no change, and 29 per cent improved (Thomas and Cooke, 1986).

Surgical Treatment

Conservative surgery. This form of therapy, carried out at either laparoscopy or laparotomy, which aims to conserve as much ovarian tissue as possible as well as the reproductive potential, has been the traditional treatment of choice in infertile women with endometriosis (Andrews, 1980). Employing microsurgical techniques and principles may improve subsequent fertility prospects (Gomel, 1980). The use of the laser in laparoscopic surgery (Feste, 1984) and in microsurgical procedures (Chong and Baggish, 1984) offers exciting prospects for the future. The role of post-operative hormonal suppression in infertile patients has been the subject of much controversy with conflicting reports both for and against.

The pregnancy rate following conservative surgery as reported in the literature varies from 30 to 75 per cent with an uncorrected pregnancy rate of about 50 per cent. The success of conservative surgery in achieving pregnancies is directly related to the severity of the disease as shown by pregnancy rates of 73 per cent, 56 per cent and 40 per cent for mild, moderate and severe degrees respectively (Buttram, 1979).

There are no available data on the annual recurrence rates after conservative surgery, but between 40 and 47 per cent of patients required a second surgical procedure for recurrence (Schenken and Malinak, 1982).

Radical surgery. This is reserved for those patients with severe symptoms and when there is no need to preserve the fertility potential, especially when other forms of treatment have failed. At surgery a total abdominal hysterectomy with bilateral salpingo-oophorectomy with resection of endometriotic lesions as completely as possible will be carried out and followed by hormone replacement therapy. Such hormone replacement therapy should be kept at a minimum as a small proportion of those patients may develop a recurrence of endometriosis related to oestrogen use. Combined oestrogen and testosterone implants may minimize the risk of recurrence due to the beneficial effects of the androgen.

Hormone Treatment

Hormonal therapy may be used for prophylactic, palliative or definitive treatment of appropriately selected patients. When used for definitive treatment, primary hormonal therapy may be particularly useful in patients with milder degrees of the disease presenting with painful symptoms and/or infertility. Use in conjunction with conservative surgery in patients with infertility may also be of immense benefit. In patients with more severe degrees of the disease, hormonal treatment may be of value.

The medical treatment of endometriosis has undergone remarkable evolution during the past four decades. The initial advocation of the use of androgens such as methyltestosterone produced some success, but with serious androgenic side-effects such as hirsutism, voice changes, breast atrophy and cliteromegaly. In addition, the risk of masculinization to the female fetus was difficult to avoid as the treatment often failed to consistently inhibit ovulation, and pregnancies occurring during treatment were occasionally observed. The use of high doses of diethylstilboestrol as advocated by Karnaky (1948), also produced intolerable adverse effects such as severe dysfunctional uterine haemorrhage, mastodynia, oedema, depression, nausea and headaches. Furthermore, prolonged high doses of oestrogens carry risks of the development of cystic glandular or adenomatous hyperplasia of the endometrium, as well as of thrombo-embolism. The use of androgens and oestrogens alone, are now only of historical interest because of the poor results, unacceptable side-effects and risks associated with their use.

More recently, hormonal therapies designed to induce decidualization (pseudo-pregnancy regimes), or to suppress ovarian function ('pseudomenopause' regimes) offered the best chance for clinical remission of endometriosis, by attempting to achieve a static endometrium, with no cyclical variations, and anovulation reminiscent of pregnancy or menopause.

The success of various hormonal therapies depends to some extent on the localization of endometriotic lesions; peritoneal and serosal implants respond better to hormonal therapy than do deep ovarian endometriomata. It would also appear that all available medical treatment regimes will only induce regression of the disease in most patients for variable periods of time, rather than induce permanent cure; this is evidenced by the high recurrence rates after hormonal therapies.

A variety of established hormonal therapies are currently available for controlling endometriosis. These include combined oestrogen–progestogen preparations, progestogen preparations and danazol. Newer hormonal preparations under clinical trials which appear to be promising include gestrinone and luteinizing hormone releasing hormone (LHRH) agonists.

Established Hormonal Treatment

Pseudo-pregnancy Regimes

Combined oestrogen–progestogen preparations. Kistner (1959) introduced the uninterrupted use of combined oral contraceptives in order to reproduce the hormonal milieu of pregnancy. In early pregnancy, hypertrophy, oedema, increased vascularity, increased glandular activity and decidualization occur in the endometrium. Later in pregnancy, the decidualized endometrium will become inactive; ectopic endometrium may thus atrophy, undergoing necrosis and resorption. The continued administration of combined oestrogen–progestogen preparations will suppress the hypothalamic release of

LHRH by a feedback mechanism, with resultant pituitary–ovarian suppression.

One of the higher dose combined oral contraceptive preparations may be administered continuously for six to nine months, starting initially with one tablet daily. If breakthrough bleeding occurs, a change to another preparation with higher oestrogen–progestogen ratio, the addition of an oestrogen preparation such as conjugated oestrogen 0.625 mg daily, or increasing the dose of the original preparation to two tablets daily may be advocated. Other side-effects may occur such as weight gain, headaches, breast enlargement and/or tenderness, nausea and depression. The risk of thromboembolism is increased, and contraindications for the use of this form of therapy are the same as those for combined oral contraception.

The reported pregnancy rates following treatment, of 20–40 per cent (Luciano and Pitkin, 1984) are not impressive when compared with those for danazol or conservative therapy. Symptomatic relief was reported to occur in up to 90 per cent of patients, but recurrence of the symptoms occurred in about one-third of the patients within one year (Kistner, 1959).

Exacerbation of endometriotic lesions or activation of quiescent lesions during the first trimester of pregnancy has been reported in some pregnant patients with endometriosis (McArthur and Ulfelder, 1965). Similarly an initial exacerbation of the symptoms of endometriosis may occur in some patients receiving pseudo-pregnancy regimes. This is probably due to the stimulatory effects of exogenous steroids causing hyperplasia of both normal and ectopic endometrium tissues.

Progestogens. A state of pseudo-pregnancy may also be effectively induced by the use of progestogenic preparations. These may be either derivatives of 19-nortestosterone such as norethisterone, norethisterone acetate, norgestrel, norethynodrel and lynoestrenol or derivatives of progesterone such as medroxyprogesterone acetate and dydrogesterone. The use of progestogens in the treatment of endometriosis may be particularly useful when the oestrogen-containing combined contraceptives are either contra-indicated or not well tolerated, and in selected patients when prophylactic or palliative long-term intermittent courses are needed.

The use of progestogens induces a hypo-oestrogenic, hyper-progestogenic state. Because oestrogens are necessary for the process of resorption of necrosed decidualized ectopic endometrial tissue (Hammond and Haney, 1978), the use of progestogens alone was considered less satisfactory than the combined oestrogen–progestogen preparations. In addition, breakthrough bleeding occurs frequently with the use of progestogens due to reduced circulating endogenous oestradiol.

Treatment with the various available progestogens may be given, either orally or as injectable depot formulations, for six to nine months. The results of treatment appear to be comparable to those reported with the combined oestrogen–progestogen preparations. Data in the literature on symptomatic relief, objective resolution, pregnancy and recurrence rates may be criticized for the lack of standardized, comparative and controlled studies, small numbers or short periods of follow-up.

Side-effects include breakthrough bleeding, weight gain, increased appetite, oedema, bloating, acne and reduced libido. Breakthrough bleeding may be helped by either increasing the dose of the progestogen used or better still by adding oestrogen compounds, if not contra-indicated, such as ethinyloestradiol 10–30 μg or conjugated oestrogen 0.625 mg daily for 21 days each month.

Following treatment with injectable medroxyprogesterone acetate depot, ovulation may be delayed for up to six to twelve months, therefore it should not be given to patients wishing to conceive.

The adverse effects of progestogens on low and high density lipoproteins (LDL and HDL) with possible consequent effects of atherogenesis and cardiovascular disease have been under investigation in recent years. Norethisterone acetate and norgestrel containing combined oral contraceptives, were found in a large multicentre study to be associated with the lowest HDL and highest LDL values (Wahl et al., 1983).

Danazol

This orally active synthetic steroid was originally synthesized by Manson et al. in 1963. It is an isoxazol derivative of 17α ethyltestosterone [17α-pregn-4-en-20-yno-(2,3-d) isoxazol-17-ol]. It has mildly androgenic (one-tenth that of testosterone) and anabolic properties.

The mechanisms of action of danazol are complex and surrounded by much controversy. The difficulties in interpreting the multitude of in vivo, in vitro and clinical studies are complicated by the fact that danazol has at least 60 metabolites, many of them being potentially biologically active (Davison et al., 1976). In reviewing the subject, Barbieri and Ryan (1981) have cited several possible modes of action for danazol which include: interference with pulsatile gonadotrophin secretion, direct inhibition of ovarian steroidogenesis by inhibiting several enzymatic processes, competitive blockage of androgen, oestrogen and progesterone receptors in the ovaries and endometrium, and suppression of sex hormone binding globulin (SHBG) levels.

The multiple effects of danazol lead to the elimination of midcycle gonadotrophin surge in pre-menopausal women, without significantly reducing the basal levels of luteinizing hormone or follicle-stimulating hormone. A hypo-oestrogenic, hypo-progestational environment also develops, with accompanying amenorrhoea, and endometrial atrophy; these effects are dose related.

The clinical use of danazol in patients with endometriosis was introduced in 1971 but it was not until several years later that it became the most widely used hormonal therapeutic agent for this condition.

For use in endometriosis, danazol may be administered orally at a dose range of 200–800 mg daily. Dmowski (1979) recommends that danazol should optimally be administered every 6 h because of its short serum half-life which is 4.5 h. Treatment should be commenced in the early follicular phase of a menstrual cycle in order to avoid the drug being taken during early pregnancy, and to minimize the problems of irregular bleeding. The dose may be titrated according to the patient's clinical response and severity of side-effects. The treatment is usually continued for six to nine months.

Danazol has been shown to be effective in cases of mild and moderate endometriosis (Low et al., 1984). It has also been shown to induce subjective symptomatic improvement in over 85 per cent of women with endometriosis (Dmowski and Cohen, 1978; Barbieri et al., 1982). Symptoms may recur, however, in approximately one-third of the patients within one year after treatment. Objective resolution and improvement of endometriotic lesions as observed at post-treatment endoscopic evaluation was noted in 70–95 per cent of patients (Dmowski and Cohen, 1975; Barbieri et al., 1982).

Pregnancy rates of 31–53 per cent in mild endometriosis and 23–50 per cent in moderate endometriosis, after treatment with danazol, were reported in a review of the literature by Schmidt (1985). An over-all uncorrected pregnancy rate of 40–50 per cent was reported by Barieri and Ryan (1981). This compares favourably with that achieved by conservative surgery alone, but comparisons with expectant management in women with mild endometriosis showed no significant difference in pregnancy rates between the two treatments which questioned the value of hormonal treatment in enhancing fertility in this group of patients (Seibel et al., 1982).

Dmowski and Cohen (1978) reported a 39 per cent recurrence rate after 37 months from completion of danazol treatment, with annual recurrences in the first, second and third years of 23 per cent, 5 per cent and 9 per cent respectively. The recurrence was delayed in the patients who conceived.

Danazol treatment is associated with a high incidence of side-effects related to its androgenic, anabolic or hypo-oestrogenic properties. The side-effects include weight gain, fluid retention symptoms, breakthrough bleeding, acne, hirsutism, oily skin, decreased breast size, deepening of voice, decreased libido, muscle cramps, mood changes, depression, emotional lability, fatigue, headaches, nausea, hot flushes and skin rash. The incidence and severity of side-effects are dose related. Some of these side-effects occur in approximately 80 per cent of women on danazol but few discontinue because of their severity.

Adverse effects of danazol therapy on lipoprotein metabolism have been reported (Fåhraeus et al., 1984). These effects included the elevation of low density lipoproteins, and the reduction of high density lipoprotein cholesterol concentrations. These effects were reversible after six months' treatment with 600 mg of danazol daily.

Danazol treatment was also reported to alter liver function and serum levels of various enzymes (Holt and Keller, 1984), so its use should therefore be contra-indicated in patients with liver disease. Patients on long-term therapy should have liver function serum enzymes and serum lipoproteins assessed.

Treatments Under Trial

Gestrinone

Gestrinone, a synthetic trienic 19-norsteroid (13-ethyl-17α-ethinyl-17 hydroxy-gona-4,9,11-trien-3-one), has been shown in recent clinical trials to be effective in the treatment of endometriosis. Gestrinone exhibits mild androgenic, marked anti-progesterone and anti-oestrogenic, as well as moderate anti-gonadotrophic properties (Azadian-Boulanger *et al.*, 1971; Raynaud *et al.*, 1975). The combined effect of these properties is to induce progressive endometrial atrophy. Gestrinone has a high binding affinity for progesterone receptors; it also binds to androgen but not to oestrogen receptors (Azadian-Boulanger *et al.*, 1984).

The endocrine effects of the therapeutic use of gestrinone in humans are similar to those of danazol in that the midcycle gonadotrophin surge is abolished although the basal gonadotrophin secretions are not significantly reduced. It also inhibits ovarian steroidogenesis as evidenced by the suppressed serum levels of oestradiol-17β and progesterone, which are maintained at the early follicular phase levels (Robyn *et al.*, 1984). Gestrinone differs from danazol, however, in that it characteristically induces a profound and progessive reduction in the serum sex hormone binding globulin (SHBG) levels by about 85 per cent, whilst the total serum concentrations of testosterone and andostenedione are reduced by about 40 per cent and 30 per cent respectively. This accounts for the five-fold increase in the free (unbound) testosterone index (Kaupilla *et al.*, 1985).

Gestrinone may be administered orally at doses of 2.5–5 mg twice weekly for six to nine months to patients with endometriosis, a dose schedule which was shown to effectively induce endometrial atrophy, achieves amenorrhoea in 85–90 per cent of patients within two months, and offers a significant reduction in steroid dosage compared with danazol which requires a minimum of 160 times higher dosage (200 mg daily) to achieve endometrial atrophy. From the early uncontrolled open studies gestrinone would appear to compare favourably with danazol, in the treatment of endometriosis, in terms of symptomatic relief and pregnancy rates (Coutinho *et al.*, 1984; Azadian-

Boulanger *et al.*, 1984; Mettler and Semm, 1984). Data on the recurrence rates are limited; in a small series of 20 patients 39 per cent were reported to have recurrence within one year (Coutinho *et al.*, 1984). The reported side-effects, occurring in up to 50 per cent of patients, included: hirsutism, seborrhoea, acne, increased weight, hair loss, voice hoarseness, cliteromegaly, breakthrough bleeding, reduced breast size, hot flushes, pruritis, nausea, muscle cramps, oedema and gastric intolerance. All these side-effects were reported to be moderate, transient and dose dependent. Gestrinone may also be administered as subdermal implants in silastic capsules at doses of 200–300 mg, sufficient to inhibit ovulation for one year, in patients requiring long-term treatment or in those with gastric intolerance to the oral preparation. The androgenic side-effects are significantly reduced by this route.

Gestrinone emerges from these reports as an effective drug which is comparable to danazol. More randomized and comparative studies are required to establish the possible role of this drug in the treatment of endometriosis.

Luteinizing Hormone-releasing Hormone Agonists

A large number of luteinizing hormone-releasing hormone (LHRH) agonist analogues has been synthesized, with various amino acid substitutions, which prolong their biological activity (Figure 1). The potency estimates for the biological activity of LHRH agonists are 50–100-times higher than that of the naturally occurring LHRH.

In pre-menopausal women the chronic administration of LHRH agonists induces desensitization of the pituitary gonadotrophin-secreting cells with resultant hypogonadotrophic hypogonadism (Schmidt-Gollwitzer *et al.*, 1981; Sandow, 1983). This reversible hypo-oestrogenic state, often referred to as reversible medical oophorectomy, may be therapeutically useful in a wide variety of sex hormone-dependent conditions including idiopathic precocious puberty (Crowley *et al.*, 1980), endometriosis (Shaw *et al.*, 1983), contraception, menorrhagia (Shaw and Fraser, 1984a) and uterine leiomyoma (Maheux *et al.*, 1985).

Surgical oophorectomy is the most effective treatment for endometriosis (Williams and Pratt, 1977) but obviously it is often not acceptable. Induction of 'medical oophorectomy' by the use of LHRH agonists was shown to be effective in the treatment of endometriosis, as reported in recent studies; LHRH agonists were administered as daily injections (Meldrum *et al.*, 1982) or intranasally (Shaw *et al.*, 1983; Shaw and Fraser, 1984b; Lemay *et al.*, 1984; Schriock *et al.*, 1985).

We (Matta and Shaw, 1987) have recently carried out a prospective, randomized study between danazol and the LHRH agonist buserelin [D-ser(TBU)^6-des-Gly-NH$_2$^{10} LHRH ethylamide], administered intranasally

	1	2	3	4	5	6	7	8	9	10	
LHRH:	Pyroglutamine	Histidine	Tryptophan	Serine	Tyrosine	Glycine	Leucine	Arginine	Proline	Glycine	Amide
Buserelin:	Pyroglutamine	Histidine	Tryptophan	Serine	Tyrosine	D-serine (TBu)	Leucine	Arginine	Proline	Glycine	Ethylamide

Figure 1. The amino acid sequence of the native LHRH and the LHRH agonist buserelin (Hoechst): [D-Ser,[10]] LHRH ethylamide

400 μg thrice daily in 62 women with endometriosis. At post-treatment laparoscopic assessment employing the Revised American Fertility Society Classification (1985), 82 per cent of 39 patients receiving buserelin, and 72 per cent of eighteen patients receiving danazol had no active residual endometriosis. The results were comparable in those with mild disease, but buserelin appeared slightly more effective in patients with moderate and severe disease, although the numbers in this sub-group were small. The two drugs appeared comparable in terms of symptomatic relief and both drugs induced significant hypo-oestrogenism, but this was more profound and sustained in the buserelin group. Buserelin was better tolerated by patients as it caused significantly fewer disturbing side-effects. Hot flushes and other mild oestrogen deficiency symptoms were the main side-effects of buserelin. LHRH agonists appear therefore to offer a new method of treatment in endometriosis. Long-term follow-up is needed to establish pregnancy and recurrence rates. Possible long-term effects of hypo-oestrogenism on bone mineral content and the cardiovascular system need to be studied before such agents could be widely used for long-term treatment in endometriosis.

Conclusions

In spite of the significant progress made recently in understanding this common condition, there remain many unanswered questions and controversial issues concerning the multiple facets of endometriosis. There is ample evidence that the disease is oestrogen-dependent but the exact role that different hormonal milieu may play in predisposing to endometriosis and in its pathogenesis is not clearly understood.

The choice of hormonal, surgical or both approaches in the treatment of patients with endometriosis remains controversial. An individualized choice based on the patient's age, parity, symptoms, fertility wishes and severity of the disease as assessed by direct visualization may offer the best approach. The failure of orthodox hormonal and conservative surgical approaches to eradicate the disease in the manner that surgical oophorectomy does reduces current interest in these treatment areas. Danazol, currently the most effective hormonal treatment available, is particularly useful for the infertile patient with mild to moderate disease, but it is expensive and has many unpleasant side-effects. New drugs under clinical trials offer hopeful alternatives in the hormonal treatment of endometriosis. Gestrinone may offer a few advantages over danazol but it has similar side-effects. More controlled comparative studies are needed to establish its possible role in future treatment choices.

Medical oophorectomy induced by the use of LHRH agonists would appear to offer an exciting new alternative; it is at least as effective as danazol and is better tolerated by patients. Comparative studies and studies into possible long-term adverse effects on bone density need to be established. It must be remembered that no hormonal treatment will cure all patients; its role, however, is predominantly to induce long-term regression of the disease. Large endometriomas and severe disease do not respond to hormonal therapy and surgery is mandatory in those patients. New techniques employing endoscopic and microsurgical techniques, possibly using lasers, many offer the best chances for maintaining the fertility prospects for those patients.

References

Acosta, A. A., Buttram, V. C., Jr, Besch, P. K., Malinak, L. R., Franklin, R. R. and Van Der Heydon, J. D. (1973). A proposed classification of pelvic endometriosis. *Obstetrics and Gynecology*, **42**, 19–25.

Andrews, W. C. (1980). Medical versus surgical treatment of endometriosis. *Clinical Obstetrics and Gynecology*, **23**, 917–924.

Azadian-Boulanger, G., Secchi, J. and Sakiz, E. (1971). Biological study of the antiprogesterone effect of R2323. *Excerpta Medica International Congress Series*, **278**, 129–133.

Azadian-Boulanger, G., Secchi, J., Tournemine, C., Sakiz, E., Vige, P. and Henrion, R. (1984). Hormonal activity profiles of drugs for endometriosis therapy, in *Medical Management of Endometriosis*, (Eds. J. P. Raynaud, T. Ojasoo and L. Martini), Raven Press, New York, pp. 125–148.

Barbieri, R. L. and Ryan, K. J. (1981). Danazol: endocrine pharmacology and therapeutic applications. *American Journal of Obstetrics and Gynecology*, **141**, 453–463.

Barbieri, R. L., Evans, S. and Kistner, R. W. (1982). Danazol in the treatment of endometriosis: analysis of 100 cases with a 4-year follow-up. *Fertility and Sterility*, **37**, 737–746.

Bayer, S. R. and Seibel, M. M. (1986). Endometriosis: clinical symptoms and infertility, in *Gonadotrophin Down-Regulation in Gynecological Practice*, (Eds. R. Rolland, D. R. Chadha and W. P. Willemsen), Alan R Liss Inc, New York, pp. 103–133.

Brosens, I. A., Koninckx, P. R. and Correleyn, P. A. (1978). A study of plasma progesterone, oestradiol-17β, prolactin and LH levels and of the luteal phase appearance of the ovaries in patients with endometriosis and infertility. *British Journal of Obstetrics and Gynaecology*, **85**, 246–250.

Buttram, V. C. (1979). Conservative surgery for endometriosis in the infertile female: A study of 206 patients with implications for both medical and surgical therapy. *Fertility and Sterility*, **2**, 117–123.

Buttram, V. C., Jr. and Betts, J. W. (1979). Endometriosis. *Current Problems in Obstetrics and Gynecology*, **11**, 11.

Cheesman, K. L., Ben-Nun, I., Chatterton, R. T. and Cohen, M. R. (1982). Relationship of luteinizing hormone, pregnanediol-3-glucoronide, and estradiol-16-glucuronide in urine of infertile women with endometriosis. *Fertility and Sterility*, **38**, 542–544.

Chillik, C. and Rosenwaks, Z. (1985). Endometriosis and in-vitro fertilization. *Seminars in Reproductive Endocrinology*, **3**, 377.

Chong, A. P. and Baggish, M. S. (1984). Management of pelvic endometriosis by means of intra-abdominal carbon dioxide laser. *Fertility and Sterility*, **41**, 14–19.

Cohen, M. R. (1976). Endoscopy, in *Recent Advances in Endometriosis, Proceedings of a Symposium, Augusta, Georgia 1975*, (Ed. R. B. Greenblatt), Excerpta Medica, Amsterdam, pp. 18–31.

Coutinho, E. M., Husson, J. M. and Azadian-Boulanger, G. (1984). Treatment of endometriosis with Gestrinone—five years experience, in *Medical Management of Endometriosis*, (Eds. J. D. Raynaud, T. Ojasoo and L. Martin), Raven Press, New York, pp. 249–260.

Crowley, W. F., Comite, F., Vale, W., Rivier, J., Loriaux, D. L., Cutler, G. B. (1980). Therapeutic use of pituitary desensitization with a long-acting LHRH agonist: a potential new treatment for idiopathic precocious puberty. *Journal of Clinical Endocrinology and Metabolism*, **52**, 370–372.

Czernobilsky, B. and Silverstein, A. (1978). Salpingitis and ovarian endometriosis. *Fertility and Sterility*, **30**, 45–49.

Davison, C., Banks, W. and Fritz, A. (1976). The absorption, distribution and metabolic fate of danazol in rats, monkeys and human volunteers. *Archives Internationales de Pharmacodynamie et de Therapie*, **211**, 294–310.

Dizerega, G. S., Barber, D. C. and Hodgen, G. D. (1980). Endometriosis: role of ovarian steroids in initiation, maintenance and suppression. *Fertility and Sterility*, **33**, 649–653.

Djursing, H., Peterson, K. and Weberg, E. (1981). Symptomatic postmenopausal endometriosis. *Acta Obstetrica et Gynecologica Scandinavica*, **60**, 529–530.

Dmowski, W. P. (1979). Endocrine properties and clinical applications of danazol. *Fertility and Sterility*, **31**, 237–251.

Dmowski, W. P. and Cohen, M. R. (1975). Treatment of endometriosis with an antigonadotrophin, danazol: a laparoscopic and histologic evaluation, *Obstetrics and Gynecology*, **46**, 147–154.

Dmowski, W. P. and Cohen, M. R. (1978). Antigonadotrophin (danazol) in the treatment of endometriosis: evaluation of post-treatment fertility and three-year follow-up data. *American Journal of Obstetrics and Gynecology*, **130**, 41–48.

Dmowski, W. P., Cohen, M. R. and Wilhelm, J. L. (1976). Endometriosis and ovulatory failure: Does it occur? Should ovulatory stimulating agents be used, in *Recent Advances in Endometriosis*, (Ed. R. B. Greenblatt) Excerpta Medica, Princeton, pp. 129–136.

Dmowski, W. P., Romaa, R. and Scommegna, A. (1980). The LUF syndrome and endometriosis. *Fertility and Sterility*, **33**, 30–34.

Doty, D. W., Gruber, J. S., Gordon, C. W. *et al.* (1980) 46 XY pure gonadal dysgenesis: a report of 2 unusual cases. *Obstetrics and Gynecology*, **55**, (**supplement 3**), 61–635.

Drake, T. S., O'Brien, W. F., Ramwell, P. W. and Metz, S. A. (1981). Peritoneal fluid thromboxane B_2 and 6-keto-prostaglandin F_1 a in endometriosis. *American Journal of Obstetrics and Gynecology*, **140**, 401–404.

El-Mahgoub, S. and Yasseen, S. (1980). A positive proof for the theory of coelomic metaplasia. *American Journal of Obstetrics and Gynecology*, **137**, 137–140.

Fähraeus, L., Larsson-Cohn, U., Ljungberg, S. and Wallentin, L. (1984). Profound alterations of the lipoprotein metabolism during danazol treatment in premenopausal women. *Fertility and Sterility*, **42**, 52–57.

Feste, J. (1984). Laser laparoscopy. *Fertility and Sterility*, **41**, 745.

Garcia, C. R. and David, S. S. (1977). Pelvic endometriosis: infertility and pelvic pain. *American Journal of Obstetrics and Gynecology*, **129**, 740–747.

Gomel, V. (1980). The impact of microsurgery on gynecology. *Clinical Obstetrics and Gynecology*, **23**, 1301–1310.

Gould, S. F., Shannon, J. M. and Cunha, G. R. (1983). Nuclear estrogen binding sites in human endometriosis. *Fertility and Sterility*, **39**, 520–524.

Groll, M. (1984). Endometriosis and spontaneous abortion. *Fertility and Sterility*, **41**, 933–935.

Halme, J., Becker, S., Hammond, M. G., Raj, M. H. G. and Raj, S. (1983). Increased activation of pelvic macrophages in infertile women with mild endometriosis. *American Journal of Obstetrics and Gynecology*, **145**, 333–337.

Halme, J., Becker, S. and Haskill, S. (1986). Altered life span and function of peritoneal macrophages: a new hypothesis for pathogenesis of endometriosis. *Society of Gynecologic Investigation, Toronto*, **Abstract 48**.

Hammond, C. B. and Haney, A. F. (1978). Conservative treatment of endometriosis. *Fertility and Sterility*, **30**, 497–509.

Haney, A. F., Muscato, J. J. and Weinberg, J. B. (1981). Peritoneal fluid cell populations in infertility patients. *Fertility and Sterility*, **35**, 696–698.

Haney, A. F., Misukonis, M. A. and Weinberg, J. B. (1983). Macrophages and infertility: oviductal macrophages as potential mediators of infertility. *Fertility and Sterility*, **39**, 310–315.

Hargrove, J. T. and Abraham, G. E. (1980). Abnormal luteal function in endometriosis. *Fertility and Sterility*, **34**, 302.

Hirschowitz, J. S., Soler, N. G. and Worstman, J. (1978). The galactorrhoea-endometriosis syndrome. *Lancet*, **i**, 896–898.

Holt, J. P., Jr. and Keller, D. (1984). Danazol treatment increases serum enzyme levels. *Fertility and Sterility*, **41**, 70–74.

Janne, O., Kaupilla, A., Kokko, E., Lantto, T., Ronnberg, L. and Vikho, R. (1981). Estrogen and progestin receptors in endometriosis lesions: comparisons with endometrial tissue. *American Journal of Obstetrics and Gynecology*, **145**, 562–566.

Jeffcoate, T. N. (1975). *Principles of Gynaecology*, (4th edition), Butterworth, London, pp. 350–364.

Jones, H. W., Jr. and Rock, J. A. (1977). Regulation of female infertility, in *Regulation of Human Fertility, WHO Symposium 1975*, (Ed. E. Diczfalusy), Scriptor, Moscow.

Karnaky, K. J. (1948). Use of stilboestrol for endometriosis: preliminary report. *Southern Medical Journal*, **41**, 1109–1111.

Kaupilla, A., Veli, I., Ronnbergh, L., Vierikko, P. and Vikko, R. (1985). Effect of gestrinone in endometriosis tissue and endometrium. *Fertility and Sterility*, **44**, 466–470.

Kistner, R. W. (1958). The use of newer progestins in the treatment of endometriosis. *American Journal of Obstetrics and Gynecology*, **75**, 264–278.

Kistner, R. W. (1959). The treatment of endometriosis by inducing pseudopregnancy with ovarian hormones: a report of 58 cases, *Fertility and Sterility*, **10**, 539–545.

Kistner, R. W. (1975). Endometriosis and infertility, in *Progress in Infertility*, (Eds. S. J. Behrman and R. W. Kistner) (2nd edition), Little Brown, Boston, p. 345.

Kistner, R. W. (1977). Endometriosis, in *Gynecology and Obstetrics*, Vol. 1, (Ed. J. Sciarra), Harper & Row, Hagerstown.

Kistner, R. W., Siegler, A. M. and Behrman, S. J. (1977). Suggested classification for endometriosis: relationship to infertility. *Fertility and Sterility*, **28**, 1008–1009.

Koninckx, P. R., Ide, P., Vandenbrouke, W. and Brosens, I. A. (1980). New aspects of the pathophysiology of endometriosis and associated infertility. *Journal of Reproductive Medicine*, **24**, 257–260.

Lemay, A., Maheux, R., Faure, N., Jean, C. and Fazekas, A. (1984). Reversible hypogonadism induced by a luteinizing hormone releasing hormone (LH-RH) agonist (buserelin) as a new therapeutic approach for endometriosis. *Fertility and Sterility*, **41**, 863–871.

Low, R. A., Roberts, A. D. and Lees, D. A. R. (1984). A comparative study of various dosages of danazol in the treatment of endometriosis. *British Journal of Obstetrics and Gynaecology*, **91**, 167–171.

Luciano, A. A. and Pitkin, R. M. (1984). Endometriosis: approaches to diagnosis and treatment. *Surgical Annual*, **16**, 297–312.

Maheux, R., Guilloteau, C., Lemay, A., Bastide, A. and Fazekas, A. (1985). Luteinizing hormone-releasing hormone agonist and uterine leiomyoma: A pilot study. *American Journal of Obstetrics and Gynecology*, **152**, 1034–1308.

Manson, A. J., Stonner, F. W., Neumann, H. C., Christansen, R. G., Clarke, R. L., Ackerman, J. H., Page, D. F., Dean, J. W., Phillips, D. K., Potts, G. O., Arnold, A., Beyler, A. L. and Clinton, R. O. (1963). Steroidal heterocycles, VII. Androstano [2,3-d] isoxazoles and related compounds. *Journal of Medicinal Chemistry*, **6**, 1–9.

Marik, J. and Hulka, J. (1978). Luteinized unruptured follicle syndrome: a subtle cause of infertility. *Fertility and Sterility*, **29**, 270–274.

Matta, W. H. and Shaw, R. W. (1987). A comparative study between Buserelin and Danazol in the treatment of endometriosis. *British Journal of Clinical Practice*, **41** **(Suppl. 48)**, 69–73.

McArthur, J. W. and Ulfelder, H. (1965). The effect of pregnancy upon endometriosis. *Obstetrical and Gynecological Survey*, **20**, 709–733.

Meldrum, D. R., Shamonki, I. M. and Clark, K. E. (1977). *Prostaglandin content of ascitic fluid in endometriosis: a preliminary report, 25th annual meeting of the Pacific Coast*, Fertility Society, Palm Springs, California.

Meldrum, D. R., Chang, R. J., Lu, J., Vale, W., Rivier, J. and Judd, H. L. (1982). 'Medical oophorectomy' using a long acting GnRH agonist: a possible new approach to the treatment of endometriosis. *Journal of Clinical Endocrinology and Metabolism*, **54**, 1081–1083.

Mettler, L. and Semm, K. (1984). Three-step therapy of genital endometriosis in cases of human infertility with lynestrenol, danazol or gestrinone administration, in *Medical Management of Endometriosis*, (Eds. J. P. Raynaud, T. Ojasoo and L. Martini), Raven Press, New York, pp. 233–247.

Metzger, D. A., Olive, D. L., Stohs, G. F. and Franklin, R. R. (1986). Association of endometriosis and spontaneous abortion: Effect of control group selection. *Fertility and Sterility*, **45**, 18–22.

Meyer, R. (1919). Uber den Staude der Frage der Adenomyosites Adenomyoma in Allgemeinen und Adenomyometitis Sarcomastosa. *Zentralblatt fur Gynakologie*, **36**, 745–759.

Morcos, R. N., Gibbous, W. E. and Findley, W. E. (1985). Effect of peritoneal fluid on *in vitro* cleavage of 2-cell mouse embryos: possible role in infertility associated with endometriosis. *Fertility and Sterility*, **44**, 678–683.

Muscato, J. J., Haney, A. F. and Weinberg, J. B. (1982). Sperm phagocytosis by human peritoneal macrophages: a possible cause of infertility in endometriosis. *American Journal of Obstetrics and Gynecology*, **144**, 503–510.

Muse, K., Wilson, E. A. and Jawad, M. J. (1982). Prolactin hyperstimulation in response to thyrotropin releasing hormone in patients with endometriosis. *Fertility and Sterility*, **38**, 419–422.

Naples, J. D., Batt, R. E. and Sadigh, H. (1981). Spontaneous abortion rate in patients with endometriosis. *Obstetrics and Gynecology*, **57**, 509–512.

Oliker, A. J. and Harris, A. E. (1971). Endometriosis of the bladder in a male patient. *Journal of Urology*, **106**, 858–859.

Olive, D. L., Franklin, R. R. and Gratkins, L. V. (1982). The association between endometriosis and spontaneous abortion. A restrospective clinical study. *Journal of Reproductive Medicine*, **27**, 333–338.

Olive, D. L., Weinberg, J. B. and Haney, A. F. (1985). Peritoneal macrophages and infertility: the association between cell number and pelvic pathology. *Fertility and Sterility*, **44**, 772–777.

Pinkert, T., Catlow, L. E. and Strauss, R. (1979). Endometriosis in the urinary bladder in a man with prostatic cancer. *Cancer*, **43**, 1562–1567.

Pittaway, D. E., Maxson, W., Daniell, J., Herbert, C. and Wentz, A. C. (1983). Luteal phase defects in infertility patients with endometriosis. *Fertility and Sterility*, **39**, 712–713.

Portuondo, J. A., Echanojauregui, A. D., Herran, C. and Ahjarte, I. (1983). Early conception in patients with untreated mild endometriosis. *Fertility and Sterility*, **39**, 22–25.

Prakash, S. J., Ulfelder, H. and Cohen, R. B. (1965). Enzyme-histochemical observations on endometriosis. *American Journal of Obstetrics and Gynecology*, **91**, 990–997.

Punnonen, R., Klemi, P. J. and Nikkanen, U. (1980). Postmenopausal endometriosis, *European Journal of Obstetrics, Gynecology and Reproductive Biology*, **11**, 195–200.

Ranney, B. (1971a). Endometriosis IV: hereditary tendencies. *Obstetrics and Gynecology*, **37**, 734–737.

Ranney, B. (1971b). Endometriosis III: complete operations. *American Journal of Obstetrics and Gynecology*, **109**, 1137–1144.

Ranney, B. (1975). The prevention, inhibition, palliation and treatment of endometriosis, *American Journal of Obstetrics and Gynecology*, **123**, 778–785.

Raynaud, J. P., Bonne, C., Bouton, M. M., Moguilewsky, M., Philbert, D. and Azadian-Boulanger, G. (1975). Screening for anti-hormones by receptor studies. *Journal of Steroid Biochemistry*, **6**, 615–622.

Revised American Fertility Society Classification of Endometriosis (1985). *Fertility and Sterility*, **43**, 351–352.

Riva, H. L., Wilson, J. H. and Kawaski, D. M. (1961). Effects of norethnodrel on endometriosis. *American Journal of Obstetrics and Gynecology*, **82**, 109–118.

Robyn, C., Delagne-Desnoeck, J., Bordoux, P. and Copinschi, G. (1984). Endocrine effects of gestrinone, in *Medical Management of Endometriosis*, (Eds. J. P. Raynaud, T. Ojasoo and L. Martini), Raven Press, New York, pp. 207–221.

Rock, J. A., Guzick, D. S., Sengos, C., Schweditsch, M., Sapp, K. C. and Jones, H. W. Jr. (1981). The conservative surgical treatment of endometriosis: Evaluation of pregnancy success with respect to the extent of disease as categorized using contemporary classification systems. *Fertility and Sterility*, **35**, 131–137.

Rock, J. A., Dubin, N. M., Ghodgaonkar, R. B., Bergquist, C. A., Erozan, Y. S. and Kimball, A. W., Jr. (1982). Cul-de-sac fluid in women with endometriosis: fluid volume and prostanoid concentration during the proliferative phase of the cycle—days 8 to 12. *Fertility and Sterility*, **37**, 747–752.

Roddick, J. W., Conkey, G. and Jacobs, E. J. (1960). The hormonal response of endometrium in endometriotic implants and its relationship to symptomatology. *American Journal of Obstetrics and Gynecology*, **79**, 1173–1177.

Sampson, J. A. (1921). Perforating hemorrhagic cysts of ovary. *Archives of Surgery*, **3**, 245–323.

Sampson, J. A. (1927a). Peritoneal endometriosis due to menstrual dissemination of endometrial tissue into peritoneal cavity. *American Journal of Obstetrics and Gynecology*, 14, 422.

Sampson, J. A. (1927b). Metastatic or embolic endometriosis due to menstrual dissemination of endometrial tissue into the venous circulation. *American Journal of Pathology*, 3, 93–109.

Sandow, J. (1983). Clinical applications of LHRH and its analogues. *Clinical Endocrinology*, 18, 571–592.

Schenken, R. S. and Malinak, L. R. (1982). Conservative surgery versus expectant management for the infertile patient with mild endometriosis. *Fertility and Sterility*, 37, 183–186.

Schmidt, C. L. (1985). Endometriosis: a reappraisal of pathogenesis and treatment. *Fertility and Sterility*, 44, 157–173.

Schmidt-Gollwitzer, M., Hardt, W., Schmidt-Gollwitzer, K., Von der Oke, M. and Nevinny-Stickel, J. (1981). Influence of the LHRH analogue Buserelin on cyclic ovarian function and on endometrium. A new approach to fertility control. *Contraception*, 23, 187–195.

Schriock, E., Monroe, S. E., Henzl, M. and Jaffe, R. B. (1985). Treatment of endometriosis with a potent agonist of gonadotrophin releasing hormone (nafarelin). *Fertility and Sterility*, 44, 583–588.

Schrodt, G. R., Alcorn, M. O. and Ibanez, J. (1980). Endometriosis of the male urinary system: a case report. *Journal of Urology*, 124, 722–723.

Schweppe, K. W. and Wynn, R. (1981). Ultrastructural changes in endometriotic implants during the menstrual cycle. *Obstetrics and Gynecology*, 58, 465–473.

Scott, R. B. and Wharton, L. R. (1957). The effects of estrone and progesterone on the growth of experimental endometriosis in rhesus monkeys. *American Journal of Obstetrics and Gynecology*, 74, 852–865.

Seibel, M. M., Berger, M. J., Weinstein, F. G. and Taymor, M. L. (1982). The effectiveness of danazol on subsequent fertility in minimal endometriosis. *Fertility and Sterility*, 38, 534–537.

Sgarlata, C. S., Hertelendy, F. and Mikhail, G. (1983). The prostanoid content in peritoneal fluid and plasma of women with endometriosis. *American Journal of Obstetrics and Gynecology*, 147, 563–565.

Shaw, R. W., Fraser, H. M. and Boyle, H. (1983). Intranasal treatment with luteinizing hormone releasing hormone agonist in women with endometriosis. *British Medical Journal*, 287, 1667–1669.

Shaw, R. W. and Fraser, H. M. (1984a). Use of a superactive luteinizing hormone releasing hormone (LHRH) agonist in the treatment of menorrhagia. *British Journal of Obstetrics and Gynaecology*, 91, 913–916.

Shaw, R. W. and Fraser, H. M. (1984b). Intranasal treatment with luteinizing hormone releasing hormone agonist in women with endometriosis. *Journal of Steroid Biochemistry*, 20, 1403 (Abstract).

Simpson, J. L., Elias, S., Malinak, L. R. and Buttram, V. C., Jr. (1980). Heritable aspects of endometriosis I: genetic studies. *American Journal of Obstetrics and Gynecology*, 137, 327–331.

Soules, M., Malinak, L. R., Bury, R. and Pointdexter, A. (1976). Endometriosis and anovulation: A coexisting problem in the infertile female. *American Journal of Obstetrics and Gynecology*, 125, 412–417.

Spangler, B. B. and Jones, H. W., Jr. (1971). Infertility due to endometriosis. *American Journal of Obstetrics and Gynecology*, 109, 850–857.

Strathy, J. H., Molgaard, C. A., Coulam, C. B. and Melton, L. J. (1982). III: Endometriosis and infertility: A laparoscopic study of endometriosis among fertile and infertile women. *Fertility and Sterility*, 38, 667–672.

Szlachter, N. B., Moskowitz, J., Bigelow, B. and Weiss, G. (1980). Iatrogenic endometriosis; substantiation of the Sampson hypothesis *Obstetrics and Gynecology*, **55 (supplement)**, 52–535.

Thomas, E. J. and Cooke, I. D. (1986). A prospective randomised double-blind placebo controlled trial of gestrinone in the treatment of minimal endometriosis, *24th British Congress of Obstetrics and Gynaecology, Cardiff*, 86 (Abstract).

Tyson, J. E. A. (1974). Surgical considerations in gynaecologic endocrine disorders. *Surgical Clinics of North America*, **54**, 425–442.

Vanrell, J. A., Balasch, J., Fuster, J. S. and Fuster, R. (1982). Ovulation stigma in fertile women. *Fertility and Sterility*, **37**, 712–713.

Vierikko, P., Kauppila, A., Ronnberg, L. and Vikho, R. (1985). Steroidal regulation of endometriosis tissue: lack of induction of 17β-hydroxysteroid dehydrogenase activity by progesterone, medroxy progesterone acetate, or danazol. *Fertility and Sterility*, **43**, 218–224.

Von Rokitansky, C. (1860). *Ztsch K Gesselsch Aerte (Wien)*, **16**, 577.

Wahl, P., Walden, C., Knopp, R., Hoover, J., Wallace, R., Heiss, G. and Rifkind, B. (1983). The effects of oestrogen/progestin potency on lipid/lipoprotein cholesterols. *New England Journal of Medicine*, **308**, 862–867.

Wardle, P. G., McLaughlin, E. A., McDermott, A., Mitchell, J. D., Ray, B. D. and Hull, M. G. R. (1985). Endometriosis and ovulatory disorder: reduced fertilization *in vitro* compared with tubal and unexplained infertility. *Lancet*, **ii**, 236–239.

Weed, J. C. and Arquembourg, P. C. (1980). Endometriosis: can it produce an autoimmune response resulting in infertility? *Clinical Obstetrics and Gynecology*, **23**, 885–895.

Wentz, A. C. (1980). Premenstrual spotting: its association with endometriosis but not luteal phase inadequacy. *Fertility and Sterility*, **33**, 605–607.

Wheeler, J. M., Johnston, B. M. and Malinak, L. R. (1983). The relationship of endometriosis to spontaneous abortion. *Fertility and Sterility*, **39**, 656–660.

Whitfield, C. R. (1986). Endometriosis, in *Dewhurst's Textbook of Obstetrics and Gynaecology for Postgraduates*, (4th edition) Blackwell Scientific, London, pp. 609–623.

Williams, T. J., Pratt, J. H. (1977). Endometriosis in 1000 consecutive celiotomies: Incidence and management, *American Journal of Obstetrics and Gynecology*, **129**, 245–250.

Ylikorkala, O. and Vünikka, L. (1983). Prostaglandins and endometriosis, *Acta Obstetrica et Gynecologica Scandinavica*, **113 Supplement** 105–107.

Functional Disorders of the Menstrual Cycle
Edited by M. G. Brush and E. M. Goudsmit
© 1988 John Wiley & Sons Ltd

CHAPTER 17

The role of improvements in communication and nutrition in the support of endometriosis sufferers

CAROLINE HAWKRIDGE
Endometriosis Society,
65 Holmdene Avenue,
London SE24 9LD

and

M. G. BRUSH
Department of Gynaecology,
United Medical and Dental Schools,
St Thomas's Campus,
London SE1 7EH

The disease process of endometriosis, its symptoms and medical treatment, have been described in the previous chapter. It outlines some of the problems a patient may have and the implications for her physical health. This chapter looks at the particular characteristics of endometriosis and its treatment which can also affect a woman's emotional and social life. By examining these effects in the context of an endometriosis 'career', it becomes possible to identify where, when and how effective communication could take place to prevent or alleviate these problems. This approach complements medical diagnosis and treatment and promotes the health of the whole person.

In a second section the role of improvements in nutrition in promoting the health of endometriosis sufferers is discussed.

Improvements in Communication

The GP Consultation

A provisional diagnosis of endometriosis is usually confirmed during a laparoscopy, rather than in a general practitioner's surgery. Laparoscopy has

279

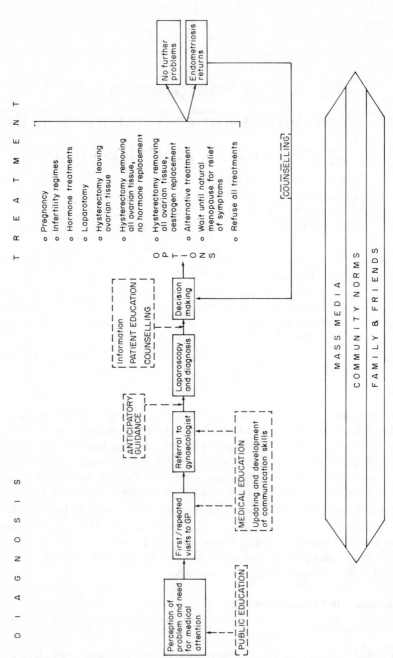

Figure 1. Outline of an endometriosis career

revolutionized the detection of many gynaecological problems including endometriosis, but it still cannot be regarded as a feasible population screening programme. Thus the question of *who* is referred for laparoscopy remains central to effective diagnosis and consultation with a GP is a very important first step in an 'endometriosis career' (see Figure 1).

For referral and diagnosis to occur, both a woman and her doctor must conclude she has a problem which warrants medical attention; she must make the initial/repeated visits and her doctor must make the decision whether or not to refer. This process requires adequate communication between both parties about symptoms and accurate perception of those at risk.

A recent survey amongst 800 members of the Endometriosis Society (Hawkridge, 1986) examined the hypothesis that communication of symptoms may be a major stumbling block in diagnosis; perhaps even greater than the problem of distinguishing endometriosis from other gynaecological disorders (e.g. pelvic inflammatory disease) which doctors already recognize. Women were asked what symptoms originally prompted them to visit their GP. Comparisons with the frequency of generally reported symptoms (see Figure 2) suggest that many women did not present 'cardinal' symptoms (after Ward, 1983) of undiagnosed endometriosis to their doctors even though they experienced them. For example, only 13 per cent were prompted to visit their doctor because of painful sexual intercourse although 55 per cent of the main sample reported this as a symptom of their endometriosis.

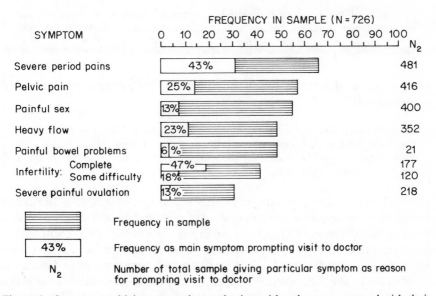

Figure 2. Symptoms which prompted consultation with a doctor compared with their reported frequency in sample

There may be several reasons for this lack of communication. Many of the symptoms of endometriosis e.g. painful periods coincide with what women (and their doctors) expect as part of the menstrual cycle. But discussions with sufferers suggest that women's experiences of 'normal' pain amongst everyday stresses and strains can also prevent them from seeking help:

'I just kept putting it (pain) down to other things i.e. PMT, problems with relationships, pressures of bringing up two young children.'

Apart from the frequent embarrassment of discussing gynaecological symptoms or undergoing a pelvic examination, many women also describe fear or experiences of being labelled 'neurotic' by their GP and not taken seriously:

'One of the problems is doctors' attitudes toward women complaining of this sort of pain—they always seem to think "She's neurotic, therefore she says she is in pain." They never think: "She is anxious because she *is* in pain!".'

While it is difficult to assess how common these feelings are, they illustrate how women's attitudes and beliefs about the (often ambiguous) symptoms of endometriosis can produce anxiety and yet fail to lead to a consultation.

Doctors' perceptions of the symptoms are also important if they are to encourage women to consult them appropriately and make an accurate diagnosis. One GP writing about endometriosis commented that:

... unless a GP is aware of the possibility of endometriosis in long suffering and oft complaining females, nothing constructive can be done. Either the patient will keep on pestering the doctor or will give up trying for medical help.' (Pirzada, 1987.)

He goes on to describe a simple questionnaire for patients with suspected endometriosis:

'Sometimes patients forget to mention certain "pointers" while at other times they may think some symptoms are insignificant . . . I would rather waste a bit more time on details than label the patient as neurotic, troublesome or a frequent offender.' (Pirzada, 1987.)

A positive, more systematic approach which encourages communication seems likely to improve early diagnosis of endometriosis. Unfortunately, it still begs the question of what are 'pointers' to the disease. Two recent studies illustrate the difficulty of providing ready answers and the need for an open mind during consultation. Several 'unorthodox' symptoms were frequently mentioned in the Endometriosis Society survey when women were asked what, *in their opinion*, were symptoms of their endometriosis (Hawkridge, 1986). For example, depression, tiredness and lethargy were reported by 63 per cent (see Figure 3). Of course, without a control group it is difficult to tell

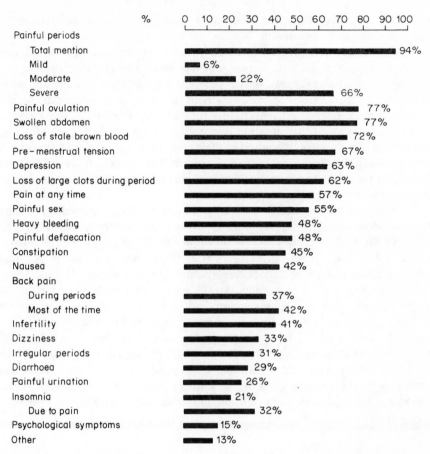

Figure 3. Symptoms of endometriosis reported in the Endometriosis Society Survey (Hawkridge, 1986). Number of women in sample = 726. (Each was asked to list *all* symptoms)

which reported symptoms are caused by endometriosis rather than other factors. Equally, some may be direct effects, while others are a response to having the disease e.g. insomnia due to pain (reported by 32 per cent). Both types of effect play an important part in a woman's physical and emotional experience of the disease, but it could still be argued that indirect effects are less relevant to a medical understanding of the disease and hence improved diagnosis. However, as yet unpublished research (Brush, 1986) which followed up over 100 sufferers reporting extreme tiredness and lethargy, found an increased incidence of thyroid auto-antibodies, which could account for these symptoms. Several patients were successfully treated with thyroxine by their GPs. This study suggests that it is premature to conclude that 'common problems' are irrelevant and underlines the artificial distinction between physical and emotional health.

Barriers to the effective communication of symptoms may partly account for the catalogue of delayed diagnosis women described in the Endometriosis Society survey. For example, only 5 per cent went to their doctors and were diagnosed in the same year that they believe their problems began; 41 per cent had to make repeated visits before they were referred to a gynaecologist. The observation that this situation is worse for young women (i.e. only 2 per cent of the sample were diagnosed in their teens although 15 per cent said that this was when they first went to their doctors and 35 per cent believed that this was when they first began to suffer) highlights the need for accurate perceptions of those at risk.

Ironically, in the absence of known causal factors, accurate medical perception of those who risk developing endometriosis is totally dependent on effective methods of diagnosis. For example, since the advent of the laparoscope it has been increasingly recognized that endometriosis is not rare amongst black women or only characteristic of women in their 30s and 40s as previously suggested (e.g. Meigs, 1949). Assertions that endometriosis is more frequent in the higher socio-economic classes (e.g. Leading Article, 1980) can be challenged on the grounds that sufferers in these groups probably have a higher level of knowledge, resources and sense of entitlement, making it more likely that they will be referred for laparoscopy and so become diagnosed. Fewer known cases amongst lower socio-economic groups is not necessarily evidence of a lower incidence. Fortunately, recent influential medical authors have argued that 'some of the myths of endometriosis need to be buried':

'It is not only a disease of private patients in affluent societies; it occurs most often before the age of 30 years and can exist after the menopause; it is not confined to thin, tense, over-achievers attempting initial conception late in life . . . it is becoming more common because women in general have greater expectations of gynaecological good health; clinicians are more aware of the clues that may lead to a diagnosis of endometriosis; and laparoscopy is more readily available universally for the early diagnosis and treatment of the disease at an early stage.' (O'Connor, 1987)

Out-of-date misconceptions of those at risk of developing endometriosis can only hinder the diagnostic process. While some groups of women suffer unnecessary delays there may be an increased probability of misdiagnosis amongst others who do not have the disease. Since endometriosis is usually a progressive disorder, a delay or failure in diagnosis has implications for a woman's physical health and fertility. Many women also feel anger and guilt, which is not necessarily directed at the medical profession!

'I deeply regret not being more assertive when possibly an earlier diagnosis could have been made. I just accepted that I was over-sensitive to pain. I was my own worst enemy.'

Much of the responsibility for diagnosing endometriosis falls on the GP as the 'gatekeeper' to hospital diagnostic services. Two GPs writing in an educational pack on endometriosis (Endometriosis Society, 1987) have responded to this challenge:

'As a general practitioner, I feel it is my duty to recognize these effects and the symptoms they produce, so that I can alleviate the sufferings of the patient at an early stage of the disease.' (Pirzada, 1987)

'Conditions such as endometriosis require mutual trust and respect between women and their doctors . . . By sharing information and listening to each other I believe women and their doctors can go some way towards healing and being healed.' (Gardner, 1987)

There is a clear need for both medical and public education to raise awareness amongst women and their doctors if communication and the provisional diagnosis of endometriosis in the surgery is to improve.

Hospital Diagnosis and Treatment

The next step in an 'endometriosis career' is referral to a gynaecologist who will usually decide to perform a laparoscopy. The patient will be required to spend one to two days in hospital. If a definite diagnosis of endometriosis is made, she may have to return for more extensive gynaecological surgery (see Figure 1).

At first glance, the emotional and social impact of surgery on a patient is generally recognized. It is accepted that patients are usually anxious about the impending operation and coping with the disruption to work, family and social commitments that hospitalization brings. In spite of this, there have been few systematic attempts to promote recovery from gynaecological surgery by offering 'anticipatory guidance'. The term anticipatory guidance has been traced back to early work in maternal and child welfare where it was defined as 'teaching the mother what to expect before she begins to worry or make mistakes' (see Janis, 1969). In a more recent definition, the Royal College of General Practitioners (1981) describes it as 'actions taken with the object of preparing a person for potentially stressful life changes'.

There are several psychological models which outline the process involved in anticipatory guidance (for a review, see Pridham *et al.*, 1979). The emphasis they place on the role of information has led to a great deal of practical research on how communication can modify the effects of surgery. For example, Wallace (1984) compared the response of patients undergoing laparoscopy who received either comprehensive information about the surgery, a booklet extolling the quality of hospital staff and equipment or routine care only. Patients receiving accurate information about their operation showed better post-operative recovery as indicated by several measures including an earlier return to eating and drinking, lower pain on a visual analogue scale and a faster return to normal activities at home. The 'placebo' leaflet about the hospital had a minimal effect on recovery with patients showing similar responses to those receiving routine care only. This supports the suggestion that creating accurate expectations is more important than information *per se*.

Other studies have tested methods of cognitive intervention which assume that a patient's pre-operative experience can be directly modified by mental exercises rather than information about impending surgery. For example, Ridgeway and Matthews (1982) considered three groups of elective hysterectomy patients. One experimental group received an information manual about the surgical procedure while the other group was given a cognitive manual which asked the reader to reappraise common worries about surgery and their own negative thoughts more positively. The control group was given general information about the ward. Interestingly, the cognitive intervention group showed less post-operative anxiety, less use of medication and were discharged earlier, but the information manual patients were more satisfied and had a greater understanding of the operation.

The development of psychological approaches to promote recovery from surgery roughly coincided with evidence that lack of information was the main reason for patient dissatisfaction with hospital experiences (Cartwright, 1964; Ley and Spelman, 1967). Subsequent research to consider ways of improving doctor-patient communication serves as a reminder that preparation for surgery can only be beneficial if it is effectively communicated.

Ley and Spelman (1967) put forward several useful recommendations for improving doctor–patient communication. These authors argue that:

'For communication to be effective the message it contains must be understood and remembered and many failures in communication are caused by simple failures of comprehension and memory.'

Based on a variety of studies, Ley and co-workers have identified three principle factors involved in patients' failure to understand:

1. The information may be incomprehensible.
2. Patients may lack the knowledge required for understanding.
3. They may be diffident about asking questions.

(for reviews see Ley, 1976 and Ley *et al.*, 1976).

Wallace (1984) found these factors equally relevant in pre-operative preparation, but also argued that the first consideration must be whether the information was actually given (even though staff might believe it had been). In a study looking at ten items of information that gynaecology ward staff reported routinely giving to patients, it was found that almost a third of the information was not actually given (Wallace, 1984).

Many of the studies of pre-operative preparation also assume that the information given is comprehensible to patients. Wallace (1984) reports that a number of preparatory leaflets would only be understood by a minority of the population. Verbal communications may be equally unsuccessful if patients do not understand medical terminology or are confused about anatomy and bodily functions. Evidence of such misconceptions has been reported (e.g. Dunkelman, 1979). Studies of gynaecology patients undergoing laparoscopy (e.g. Wallace, 1979; Reading, 1981) confirm other reports that patients are reluctant to ask questions which might remedy their confusion or ignorance (Cartwright, 1964; Ley and Spelman, 1967; Fletcher, 1980).

Inevitably patients forget much of what they have been told and research suggests that this happens almost immediately. Several methods for improving patients' recall have been explored with positive results (Ley, 1976). Stating important information first and repeating it helps patients to remember it. Explicit categorization is another useful technique. Giving patients specific rather than general advice also encourages remembering because specific advice is regarded as more important. A hospital study exploiting these methods showed that patients' understanding can be increased and that this leads to greater satisfaction and compliance (Ley et al., 1976).

Other studies have argued for the importance of writing down information for patients (e.g. Gauld, 1981) and this appears to be increasingly popular. However, there are dangers in being tempted to use leaflets exclusively, especially as a time-saving device. Unless leaflets are used in addition to face-to-face contact, they only allow one-way communication from author to reader. The messages cannot be revised and there is no opportunity for feedback about whether they have been received and/or understood. Messages cannot be repeated if and when necessary. The reader can not seek clarification or check whether meanings are shared.

These limitations are especially important when patients have unknown fears and expectations. For example, laparoscopy is an exploratory operation and it seems likely that many patients will be worried about a serious diagnosis. However, it is less obvious that patients might worry about *not* being diagnosed. This situation can appear to deny their experience of the symptoms and request for help unless there is an opportunity for discussion:

'Feeling of panic, lack of confidence—and being told the pain was in my mind.'

This is not to say that leaflets which describe a complicated disease such as endometriosis and/or some of its treatment are not very useful. Basing the material on discussions with sufferers can help to ensure that it addresses common beliefs and expectations and avoids misunderstandings. This is important in a condition such as endometriosis where confusion about the disease process has led to worrying beliefs about 'bleeding inside' and the possibility of cancer which is often associated with 'growths'. Information that can be passed on to family and friends can help avoid feelings of isolation amongst patients who have probably will not have heard of the disease before. Even when patients can explain their problem people may find it hard to believe without the 'evidence' of a leaflet:

'I thought that there was only me that suffered from this as no one had ever heard of it before. When they ask me what's wrong when I don't look well and I try to explain, they look at me as though to say I'm silly. No one really knows what we go through.'

The treatment of endometriosis depends on several things, including the severity of the disease, the problems it is causing, a patient's age and any wishes to have or complete a family. The current range of treatments is listed in Figure 1. Paradoxically, pregnancy can alleviate the condition but 40 per cent of sufferers experience infertility. In both cases, a woman (and her partner) are faced with difficult emotional dilemmas and choices. The main drug treatments (e.g. danazol, norethisterone and dydrogesterone) usually have depressing side effects (e.g. weight gain and masculinization) and taking a six to nine month course requires considerable persistence. Further surgery may also be recommended. Whether it is a laparotomy to remove endometrial cysts or a hysterectomy, it will involve many of the psychological concommitants described earlier. The debate about hysterectomy resulting in loss of libido and depression continues (e.g. Kincey and McFarlane, 1984) while endometriosis patients face the further argument about the benefits of removing healthy ovaries and controlling circulating oestrogens with hormone replacement therapy (e.g. Studd, 1986). There are also a whole range of alternative and complimentary medicines which endometriosis sufferers have found useful. However, the natural menopause is the only 'more or less' guaranteed cure (see O'Connor, 1987) and few patients are old enough to choose to wait.

Many of the options outlined above require 'life' decisions which cannot readily be reversed. Furthermore, current treatments of endometriosis do not have high success rates and patients often have to persevere, trying different alternatives. An uncertain outcome often combines with false expectations of cure to produce anxiety and depression. Whatever course women choose to take they will need adequate information, counselling and an opportunity to review their progress. Although a particular treatment may be advocated in view of the patient's physical health, a counselling approach which helps the person explore her thoughts and feelings, reach an understanding of her strengths and then use them to make appropriate decisions and actions will also help women cope more effectively. Recognition of the emotional and social impact of different regimes and the need to maintain the patient's self esteem are vital to treatment which aims to prevent or alleviate the problems caused by endometriosis rather than simply replace them with new or even additional ones.

Nutritional Support in Endometriosis

As discussed earlier surgical and/or medical treatment of endometriosis may be very effective in many cases but there are the inevitable exceptions. These may be due to a variety of factors including the widespread nature of the endometriosis, often with extensive adhesions, making it impossible to remove it, locations such as the gut wall, which pose difficult problems for the surgeon, and inability to tolerate medical treatment, especially danazol and progestogens. Any lack of extended post-operative medical care may lead to a state of chronic ill health characterized by pain and increasing debility.

It is well known that most pain-killers have unpleasant and sometimes dangerous side-effects when used in the amounts necessary to control the pain from endometriosis. Large amounts of aspirin have gastro-intestinal side-effects, and the toxicity of long-term use of paracetamol is well known. Stronger pain-killers related to morphine have CNS depressant effects with consequent drowsiness and interference with quality of life. Therefore, any natural compounds with painkilling properties will be of potential value as will any natural anti-inflammatory treatment.

This section will discuss several preparations which have anti-inflammatory properties including selenium and various essential fatty acid preparations. Also the current position regarding DL-phenylalanine which has pain-relieving properties will be considered.

Anti-inflammatory Treatments

Evening primrose oil (EPO). The use of EPO in premenstrual syndrome is fully discussed in Chapter 5. Its use is being explored in a variety of other conditions (Horrobin, 1982) and a number of further studies have been undertaken since that time. It has become clear that EPO can exert general anti-inflammatory effects, probably due to its ability to increase the synthesis of prostaglandin E_1 and thereby tend to correct the ratio of '1' series to '2' series prostaglandins. This is beneficial in view of the known role the '2' series prostaglandins in certain inflammatory processes. It has been used on an open basis by endometriosis sufferers belonging to the Endometriosis Society and useful relief has been reported. The usual dose is three 500 mg capsules twice daily after food (see also p. 79). A double-blind study to follow up this encouraging first report, will shortly be commenced with the support of the Endometriosis Society.

Unfortunately, biochemical studies of these processes are at an early stage and little definitive data is, so far, available.

Others oils containing essential fatty acids. There are now at least two other vegetable oils which are rich in essential fatty acids and, in particular, have a high content of γ-linolenic acid (GLA). These are blackcurrant seed oil and borage seed oil (see pages 78–79 for details). It is reasonable to assume that use of these oils would tend to correct the ratio of the '1' series prostaglandins to the '2' series prostaglandins and would have an anti-inflammatory action similar to that of evening primrose oil. So far, no reports of the use of these oils in the management of endometriosis have been given, but in view of the high concentration of GLA involved, first results will be awaited with interest.

Selenium. Selenium is a trace element which has received increasing interest in recent years, especially with regard to Keshan disease, a cardiomyopathy which occurs in a severely selenium deficient rural area of China (Keshan Disease Research Group of the Chinese Academy of Medical Sciences, Beijing, 1979a,b; Chen *et al.*, 1980). Isolated instances of selenium deficiency cardiomyopathy attributed to eccentric nutrition or iatrogenic causes have also been reported (Collip and Chen, 1981; Johnson *et al.*, 1981; Van Rij *et al.*, 1979).

It is also known from animal studies that selenium may have useful anti-inflammatory effects (Roberts, 1963a,b) and may enhance the immune response (Spallholz *et al.*, 1973a,b, 1974; Norman and Johnson, 1976; Sheffy and Schultz, 1978; Shackelford and Martin, 1980).

High levels of the selenium-containing enzyme, glutathione peroxidase, are found in peritoneal exudate cells in animals, and phagocytic cells of selenium-deficient rats could ingest yeast cells *in vitro* but not kill them (Serfass and Ganther, 1975, 1976). These findings were confirmed in selenium-deficient cattle by Boyne and Arthur (1979).

Little research has, so far, been carried out on the use of selenium in the management of inflammatory conditions and situations where immunological status is poor. However, for some years preparations containing selenium and, in particular, a commercial preparation of selenium yeast and vitamins A, C and E (Selenium ACE), has been used empirically as an adjunctive treatment in rheumatic disease and in endometriosis, and useful results on an open basis have been observed. At a dose of one capsule of Selenium ACE twice daily this gives a total of 200 μg selenium and 3000 i.u. vitamin A, 180 mg vitamin C and 90 i.u. vitamin E daily. The use of selenium in organic form, obtained from yeast cultured with selenium, appears to increase bioavailability and is acceptable to all except those with a known sensitivity to yeast. In the latter case, an inorganic form of selenium may be substituted.

Natural Pain-killing Agents

The most promising natural pain-killing method involves the use of the natural amino acid, DL-phenylalanine (DLPA), taken in large amounts. This is thought to enhance the natural pain-killing mechanisms mediated by endorphins and has the great advantages of having an extremely low toxicity and freedom from the build-up of tolerance.

The original studies on phenylalanine in the management of pain were carried out using D-phenylalanine (DPA) (Ehrenpreis *et al.*, 1978a,b, 1981; Budd, 1983; Balagot *et al.*, 1983), but later workers have found that DL-phenylalanine is equally effective and has a greater nutritional value due to its content of the L-form of phenylalanine. The studies of Ehrenpreis *et al.* (1978b) and some later workers were mainly concerned with the relief of pain caused by various types of arthritic conditions, with results from good to excellent, but other conditions, such as migraine and neuralgia, also showed benefits.

The mechanism of action of DPA and DLPA is thought to involve the inhibition of the enzymes which normally rapidly inactivate the endorphins, the natural pain-killing mechanism of the body. These enzymes include carboxypeptidase A and enkephalinase. When inhibition of these degradative enzymes has been achieved, the endorphins can give a much more prolonged pain-killing action. It is interesting to note that Ferreira and Nakamura (1979) showed that enkephalins can block the inflammatory effects of prostaglandins, thus giving a further mechanism of action for pain relief by endorphin-like substances.

Further relevant studies (Cheng and Pomeranz, 1980; Hyodo *et al.*, 1983) show that D-phenylalanine can enhance the analgesic effect of acupuncture. This is consistent with the evidence suggesting that at least part of the mode of action of acupuncture involves the release of endorphins (Mayer *et al.*, 1977; Clement-Jones *et al.*, 1980; Nakano and Ikezono, 1981).

As there is a large inflammatory component to the pain experienced by chronic endometriosis sufferers, one of us suggested that members of the Endometriosis Society, the British self-help group, might like to try DLPA. Some members have done so with considerable benefit, although not in all cases. In a few cases, the sufferer has been able to identify two components to her pain and has noted improvement in only one of them. The only side-effect reported is one case of marked indigestion leading to cessation of treatment.

The original dosage recommendations of the USA workers were two 375 mg DLPA tablets three times daily before meals but, in our experience, some women need to start with one tablet twice daily and work up to the higher dose in gradual steps. Once the correct dose is reached, relief should start within a few days. The action of DLPA can be prolonged and effects may persist for two to three weeks after cessation of treatment in some cases. This may help reduce the cost of treatment by allowing an intermittent dose schedule for some women. It has been suggested that for the most effective use of DLPA, vitamins C and B_6 should be taken as well. There appear to be no contraindications to taking other common analgesics, such as aspirin and anti-prostaglandin drugs as well as DLPA and, in some cases, this may be advantageous. The usual cautions regarding long-term use of aspirin and anti-prostaglandin drugs will of course still apply.

References

Balagot, R. C., Ehrenpreis, S., Kubota, K. and Greenberg, J. (1983). Analgesia in mice and humans by D-phenylalanine: relation to inhibition of enkephalin degradation and enkephalin levels, in *Advances in Pain Research and Therapy*, Vol. 5, (Eds. J. J. Bonica, J. C. Liebeskind and D. G. Albe-Fessard) Raven, New York, pp. 289–293.

Boyne, R. and Arthur, J. R. (1979). Alterations of neutrophil functions in selenium deficient cattle. *Journal of Comparative Pathology*, **89**, 151–158.

Brush, M. G. (1986). (in preparation).

Budd, K. (1983). Use of D-phenylalanine, an enkephalinase inhibitor, in the treatment of intractable pain, in *Advances in Pain Research and Therapy*, Vol. 5, (Eds. J. J. Bonica, J. C. Liebeskind and D. G. Albe-Fessand), Raven, New York, pp. 305–308.

Cartwright, A. (1964). *Human Relations and Hospital Care*, Routledge and Kegan Paul, London.

Chen, X., Yang, G., Chen, J., Chen, X., Wen, Z. and Ge, K. (1980). Studies on the relations of selenium and Keshan disease. *Biological Trace Element Research*, **2**, 91–107.

Cheng, R. S. and Pomeranz, B. (1980). A combined treatment with D-amino acids and electro acupuncture produces a greater analgesia than either treatment alone; naloxone reverses these effects. *Pain*, **8**, 231–236.

Clement-Jones, V., McLoughlin, L., Tomlin, S., Besser, G. M., Rees, L. H. and Wen, H. L. (1980). Increased beta-endorphin but not metenkephalin levels in human cerebrospinal fluid after acupuncture or recurrent pain, *Lancet*, **ii**, 946–949.

Collip, P. J. and Chen, S. Y. (1981). Cardiomyopathy and selenium deficiency in a two-year-old girl. *New England Journal of Medicine*, **303**, 1304–1305.

Dunkelman, H. (1979). Patients' knowledge of their condition and treatment: How it might be improved. *British Medical Journal*, **2**, 311–314.

Ehrenpreis, S., Balagot, R. C., Comaty, J. E. and Myles, S. B. (1978a). Naloxone reversible analgesia in mice produced by D-phenylalanine and hydrocinnamic acid, inhibitors of carboxypeptidase A, in *Advances in Pain Research and Therapy*, Vol. 3, (Eds. J. J. Bonica, J. C. Liebeskind and D. G. Albe-Fessad), Raven, New York, pp. 479–488.

Ehrenpreis, S., Balagot, R. C., Myles, S., Advocate, C. and Comaty, J. E. (1978b). Further studies on the analgesic activity of D-phenylalanine (DPA) in mice and humans, in *Endogenous and Exogenous Opiate Agonists and Antagonists*, (Ed. E. L. Way), Pergamon, Elmsford, New York, pp. 379–382.

Ehrenpreis, S., Greenberg, J., Kubota, K. and Myles, S. (1981). Analgesic properties of D-phenylalanine, bacitracin and puromycin in mice: relationship to inhibition of enkephalinase and beta-endorphinase, in *Advances in Endorphins and Exogenous Opioids*, (Eds. H. Takagi and E. J. Simon), Kodansha-Elsevier, Tokyo, pp. 279–281.

Ferreira, S. and Nakamura, M. (1979). II—Prostaglandin hyperalgesia: the peripheral analgesic activity of morphine, enkephalins and opioid antagonists. *Prostaglandins*, **18**, 191–200.

Fletcher, C. (1980). Listening and talking to patients. I: The problem. *British Medical Journal*, **281**, 845–846.

Gauld, V. A. (1981). Written advice: Compliance and recall, *Journal of the Royal College of General Practitioners*, **31**, 553–556.

Gardner, K. (1987). I don't know what this pain is due to, in: *Endometriosis: an Educational Pack for GPs*, (Ed. Anon), The Endometriosis Society, Coventry.

Hawkridge, C. (1985). *An Examination of Patient Education for Women Education for Women Undergoing Hysterectomy*. Unpublished dissertation, Diploma in Health Education, Leeds University.

Hawkridge, C. (1986). A Survey amongst 800 Members of the Endometriosis Society, UK. *Proceedings of Endometriose 86: Symposium International, France*, (in press). Karger Basle.

Horrobin, D. F. (Ed.) (1982). *Clinical Uses of Essential Fatty Acids*, Eden, Montreal.

Hyodo, M., Kitade, T. and Hosoka, E. (1983). Study on the enhanced analgesic effect induced by phenylalanine during acupuncture analgesia in humans, in *Advances in Pain Research and Therapy*, Vol. 5, (Eds. J. J. Bonica, J. C. Liebeskind and D. G. Albe-Fessard), Raven, New York, pp. 577–582.

Janis, I. L. (1969). *Stress and Frustration*, Harcourt Brace Jovanovich, New York.

Johnson, R. A., Baker, S. S., Fallon, J. T., Maynard, E. P., Ruskin, J. N., Wen, Z., Ge, K. and Cohen, H. J. (1981). An occidental case of cardiomyopathy and selenium deficiency. *New England Journal of Medicine*, **304**, 1210–1212.

Keshan Disease Research Group of the Chinese Academy of Medical Sciences, Beijing (1979a). Observations on effect of sodium selenite in preventing Keshan disease. *Chinese Medical Journal*, **92**, 471–476.

Keshan Disease Research Group of the Chinese Academy of Medical Sciences, Beijing (1979b). Epidemiologic studies on the etiologic relationship of selenium and Keshan disease. *Chinese Medical Journal*, **92**, 477–482.

Kincey, J. and McFarlane, T. (1984). Psychological aspects of hysterectomy, in *Psychology and Gynaecological Problems*, (Ed. A. Broome and L. Wallace), Tavistock, London, pp. 142–160.

Leading Article (1980). Endometriosis—continuing conundrum, *British Medical Journal*, **281**, 889–890.

Ley, P. and Spelman, M. S. (1967). *Communicating with the Patient*, Staples Press, London.

Ley, P. (1976). Towards better doctor-patient communications, in *Communication Between Doctors and Patients* (Ed. A. E. Bennett), Oxford University Press, Oxford.

Ley, P., Bradshaw, P. W., Kincey, J. A. and Atherton, S. T. (1976). Increasing patients' satisfaction with communications. *British Journal of Social Clinical Psychology*, **15**, 403–413.

Mabbett, L. (1986). The Emotional Apsects of Endometriosis, *Proceedings of Endometriose 86: Symposium International, France*, (in press). Karger, Basle.

Mayer, D. J., Price, D. D. and Rafii, A. (1977). Antagonism of acupuncture analgesia in man by the narcotic antagonist naloxone. *Brain Research*, **121**, 368–372.

Meigs, J. V. (1949). Medical treatment of endometriosis and significance of endometriosis. *Surgery Gynaecology and Obstetrics*, **89**, 317.

Nakano, S. and Ikezono, E. (1981). Effects of electro acupuncture on the levels of endorphins and substance P in human lumbar CSF, in *Advances in Endogenous and*

Exogenous Opioids, Ed. J. Takagi and E. J. Simon), Kodansha-Elsevier, Tokyo, pp. 312–314.

Norman, B. B. and Johnson, W. (1976). Selenium responsive disease. *Animal Nutrition and Health*, **31**, 6.

O'Connor, D. T. (1986). Endometriosis in *Current Reviews in Obstetrics and Gynaecology*, (Eds. A. Singer and J. Jordan), Churchill Livingstone, London.

Pirzada, B. I. (1987). Endometriosis as seen by a general practitioner, in *Endometriosis: an Educational Pack for GPs* (Ed. Anon), The Endometriosis Society, Coventry.

Pridham, K. F., Hansen, M. F. and Conrad, H. H. (1979). Anticipatory problem solving: models for clinical practice and research, *Sociology of Health and Illness*, **1**, 177–194.

Reading, A. E. (1981). Psychological preparation for surgery: patient recall of information. *Journal of Psychosomatic Research*, **25**, 57–62.

Ridgeway, V. and Matthews, A. (1982). Psychological preparation for surgery: a comparison of methods. *British Journal of Clinical Psychology*, **21**, 271–280.

Roberts, M. E. (1963a). Anti-inflammation studies. I. Anti-inflammatory properties of liver fractions. *Toxicology and Applied Pharmacology*, **5**, 485–499.

Roberts, M. E. (1963b). Anti-inflammation studies. II. Anti-inflammatory properties of selenium. *Toxicology and Applied Pharmacology*, **5**, 500–506.

Royal College of General Practitioners (1981). Prevention of Psychiatric Disorders in General Practice. *Report of a Sub-Committee of the RCGP Working Party on Prevention, Report from General Practice 20*, Royal College of General Practitioners, London.

Serfass, R. E. and Ganther, H. E. (1975). Defective microbicidal activity in glutathione peroxidase-deficient neutrophils of selenium-deficient rats. *Nature*, **255**, 640–641.

Serfass, R. E. and Ganther, H. E. (1976). Effects of dietary selenium and tocopherol on glutathione peroxidase and superoxide dismutase activities in rat phagocytes. *Life Sciences*, **19**, 1139–1144.

Shackelford, J. and Martin, J. (1980). Antibody response of mature male mice after drinking water supplemented with selenium. *Federation Proceedings*, **39**, 339.

Sheffy, B. E. and Schultz, R. D. (1978). Influence of vitamin E and selenium on immune response mechanisms. *Cornell Veterinarian*, **68, Supplement 7**, 89–93.

Spallholz, J. E., Martin, J. L., Gerlach, M. L. and Heinzerling, R. H. (1973a). Immunologic responses of mice fed diets supplemented with selenite selenium. *Proceedings of the Society for Experimental Biology and Medicine*, **143**, 685–689.

Spallholz, J. E., Martin, J. L., Gerlach, M. L. and Heinzerling, R. H. (1973b). Enhanced IgM and IgG titers in mice fed selenium. *Infections and Immunity*, **8**, 841–842.

Spallholz, J. E., Heinzerling, R. H., Gerlach, M. L. and Martin, J. L. (1974). The effect of selenite, tocopherol acetate and selenite, tocopherol acetate on the primary and secondary immune responses of mice administered tetanus toxoid or sheep red blood cell antigen. *Federation Proceedings*, **Abs. 33**, 694.

Studd, J. W. W. (1986). Oestradiol and Testosterone Implants After Hysterectomy for Severe Endometriosis, *Proceedings of Endometriose '86: Symposium International, France*, (in press). Karger, Basle.

Van Rij, A. M., Thomson, C. D., McKenzie, J. M. and Robinson, M. F. (1979). Selenium deficiency in total parenteral nutrition. *American Journal of Clinical Nutrition*, **32**, 2076–2085.

Wallace, L. (1979). Psychological adaptation of women undergoing laparoscopy for

infertility investigations and sterilization in *Psychology and Obstetrics and Gynaecology*. Proceedings of the British Psychology Society Conference, London.
Wallace, L. (1984). Psychological preparation for gynaecological surgery, in *Psychology and Gynaecological Problems* (Eds. A. Broome and L. Wallace) Tavistock, London, pp. 161–189.
Ward, G. D. (1983). Endometriosis: an overview. *British Journal of Clinical Practice*, **Symposium supplement, 24**, 34–36.

Index

297